GALEN ON HUMAN PHYSIOLOGY

Galen of Pergamum, known as 'the prince of medicine', is an important figure not only for the history of medicine but also for ancient philosophy, history of ideas and cultural history. In this book, Aistė Čelkytė explores Galenic physiology and examines how this highly influential figure theorised the unity of the multi-part, ever-moving and ever-changing human body. She approaches this question by first studying how Galen 'takes the body apart', that is, the different divisions of the body into parts that he proposes, and then how he 'puts it back together', that is, his use of philosophical tools to posit the vital unity among these parts. She then looks at Galen's theorisation of human nature, his understanding of parthood, the hierarchies between the parts that underpin vital functions, the 'mechanisms' that make the body *one* and Galen's understanding of the body as a multifaceted but unified whole.

AISTĖ ČELKYTĖ is a postdoctoral fellow at the Centre for the Arts in Society (LUCAS) at Leiden University and a researcher at Vilnius University. She is the author of *The Stoic Theory of Beauty* (2020).

GALEN ON HUMAN PHYSIOLOGY

Taking the Body Apart and Putting it Back Together Again

AISTĖ ČELKYTĖ

Leiden University

CAMBRIDGE
UNIVERSITY PRESS

CAMBRIDGE
UNIVERSITY PRESS

Shaftesbury Road, Cambridge CB2 8EA, United Kingdom

One Liberty Plaza, 20th Floor, New York, NY 10006, USA

477 Williamstown Road, Port Melbourne, VIC 3207, Australia

314–321, 3rd Floor, Plot 3, Splendor Forum, Jasola District Centre, New Delhi – 110025, India

103 Penang Road, #05-06/07, Visioncrest Commercial, Singapore 238467

Cambridge University Press is part of Cambridge University Press & Assessment, a department of the University of Cambridge.

We share the University's mission to contribute to society through the pursuit of education, learning and research at the highest international levels of excellence.

www.cambridge.org
Information on this title: www.cambridge.org/9781009435819

DOI: 10.1017/9781009435833

When citing this work, please include a reference to the DOI 10.1017/9781009435833

First published 2025

A catalogue record for this publication is available from the British Library

Library of Congress Cataloging-in-Publication Data
NAMES: Čelkytė, Aistė author
TITLE: Galen on human physiology : taking the body apart and putting it back together again / Aistė Čelkytė.
DESCRIPTION: Cambridge ; New York, NY : Cambridge University Press, 2025. | Includes bibliographical references and index.
IDENTIFIERS: LCCN 2025004178 (print) | LCCN 2025004179 (ebook) | ISBN 9781009435819 hardback | ISBN 9781009435826 paperback | ISBN 9781009435833 epub
SUBJECTS: LCSH: Galen | Human physiology–History | Medicine, Greek and Roman
CLASSIFICATION: LCC R126.G8 C45 2025 (print) | LCC R126.G8 (ebook) | DDC 610.938–dc23/eng/20250408
LC record available at https://lccn.loc.gov/2025004178
LC ebook record available at https://lccn.loc.gov/2025004179

ISBN 978-1-009-43581-9 Hardback

Contents

Acknowledgements

Most of the work for this study was carried out in the context of the project *Human Nature: Medical and Philosophical Perspectives in the Work of Galen of Pergamum* funded by NWO (De Nederlandse Organisatie voor Wetenschappelijk Onderzoek) at Utrecht University. I would like to thank my colleagues there, Julia Trompeter, Robert Vinkesteijn, Clarine Rijpstra-van Daal and especially the principal investigator of the project Teun Tieleman for discussions, feedback and for reading many Galenic texts together. I am also grateful to a number of scholars who discussed Galen with me over the years, especially Jim Hankinson, Julien Devinant, Peter Singer, Philip van der Eijk, Albert Joosse, Matyáš Havrda, Aileen Das, Caroline Petit, Helen King, David Kaufman, Inna Kupreeva, Orly Lewis, Riccardo Chiaradonna, Vilius Bartninkas and Elvira Wakelnig. I would also like to thank Svetla Slaveva-Griffin and Sean Coughlin for sharing drafts of their work with me. Versions of parts of this work were presented at various events at Leuven, Hokkaido, Edinburgh, Utrecht, Austin, London, Berlin and Leiden as well as the *Animalia* Network and CAW (Centrum voor Antieke Wijsbegeerte) reading seminar, and I am extremely grateful for comments, critiques and ensuing conversations with those audiences. This work would not have been possible without the support of my colleagues at Leiden, especially: Tazuko ban Berkel, Casper de Jonge, Ineke Sluiter, Bert van den Berg, Bob van Velthoven, Glyn Muitjens and others. I would also like to thank George Boys-Stones and Luca Castagnoli for bearing with my early ventures into philosophical and physiological problems in Galen. Finally, I am grateful to the anonymous reviewers for their comments and suggestions.

Note to Reader

Abbreviations for Greek and Latin authors follow H. G. Liddell, R. Scott and H. S. Jones. 1996 (1940). *A Greek–English Lexicon*, 9th edn. Oxford: Oxford University Press, as well as P. Glare (ed.). 1982. *Oxford Latin Dictionary*. Oxford: Oxford University Press. Other abbreviations are as follows.

Boys-Stones	G. R. Boys-Stones (ed.). 2018. *Platonist Philosophy 80 BC to AD 250: An Introduction and Collection of Sources in Translation*. Cambridge: Cambridge University Press.
CMG	1907 (various editions). *Corpus Medicorum Graecorum*. Leipzig and Berlin: Teubner; Akademie Verlag; De Gruyter.
DK	H. Diels and W. Kranz (eds.). 1951–2. *Die Fragmente der Vorsokratiker*. 6th edn. 3 vols. Berlin: Weidmann.
K	K. G. Kühn (ed.). 1821–33. *Claudii Galeni Opera Omnia*, 22 vols. Leipzig: Knobloch.
Littré	É. Littré (ed.). 1839–61. *Oeuvres complètes d'Hippocrate*, 10 vols. Paris: J. B. Baillière.
LS	A. A. Long and D. Sedley (eds.). 1987. *The Hellenistic Philosophers*. 2 vols. Cambridge: Cambridge University Press.
von Staden	H. von Staden. 1989. *Herophilus: The Art of Medicine in Early Alexandria*. Cambridge: Cambridge University Press.
SVF	J. von Arnim (ed.). 1903–5. *Stoicorum veterum fragmenta*. 3 vols. Leipzig: Teubner.

Galen's works are referenced in accordance with critical editions as well as C. G. Kühn. 1821–1833. *Claudii Galeni Opera Omnia*. Leipzig (reprinted Cambridge: Cambridge University Press, 2011). The titles of Galen's treatises are abbreviated following R. J. Hankinson (ed.). 2008. *The Cambridge Companion to Galen* (Cambridge: Cambridge University Press), appendix 1. The titles referenced in this study are cited as follows.

AA	*De anatomicis administrationibus*
Adv. Jul.	*Adversus Julianum*
Aff. Dig.	*De proprium animi cuiuslibet affectuum dignotione et curatione*
Ars. Med.	*Ars medica*
Art. Sang.	*An in arteriis sanguis contineatur*
CAM	*De constitutione artis medicae*
Caus. Puls.	*De causis pulsuum*
Caus. Resp.	*De causis respirationis*
CC	*De causis contentivi*
Comp. Med. Loc.	*De compositione medicamentorum secundum locos*
Cur. Rat. Ven. Sect.	*De curandi ratione per venae sectionem*
Diff. Feb.	*De febrium differentiis*
Diff. Puls.	*De differentiis pulsuum*
Foet. Form.	*De foetuum formatione*
Hipp. El.	*De elementis ex Hippocrate*
Hipp. Epid.	*In Hippocratis epidemiarum*
Hipp. Prog.	*In Hippocratis prognosticum*
Hipp. Vict.	*In Hippocratis de salubri victus ratione*
HNH	*In Hippocratis de natura hominis*
Inaeq. Int.	*De inaequali intemperie*
Inst. Log.	*Institutio logica*
Inst. Od.	*De instrumento odoratus*
Lib. Prop.	*De libris propriis*
Loc. Aff.	*De locis affectis*
Marc.	*De marcore*
MM	*De methodo medendi*
MMG	*Ad glauconem de methodo medendi*
Morb.	*De moribus*
Morb. Diff.	*De morborum differentiis*
Mot. Dub.	*De motibus dubiis*
Nat. Fac.	*De naturalibus facultatibus*
Nerv. Diss.	*De nervorum dissectione*
Opt. Corp. Const.	*De optima corporis nostri constitutione*
PHP	*De placitis Hippocratis et Platonis*
Plat. Tim.	*In Platonis timaeum*
Praes. Puls.	*De praesagitione ex pulsibus*
Prop. Plac.	*De propriis placitis*
Protr.	*Protrepticus*
Puer. Epil.	*Puero epileptico consilium*

QAM	*Quod animi mores corporis temperamenta sequuntur*
San. Tu.	*De sanitate tuenda*
Sem.	*De semine*
Subf. Emp.	*Subfiguratio empirica*
Symp. Caus.	*De symptomatum causis*
Symp. Diff.	*De symptomatum differentiis*
Temp.	*De temperamentis*
Thras.	*Thrasybulus sive utrum medicinae sit an gymnasticae hygiene*
Trem. Palp.	*De tremore, palpitatione, convulsione et rigore*
UP	*De usu partium*
Us. Puls.	*De usu pulsuum*
Ut. Resp.	*De utilitate respirationis*
Ven. Sect. Er.	*De venae sectione adversus Erasistratum*

Introduction

I.1 Vital Unity in Galen

ἐκ δέ νυ Φοίβου
ἰητροὶ δεδάασιν ἀνάβλησιν θανάτοιο.

Callimachus, *Hymn to Apollo*[1]

Callimachus' *Hymn to Apollo* mentions medicine very briefly, but a couple of short lines are enough to make two points: medicine is a divinely bestowed expertise and the goal of this expertise is to postpone death. Both of these points are echoed in the works of Galen of Pergamum, whom Andreas Vesalius famously called the 'prince of medicine'. As the moniker indicates, Galen was one of the most significant figures in the history of medicine in Europe and the Middle East, and his very large extant corpus is replete with information about ancient understandings of the body and its vital functions.

Galen is not, however, only a medical writer. Although he has much to say about treating of wounds, setting bones and curing fevers, his philosophical education and philosophical interests are also prominent in his attempts to theorise the human body and its nature. Arguably, his medical and philosophical interests often go together, informing each other in profound ways. Just like doctors in Callimachus' hymn receive their knowledge from Apollo, so he builds his understanding of human nature on studying divine matters. Galen showed considerable interest in the questions pertaining to divine design and teleology, and he was not averse to exploring more general connections between religious practices and medicine.[2] However, it is the more philosophical topic of the divine design that proves to be a key commitment and the crucial point of contention in

[1] *Ap.* 2.45–6.
[2] For Galen's theological views and his relationship with religions more generally, see Tieleman (2005, 2016) and Walzer (1949). On Galen's view on prophecy in medicine, see van Nuffelen (2014).

polemics, not the notion of divinity and attendant practices informed by broader culture. Throughout his works, Galen describes himself as firmly committed to the ancient version of creationism,[3] in the sense that he is convinced that the world was designed by the benevolent designer. One of the constant refrains and motifs of his monumental *On the Usefulness of Parts* is the remarkable efficiency of the design of the body,[4] which renders it a cohesively functioning entity.[5]

However, the entanglement of medicine and philosophy is even more palpable in what Callimachus describes as the goal of medicine: the knowledge of how to postpone death, in other words, the knowledge of preserving and extending vitality. This preoccupation is a dominant theme in Galen, not just in the sense of practical medical knowledge but also in the sense of seeking to understand the human nature so that medical practice can be informed and improved by it. What is the vitality that doctors must learn to preserve, under the divine tutelage? If doctors are to do their job, this question requires a non-abstract answer: it requires identifying and locating the vitality in the body. What is it exactly in the body that must be preserved in order to keep a patient alive and healthy?

Galen has much to say about various parts and elements constituting the body and their significance. In fact, perhaps a bit too much: his tendency to posit multiple body constituents without providing an explanation of how they are all related has been noted in the scholarship.[6] This volume is a study of how Galen theorises the relationship between a part and the whole. It looks at different classifications of body parts that he makes, the definitions of parthood, the way he constructs the relationship between different parts and the different roles he assigns to the parts. In short, it is a study of how Galen takes the body 'apart', not in an anatomical but in a conceptual way informed by anatomy, and then puts it back together again into a single entity that breathes, eats, moves and interacts with its environment.

In as much as it is a study of parts and wholes, this work concerns Galen's engagement with metaphysics. The relationship between parts

[3] Sedley (2007) is an extensive study of the origins and various aspects of this tradition. Although the monograph is primarily focused on the philosophers from the Archaic to the Hellenistic periods, it also contains an epilogue on Galen who 'exploits, and advances the pagan creationist tradition like no one before him, and so with all the skill and insight of a practicing scientists' (243).

[4] In *On My Own Books* (*Lib. Prop.* 3.12 (143, 24–144, 6 Boudon-Millot=19.20–21K)), Galen describes this treatise as written in Aristotelian, as well as medical, traditions. It thereby resembles a treatise written by Aristotle himself, namely *Parts of Animals*, although Galen claims he corrects Aristotle's errors. See Hankinson (1998: 386–8).

[5] Hankinson (1989).

[6] Van der Eijk (2020: 64).

and wholes was a preoccupation of the ancient Greek and Roman philosophers, and Galen's reflection on the topic is well-entrenched in this tradition.[7] He presents himself as a follower of Plato.[8] However, he also adopts many elements of the Peripatetic tradition, which shapes his understanding of human nature in formative ways.[9] Oftentimes, he associates his stance with a tradition to which he assigns many fairly different philosophical schools. For example, in his attack on the atomist style of monism (in the sense of positing only one type of matter as fundamentally composing the body),[10] he contrasts it with the four-element theory, which he attributes not only to Hippocrates but also to an array of respectable philosophers, especially Aristotle and Chrysippus.[11] This approach is part of Galen's broader project of refuting mechanistic physiology. Such a confluence of popular philosophical influences is not

[7] Sextus Empiricus dedicates a section of his *Against Professors* to refuting *tout court* theories of parthood (*M* 9.331–58). Recent scholarship showed that Plato (Harte 2002) and Aristotle (Koslicki 2008) offer philosophically complex reflections on parthood; see also Barnes (1988), which lays important ground for examining this topic, and Holmes (2020), which argues that the notion of *sumpatheia* is a lens through which ancient mereological views are developed.

[8] For broader discussions, see de Lacy (1972) and Singer (1991, 2014: 18–20); for specific dialogues, see Das (2020: 3–5); Vegetti (2000) and Vinkesteijn (2022) on the *Timaeus*; on the *Phaedrus*, see Rocca (2006), Rosen (2013) and Tieleman (2020), see also Chapter 2. During Galen's lifetime, the prevalent version of Platonism was the so-called Middle Platonism, see Chiaradonna (2009) for his interaction with the tradition.

[9] See van der Eijk (2009), Singer (2014: 20–38) and Vinkesteijn (2022). See also Gottschalk (1987: 1166–71), Kovačić (2001) and Moraux (1984). Holmes (2020: 77) points out that Aristotle (unlike Plato, who is preoccupied with mathematical unity) had important vitalist commitments when it comes to unity. Aristotelian thought certainly forms a crucial background to Galen's thought, but it is also worth noting that Galen's work deals with medical realities and is circumscribed by practical goals.

[10] Galen's attack on this type of monism and commitment to pluralist element theory are explored in the scholarship fairly extensively, see, for example, Hankinson (2017a) and Kupreeva (2014); see also Caston (1997). Material monism is common to many Presocratics, especially Ionians, see Barnes (1982: 38–44); and it has been pointed out in the scholarship that atomism, which posits the existence of the many by definition, has some important connections to the monist arguments concerning the unity of matter, see Sedley (2008). A useful way of systematising and clarifying what is at stake has been proposed by Patricia Curd who distinguishes three types of monism in ancient philosophy: material monism, which posits a single kind of matter that constitutes everything in the world; numerical monism, which advocates for the existence of a single entity in the world; and, finally, predicational monism, which maintains that each existing entity can only hold one predicate about what it is, and this predication must be non-marginal (1998: 65–6). See also Barnes (1982: 155–302) and Makin (2014).

[11] *Hipp. Elem.* 5.14 de Lacy (1.451K) and 9.20 de Lacy (1.486K), respectively. Chrysippus is an interesting case, because Galen chooses him as the representative of cardiocentrism that he attacks in *PHP*. Although Chrysippus often serves as a target, Galen is nonetheless influenced by Stoicism in several respects, see Tieleman (2009); see also Lloyd (2008). On Galen's claim that he inherits his physics from Hippocrates, see Hankinson (2008a).

unusual for someone writing in the second century CE,[12] which makes Galen's work a product of its time too. This is not to say that Galen ought to be studied as just another eclectic late Platonist. Unlike many of his contemporary philosophers, Galen grounds his views on the vitality and the unity of the human body in a minute physiological and anatomical detail. On one striking occasion, he criticises the focus of the contemporary philosophers on the *kosmos*, arguing that the puzzles of the human body are no lesser. In the treatise *On the Formation of the Embryo* he argues that the study of motion need not concern itself with cosmology alone, and the body presents equally wonder-worthy phenomenon.

Having rebuked the Epicureans for rejecting the notion of the benevolent designer, Galen goes on to consider the question of how the design takes place, viz. what its substance is. First, he discusses the possibility that the gods, having constructed the seeds of animals and plants in a way that allows them to grow and function on their own, depart and let these processes take place by themselves, referencing philosophical and scientific ideas.[13] However, he is concerned that it is not possible for the moisture found in the act of generation to carry out so many complex actions over a long period of time without an error. Without attempting to find a resolution, Galen moves on to what he calls an even more astonishing matter, namely, that no one of those who write on *phusiologia* either observed or investigated how that which is happening throughout entire life and is seen by all of us happens. He specifies his point by raising a question of what is at work in the activities (ἐνεργεῖαι) of the body parts.[14]

It is important to note that Galen is not merely rejecting 'philosophical' enquiry in favour of a medical one. On some occasions, Galen contrasts medical practice and overtly abstract philosophical theory, thus clearly suggesting that these are distinct, and the former can be done without the latter,[15] but it is not entirely the case here. He goes on to list various attempts to theorise muscle motion and the shortcomings of these

[12] In terms of cultural history, this is the so-called Second Sophistic period. For seminal studies, see Schmitz (1997) and Swain (1996); also articles in Bowersock (1974). For a discussion of Galen in particular and the Second Sophistic, see Kollesch (1981) and von Staden (1995, 1997a).

[13] See Berryman (2009: chapter 6, esp. pp. 208–9) reading the passage against the background of developments in mechanics.

[14] *Foet. Form.* 6, 6 Nickel (4.689K): ἔτι δὲ θαυμαστότερον, ὃ διὰ παντὸς τοῦ βίου γιγνόμενον ἁπάντων ἡμῶν ὁρώντων οὐδεὶς τῶν τὴν φυσιολογίαν ἀπαγγελλομένων οὔτε κατενόησεν οὔτ' ἐζήτησεν, ὅπως γίγνεται. τί δὲ τοῦτ' ἔστι τὸ κατὰ τὰς ἐνεργείας τῶν μορίων. On the notion of activities, see Debru (2008: 265–6). Also important here is the Aristotle-derived methodology, starting with what is evident to the senses and examining the non-evident essence or function of the organ, see Tieleman (2008: 56–8).

[15] For example, in *Prop. Plac.* 7.3–4 (86 Lami Garofalo).

theories.[16] First is the theory – rejected by himself and most other doctors – that each muscle is like an animal. He then notes that the theory he himself espouses, which states that the nerves move muscles, faces some difficulty in explaining the presence of some very small nerves in the muscles, not to mention the fact that people and animals seem to know which muscles to move without being aware of them.[17] Galen wraps up this discussion by noting that the question of the soul constructing the animal is problematic, with a single exception: it is clear that a providential creator designs human bodies.[18] Although the problem of muscle motion is informed by medical enquiries, Galen clearly aims to present it as belonging together with more standard questions about the mind-body relationship. When he introduces the problem, he uses the example of the finger bones and joints being moved in a variety of ways to show that the nature of muscle motion is unclear, adding that those who wish to understand the nature of the universe and the heavenly bodies ought to concern themselves with this problem instead.

The point Galen makes here is quite striking. He argues that two seemingly different types of enquiries, into the soul and *kosmos* on the one hand and into muscle motion on the other, belong together. Both of them belong to the broad discipline of *phusiologia*. Such grouping can be motivated by the view that *phusiologia* is a study of the primary elements.[19] Both investigations reveal comparable insights about nature, or at least, the investigators of the nature of the muscle motion are not missing out on any profound insights. In fact, Galen's phrasing, presenting one investigation as preferrable, suggests that working out the activities of the body parts might be a more sensible way of studying nature. From these passages alone, *phusiologia* emerges as a highly distinctive kind of specialisation, combining both medical and philosophical elements. With this point,

16 A comparison with such texts as Plutarch's *Virt. Mor.* 442D is enlightening. The latter states that pneuma, sinews, bones and other parts, although irrational, spring to action when prompted by the ʻορμή sent by the reasoning part, and uses this as evidence for dualism. Galen's exposition of the difficulties that arise when attempting to account for the details of motion sounds like a fair reprimand to those who, like Plutarch, would use such examples to establish their point, without seeing that his illustration raises more problems than it answers. Of course, we could say that for the sake of Plutarch's argument, it is enough to know *that* body parts move at will or rational reflection. Yet, as Galen will show, there is more than one theory for accounting how the motion at will takes place in the body; some theories would lend support for their arguments, and some would not.

17 *Foet. Form.* 6, 7–16 Nickel (4.690–3K); see also Chapter 4 on the nervous system.

18 *Foet. Form.* 6, 16 Nickel (4.693K); see also Gill's discussion of this section of the treatise too, pointing out that, interestingly, Galen does not discuss Platonic dualism as an option here, that is, that an embryo is produced by immaterial soul and matter (2010: 134–5).

19 As stated in *MM* 2.5 (10.107K).

Galen is engaging in and aiming to modify the discourse with a complex history that existed long before his lifetime.

I.2 *Phusiologia*

In the Archaic and Classical periods, the ancient Greek term *phusiologia* primarily referred to the study of nature as whole and included the thought of Presocratic philosophers.[20] Galen's contrast between those who claim to be *phusiologoi* and those who study of muscle motion also invokes the primarily philosophical association of the term. It seems that Galen is arguing for a new, medical concept of *phusiologia*, but the term entered medical vocabulary before his time as denoting a branch of medicine.[21] Galen himself ascribes the discovery of its principles to Hippocrates and a number of philosophers who respected his authority, including Plato, his successors Speusippus and Xenocrates, Aristotle and Theophrastus as well as the Stoics Zeno and Chrysippus.[22] He singles out the Peripatetic tradition for being in particular agreement with Hippocratic principles of *phusiologia* (τὰς Ἱπποκράτους ἀρχὰς τῆς φυσιολογίας) and claims to have demonstrated this point in other treatises, including *On the Elements According to Hippocrates*, *On Mixtures*, its sequel *On Anomalous Dyskrasia*, *On the Best Constitution of the Body* and *On the Natural Capacities*.[23]

[20] Nutton (2012b: 28). It is also worth noting that the distinction between philosophy and medicine is by no means sharp in antiquity, see Frede (1987: 227–34, 243–4). For medicine-related interests of various Presocratics, see Longrigg (1993: 26–81). See also papers in Vasallo (2017), showing the range of the Presocratic 'physiological' endeavours.

[21] A quite different question is whether Galen was read in this way by his contemporaries and successors; see Slaveva-Griffin (manuscript in preparation, chapter 1) for the argument that Galenic texts mark the point at which *phusiologia* became increasingly medicalised and understood as a medical undertaking.

[22] *MM* 1.2 (10.10K). The context here is an attack on Thessalus the Methodist for criticising such famous doctors as Diocles, Praxagoras and especially Hippocrates. In a long and rhetorically charged rebuke, Galen invokes the authority of philosophers to show that no respected figure disagrees with Hippocrates. He is not charitable to the Methodists. For a more in-depth study of the methods of this school, see Frede (1987: 261–78) and Tecusan (2004); see also Salas (2020a) for the argument that Galen's definition of disease probably originated in connection to this tradition, which shows that he was more indebted to the Methodists than his criticism of their understanding of medicine would lead one to believe. Regarding the question of how the Stoic views fit into the Galenic theory, and how compatible they actually are with Aristotelianism, see Gill (2010: 76–84).

[23] *MM* 1.2 (10.15K); see also *MM* 1.2 (10.17K) for the claim that Hippocratic *phusiologia*, and all the aforementioned philosophers (on the grounds of *phusiologia*), showed that considering the nature of the body overall is necessary for curing any disease; see also Jouanna (2013: 308). See Hankinson (2008a: 2011–17) for a discussion of how Galen makes the elemental theory 'Hippocratic' in this work; see also Hankinson (2016: 243–7). There are some commonalities in the treatises that Galen lists as propounding the Hippocratic *phusiologia*: the theory of the four qualities – the hot, the cold,

These treatises are also polemical, dominated by disagreements with various Hellenistic doctors as well as their followers. Especially prominent are the disagreements with the Epicurean-inspired forms of atomism that play a prominent role in *On the Natural Capacities* and *On the Elements According to Hippocrates.* Ultimately, Peripatetic tradition is significant to Galen not only because of the claims it makes but also because it represents an alternative to popular but quite incorrect way of theorising bodily functions.[24]

Despite significant pedigree, the term *phusiologia* shows up relatively rarely in Galenic corpus, and even when it does, it is fairly ambivalent: on the one hand, *phusiologia* is not necessary and, in certain cases, even distracting. On the other hand, it can be useful.[25] One of the more detailed discussions unpacking this notion occurs in *On the Constitution of the Art of Medicine*, and it is a good example of how Galen muddles the concept in the analysis that is meant to clarify the matters. Here, he makes a distinction between theoretical and productive arts, raising the question of which category medicine belongs to. He distinguishes arithmetic, astronomy and *phusiologia* from such arts as dancing or house building. While the latter are concerned with their action (whether producing a result or not), the *telos* of the former is to investigate the nature of the object.[26] Having noted that it is not hard to figure out which category

the dry and the wet – and their mixtures play a prominent role in all of them. However, there is little sign of systematic attempt to establish *phusiologia* as the investigation of elements. Of all these treatises, only the very first and the very last contain cognates of *phusiologein* (*Hipp. Elem.* 5.4 de Lacy (1.449K); 9.21 de Lacy (1.486K); *Nat. Fac.* 1.14 (133, 22 Helmreich=2.245K); 2.4 (165, 14 Helmreich=2.88K) and (166, 21–22 Helmreich=2.90K)), and of these two, only the *On the Elements According to Hippocrates* provides an extensive theoretical discussion of the primary elements.

24 In *Nat. Fac.* 2.4 (168, 9–14 Helmreich=2.92–3K), Galen claims that Erasistratus has no connection to the Peripatetic *phusiologia.* According to him, this tradition originates with Hippocrates and then is advocated by Aristotle and the Stoics. See also Berryman (2009: 178).

25 Nutton (2012b: 30–1). Interestingly, pseudo-Galenic texts (following the tradition of Hippocratic rationalism) appear to be more enthusiastic about its importance than Galen himself. Arguably, this might be owing to the fact that such texts as *Def. Med.* 11 (19.351K) use it as a distinctly medical term, while Galen uses it in a way that reflects its philosophical heritage. In order to *phusiologein*, one has to engage in questions that go beyond medical concerns and interests. See Singer (2014) for a discussion of Galen's ambivalent relationship with philosophy.

26 *CAM* 1, 1 Fortuna (1.227K): Ἐπειδὴ τῶν τεχνῶν ἔνιαι μὲν ἐν μόνῳ τῷ θεωρῆσαι τὴν φύσιν ὧν ἐπισκοποῦνται πραγμάτων ἔχουσι τὸ τέλος, ὡς ἀριθμητικὴ καὶ ἀστρονομία καὶ φυσιολογία. This distinction of course predates Galen, it can already be found in Plato's *Statesman* 258D–E. Aristotle's *Metaphysics* 6.1 (1025b25–7) classifies ἡ φυσική, the study of those substances that contain the principle of motion and rest within themselves, as a theoretical science (rather than practical or productive).

medicine belongs to, he goes on to state that it is clearly a productive art, as its results can be shown.[27]

There is a clear and fairly sharp distinction between *phusiologia* and medicine. It seems like these are fundamentally different *types* of arts. However, the sharp distinction becomes much more blurry as the treatise progresses. Soon thereafter, for example, Galen notes that medicine requires the knowledge of simple parts: their substance (*ousia*), construction (*diaplasis*), size, number and combination with each other (*sunthesis*).[28] Although this requirement pushes medicine close to the theoretical sciences according to his own conditions set for each category, Galen keeps on developing the house-building simile without acknowledging the blurring distinction.

Furthermore, the simile changes from building the house to knowing what it is. He compares wishing to know the constitution of a human body to wishing to know precisely what kind of a thing an existing house is.[29] Galen avoids using the term 'nature' here, but such an investigation would be at least adjacent to investigating nature, if not identical to it. He adds that a person, wishing to understand some particular house, would use the methods of dialysis and analysis, just like the human body is known by anatomy. He goes on to compare the perspective of the house builder with that of god and nature and – intentionally or accidentally – distances medicine further from house building by identifying those with an interest in medicine with the examiners of the house, not its builders.[30] Thus Galen's simile elucidating the nature of medical art goes askew, but it illustrates very well the uneasiness in his treatment of the concept of *phusiologia*.

On the one hand, there is more to medical activities than *phusiologein*; medicine also involves a crucial practical component. In fact, practice is surely the very point of medicine. Presumably, Galen would not object to the claim that medicine that does not produce any results is not medicine at all; in that case, it would be more proper to call it *phusiologia*. On the other hand, not investigating what the body is, how it is constituted and how it functions seems hardly an option for medical practitioners as Galen describes them here. This ambivalence about *phusiologia* as an area of

[27] *CAM* 1, 7 Fortuna (1.229K). [28] *CAM* 2, 2 Fortuna (1.230–1K).

[29] *CAM* 2, 3 Fortuna (1.231K): Ὥσπερ οὖν ὁ τὴν ἤδη γεγενημένην οἰκίαν ὁποία τίς ἐστιν ἀκριβῶς γνῶναι βουλόμενος.

[30] *CAM* 2, 4 Fortuna (1.231K).

interest to medicine mirrors Galen's multifaceted engagement with rationalist and empiricist traditions of medicine.

I.3 Empiricism, Rationalism and *Phusiologia*

Galen's engagement with the two traditions has been at the forefront of Galenic scholarship for a while,[31] but its parallels with *phusiologia* are rarely noted. The practitioner of medicine that Galen portrays in this passage is a rationalist. The practitioners of this Hellenistic school of thought identify their intellectual pedigree with the Hippocratic tradition, and the distinguishing aspect of this tradition is the emphasis on the theoretical understanding of the body *qua* the principles underpinning the functioning of the entire natural world. In other words, the rationalists are committed to the belief that the theoretical knowledge of human nature including the causal principles that govern it, is necessary for a successful medical practice.[32] This view is also reflected in the aforementioned passage. The commitments of the rationalist doctors appear very distinctive when they are contrasted with the commitments of empiricists.

Medical empiricism is a more striking stance, since the members of the sect make experience, either personal or commonly accumulated, the grounds for medical practice. This is not to say that the dichotomy between the rationalists and the empiricist is straightforward. While rationalists' medical practice links them with philosophical discussions of the natural world, human nature and the principles that govern both, the empiricists do share substantial ties with philosophy too, primarily sceptic epistemology.[33] In order to account for their methodology that prioritises experience over any type of theoretical explanation, the empiricists, perhaps somewhat paradoxically, built sophisticated epistemological accounts about sign inferences as well as such methods as 'transition to the similar' that allows them to postulate similarities between different medical cases without committing to any view about the underlying causes.[34]

[31] Important work is collected in Frede (1987); see especially 'The Ancient Empiricists' (chapter 13) and 'On Galen's Epistemology' (chapter 15); see also Hankinson (2022a) and Kupreeva (2022).

[32] See Allen (2001: 93–4) and Hankinson (1998: 306–18).

[33] This is not to say simply that the empiricists are sceptics. Sextus Empiricus famously eschews the empiricists from the association with Pyrrhonism in favour of Methodism (*PH* 1.236; see also Allen (2001: 89–99). At the same time, it is worth noting that some empiricists might have had more affinity with Pyrrhonism than others; see the discussion in Frede (1987: 248–60).

[34] Allen (2001: 107–22); Hankinson (1998: 312–16); it is also worth noting that empiricists, like almost all the other large schools, were not monolithic. See Hankinson (1998: 317–18) for the

Galen himself, as a self-styled follower of Hippocrates, has strong affinities with rationalism,[35] although his attitude towards the rival empiricism is also far from critical. He praises empiricists for their systematic and consistent approach to medical methodology.[36] The strength of this method lies, according to Galen, in successful therapeutic practice. He even goes so far as to argue that it is better for doctors to be empiricists rather than follow a flawed rational method.[37] The theoretical understanding of the constitution of the body, therefore, is clearly not absolutely necessary for medical practice and, consequently, an experience-based approach is an attractive alternative in principle.[38]

Having said that, Galen himself identifies with the rationalist tradition. The affinity to this tradition is evident in his methodology, as the theoretical notion of demonstration is key for fashioning his own approach to the study of the body.[39] The reason for that emerges in his discussions of complex illnesses. When an illness is a matter of a single pathological condition, either the rationalist or the empiricist method will do. When more than one condition is present in a patient, an empiricist doctor will be ill-equipped to determine the proper treatment and only rational methods can offer a solution.[40] He also rebukes empiricists for their advice to turn away from *phusiologia* and not try to understand human nature the way philosophers do, going all the way to the primary elements by means of reason.[41] Ultimately, Galen approves of the principles of both

argument that such figures as Menodotus and Heraclides of Tarentum might be examples of the more moderate version of empiricism, admitting some usefulness of theory.

35 For example, in *MM* 5.10 (10.347K), he writes that empiricists discover by experience what 'we' find by indication, see also *MM* 3.7 (10.204K). He repeats the claim he made earlier in the treatise, that both rationalists and empiricists have a way of figuring out what treatment would work, although neither has a way to find everything in *MM* 3.1 (10.159K); see also *MM* 13.6 (10.896K) for a similar claim in the context of pharmacology. Galen also criticizes both in *On the Therapeutic Method*, although the general aim of his critique in both cases is specific practices rather than their respective principal methods.

36 *MM* 1.4 (10.32K).

37 *MM* 13.16 (10.916K). See also Frede (1987: 235–7).

38 Frede (1987: 295). Galen's own methods also place great importance on experience. On the difference between the empiricist and Galenic use of experience, see van der Eijk (2005: 292).

39 As the key treatise, *On Demonstration*, is not extant (though see Havrda 2015), this method has been well studied on the basis of the other works that are extant; see, for example, Lloyd (1996); Morison (2008: 69–75) and Tieleman (1996, 2022).

40 *MM* 10.10 (10.707K). See also *MM* 3.2 (10.173K) for the same argument in a pharmacological context. Another interesting case is diagnostics by taking into account customs of a patient in *MM* 9.16 (10.655K). Here, Galen argues that experience of a patient can only tell an empiricist how a certain practice affected the person so far, not what accumulated effects of that practice might be in the future. Thus, the inability to calculate the effects of some practice by reason raises the possibility of prescribing something harmful. See also Hankinson (1998: 309–11) for a discussion of the same kind of argument in Galen's *On Medical Experience*.

41 *MM* 2.5 (10.107K): ἄχρι τῶν πρώτων στοιχείων ἀνιόντες τῷ λόγῳ.

empiricism and rationalism, but he finds the methods of the latter to be superior, while being acutely aware of the potential pitfalls of practicing rationalism, that is, erroneous misapplications of reasoning.

Galen's approach to the disagreement between the rationalists and the empiricists sheds light on his ambivalent approach to *phusiologia*. As the study of the nature of things, *phusiologia* is a distinctly rationalist undertaking. Furthermore, it has a certain philosophical heritage, and Galen uses the word in relation to specific philosophical schools on some occasions.[42] *Phusiologia*, therefore, has all the same advantages and shortcomings as any other rationalist undertaking in medicine: it can be illuminating but it also entails the risk of reasoning errors. Galen is also wary of the theoretical (or 'philosophical') discussions that venture off too far from medical issues.[43] Despite all of these pitfalls, rationalism still remains the preferable methodology because it has significant advantages when applied well. The same could be said of *phusiologia*, because, despite his hesitancy, Galen does not avoid it entirely. In fact, as Vivian Nutton points out, 'his practice as described in his own writings could easily be viewed by outsiders as a typically Hippocratic "physiological" exposition of the basic principles that govern the bodily universe. Galen frequently refers to mixtures, humours and so on to support conclusions reached by observation, experiment or logic, or, at the very least, to exclude ideas of others that he considered erroneous.'[44] The reasons that prevent him from unilaterally advocating for rationalism are also, presumably, reflected in his ambivalence towards *phusiologia*. The study of *phusiologia*, therefore, has some complications owing to the way Galen conceptualises this area of study, but it does not follow that it cannot be done.

In this work, I use the term 'physiology' to refer to Galen's examinations of the body parts and their activities (ἐνεργεῖαι), following his use of the term in the aformentioned passage of *On the Formation of the Embryo*. In other words, 'physiology' here denotes the study of how the body parts are constituted, what principles govern their activities, how those activities contribute to the functioning of the body as a whole and, in some cases, what the design of the body indicates about the construction of the world. This physiology is neither comparable to the modern notion of 'physiology' nor the exact equivalent of ancient *phusiologia*, but the area of study that Galen thinks *phusiologoi* would be better off studying in any case. It concerns the body parts and their activities, as well as the activities of

[42] Nutton (2012b: 31). [43] *PHP* 9.7.9 de Lacy (5.779–80K). [44] Nutton (2012b: 32).

different parts 'working together' in order to produce systems that maintain vitality.[45]

This volume studies Galen's contribution to this area with a bipartite focus, which reflects his interests in both pluralising and unifying the body and its functions. First, it focuses on the notion of parthood and the many ways in which Galen divides up the body into parts. In doing so, he conceptually takes the body apart, thus pluralising it. Second, it studies the vital processes that these parts are responsible for, such as respiration or nutrition. The full execution of these processes requires multi-organ involvement and, thus, in his attempts to come up with a robust account of these processes, Galen 'puts the body back together', unifying it. I use this methodological cycle to frame the discussion in each of the chapters and in the book overall.

I.4 Parts

The focus on diverse notions of parthood is another methodological pillar of this study. There are many different ways of dividing the body and even more ways of conceptualising these divisions. For example, the most obvious is the division into large visible limbs, such as a hand, a leg, an eye and so on.[46] This taxonomy, however, does not seem to play a major role in Galen's thought. In this work, I focus on those divisions into parts that are more theory-laden and play some role in theorising human nature.

The discussion is especially centred around those parts whose ἐνεργεῖαι Galen theorises most extensively. Before delving into a further discussion of the different divisions of such parts, it is worthwhile to make a note about the translation of this term. It can be translated as both 'activities' and 'functions'. It has been pointed out that Galen's ἐνεργεῖαι differ from contemporary 'functions' and therefore 'activities' is a more suitable option.[47] A lot of recent scholarship use the latter, and I adopt it in this work as well. However, I also talk of the 'functioning' of physiological

45 I use the term 'vitality' to refer to the term ἡ ζωή. Galen uses it when describing vital processes and the parts that carry them out; damage to, for example, respiration, constitutes the threat to 'life itself' (αὐτην τὴν ζωὴν), *Ut. Resp.* 1.1 (80 Furley and Wilkie=4.470K); see also *MM* 9.10 (10.637K); *UP* 6.2 (1.302, 5–7 Helmreich=3.414K). A very similar use in Debru (2008: 263). See also Debru (1996: 258) for the claim that Galen's account of breathing ultimately involves elements and preoccupations that do not exactly correspond to the modern areas of anatomy, physiology or pathology.

46 *UP* 1.8 (1.13, 9–11 Helmreich=3.18K); *Inaeq. Int.* 1 (7.734–5K); *Loc. Aff.* 6.6.5 Brunschön (8.440K).

47 Furley and Wilkie (1984: 61).

systems and the body as a whole, and I argue that there is an ever-present preoccupation with the functionalist understanding of parts and their significance.

When it comes to grouping parts into different categories, the most common taxonomy in Galen's texts is the division of a body into structured and homoeomerous parts.[48] This seemingly simple division is ubiquitous. Apart from the Peripatetic influence (already discussed in scholarship), I argue that Galen understands this division against a certain Hippocratic background too. The frequency with which Galen uses it suggests that it is significant, and the concluding part of this volume presents an argument that this division is fundamental for a Galenic understanding of the human body, and therefore it plays a role in most discussions.

On a few occasions, Galen also introduces what he calls the Hippocratic division of a body into solids, fluids and pneumata.[49] This higher-order division of parts not only plays a crucial role in pathology but also encompasses the famous Galenic humoral theory, incorporating it into a general account of human functioning. The upshot of this taxonomy is the division of tissues into types, according to what could be called texture or viscosity. The textural properties (themselves pre-determined by their respective mixtures) determine how different types of tissues in a body interact with each other, including the speed with which certain pathological or therapeutic changes take place. This theory plays an especially important explanatory role in Chapter 3.

A more generally applicable division of the body can also be found in Galen's description of diagnoses and treatments of fevers. Key to a successful treatment of a fever is the preservation of the three central physiological systems underpinned by the organs governing them: the brain, the heart and the liver. Galen explains that the continuous functioning of these parts ensures the maintenance of life and therefore their preservation ought to be prioritised in medical treatments.[50] Thus, the fever conditions show that these are the main parts of a human being for all (medical) intents and purposes. These three systems, therefore, form the cornerstones of Galenic physiology. They correspond to the tripartite soul system that Galen

48 See the list of passages in Chapter 1, note 48.

49 *Trem. Palp.* 5 (7.596–7K); see also *Diff. Feb.* 2 (7.277K) and *Caus. Puls.* 4.10 (9.176–7K). Interestingly, a slightly different formulation can be found in *MM* 11.1 (10.737K), where the three elements are pneumata, truly solid parts and fleshy parts. See Hipp. *Epid.* 6.8.7 (5.346, 5–6 Littré); Flemming (2000: 95–6) approaches ancient medical tradition in general as concerned with these three kinds of substances.

50 *MM* 9.10 (10.635–8K).

inherits from Plato. The physiological domains of the three souls are the nervous system, the cardiac/pneumatic system and the vegetative system. The activities of these systems are fundamentally different in nature. While the nervous system is in charge of voluntary motion and perception, thus enabling rational activities, the cardiac/pneumatic and the vegetative systems are in charge of cardiac activities that maintain the innate heat and nutritive activities underlying growth and healthy functioning respectively. Together, they constitute a kind of unity that underpins the maintenance of vitality, so that serious damage to any one of these systems will inevitably result in lethal damage to the others. Galen never explains explicitly how these systems form such a closely intertwined and unified common system. At the same time, the underlying unifying concepts, assumptions and theoretical devices can emerge from a systematic study of the relevant material in his oeuvre.

I.5 Chapter Descriptions

The chapters of this volume build on one another. The study starts with a general discussion of the ways in which Galen divides up the body into parts. The chapter analyses the conception of parthood by focusing on the two claims that, when taken together, amount to a very idiosyncratic view. First, Galen claims that the loss of a bone results in a complete loss of voluntary motion in the limb. Second, he also claims that the loss of a stomach is not vital and does not impede the ability of the body to be nourished. Not all parts, therefore, are created equal. Having analysed several of Galen's divisions of parts, the chapter concludes that he theorises parthood in relative terms, in reference to the functional role the part plays in a bodily process. Furthermore, the organic functionality of the body is tied to and determined by the three central systems: the nutritive, the cardiac and the nervous. Their significance manifests itself via three processes they govern: nutrition and growth, breathing, and voluntary motion and perception, respectively. The following three chapters are structured around answering the question of why and how each of these processes constitute the vitality of the human body.

Chapter 2 focuses on the domain of the vegetative soul, comprising nutrition and growth. The vegetative capacities are the most fundamental, but also the simplest activities that distinguish organic from inorganic life. They are present not only in animals but also in plants. This chapter examines the central vegetative system consisting of the liver, the veins and their supporting organs, as well as the vegetative capacities present in all the tissues that are subservient to this system. The chapter not only discusses the relationship between the central parts and capacities in the rest of the body, but also examines the ways in which these capacities manifest themselves, arguing they represent Galen's attempts to grapple with the notion of basic vitality, which in later terminology became known as the organic life. The key problem is the extent of the capacities: although their primary domain is nutrition and growth, they are also called 'demiurgic', a term with significant philosophical pedigree and implications, in an embryological context. The chapter delineates the scope of the vegetative domain by examining the process of nutrition, Galen's description of the vegetative capacities and his conceptualisation of 'demiurgic' acts.

If Chapter 2 addresses the notion of the basic vitality, Chapter 3 deals with the cardiac system that underpins the more complex animal vitality. The key process governed by the cardiac system is breathing, and the chapter begins with a discussion of different types of breathing, as well as the anatomy that underpins those types, before moving on to Galen's explanation of why deprivation of breath leads to death. Key to the process of breathing is pneuma, and he distinguishes three types: the vital, which is important for respiration, the psychic, which plays a role in perception, and the natural pneuma, whose existence is uncertain. Given that the account of breathing already covers the role of the vital pneuma, the discussion moves on to the role of the other two types: the super-refined psychic and the most turgid natural pneuma. The account of the latter is elusive, but, I argue, Galen's approach to the question of its existence shows a tendency to adopt a pattern. The properties of the natural pneuma are linked to the activities of the nutritive system, just like the properties of the vital and the psychic pneumata are linked to the cardiac and the nervous systems, respectively. In addition to discussing the three types of pneuma and their activities, the chapter also introduces yet another Galenic division of the body into solids, fluids and pneumata. This division according to texture and movement of tissues offers an important glimpse into how Galen conceives of the interaction between parts. Moreover, the rapid alteration in the pneumatic tissues underpins the physiological understanding of animal vitality.

Chapter 4 is devoted to the final and, in a certain sense, most complex physiological domain, the nervous system, in charge of three activities: voluntary motion, pain and perception. Unlike the motion of the cardiac and nutritive system, called motions 'by nature', the motion of this system is voluntary. This physiological domain, thus, is the one that enables the exercise of control, and the discussion in this chapter is focused on delineating the extent and the nature of this control. Key to this control is the role of nerves. Building his understanding against the background of the discoveries of the Alexandrian Herophilus, Galen presents an extensive discussion of the anatomy of nerves. His descriptions of the different types of nerves are more elaborate than his discussions of veins and arteries, but their typology shares similarities with pneumata. Most notably, sensory nerves and the psychic pneuma, both of which play an important role in perception, are much finer in texture than their counterparts responsible for vital activities. Thus emerges one of the patterns that Galen uses to classify body parts belonging to different systems.

Starting from the motor nerves responsible for voluntary motion, the chapter examines the anatomy that enables these nerves to exercise control over muscles and bones. I also argue that, in the context of the bodily motions overall, the role of voluntary motion is relatively small. Subsequently, I discuss Galen's account of pain, arguing that the primary phenomenon takes place in the tissues, and nerves simply enable the sensation; the fundamental mechanism of this phenomenon is the same as the one found in sense perception (covered in Section I.6) and in the internally directed sensation, such as hunger, discussed in Chapter 2. Galen, thus, applies the same model of the perceptive capacity of nerves to explain different phenomenon. The nervous tissues present a number of problems when it comes to accounting for perception, but this chapter especially focuses on the problem of the inherent sensitivity of the tissue. In a rare critique of Herophilus, Galen rejects his finding of the inherent sensitivity of the tissue, which, I argue, is important in explaining his hesitation towards accepting more physicalist understanding of psychic properties.

The final chapter is dedicated to the ways in which Galen unifies the discrete parts and systems into a single unified entity, especially focusing on the tripartition. The adoption of the Platonic tripartition is, at least in one important way, puzzling. Originally, the tripartition of the souls helped to explain the psychological conflict; Galen, however, is strongly committed to the physiological tripartition, and, in fact, the discussions in the previous chapters show that he does indeed make the three physiological systems fairly discrete. But the body is also obviously a unified entity, and this chapter explores Galen's theorisation of the grounds of its unity. Starting with anatomical unity, the chapter moves on to discuss the material flux into and out of the body that the three central systems control. Galen posits the persistence of identity through this material change with a reference to the form. The following discussion shows Galen's complex relationship with this notion. Like some of his contemporary Middle Platonists, Galen adopts the Stoic idea that the formal cause is subordinate and instrumental to the cause from the maker, the efficient and the final causes. The proper explanation, thus, lies not with the form of the body but its design, especially the purpose of the design. Finally, I argue the notion of a cohesive cause, which Galen uses to theorise such processes as respiration and pulse, can account successfully for vitality, giving an elegant way for unifying vital activities and the parts performing them into a single unified whole.

The Conclusion summarises the findings by explaining the key motivations and claims behind the Galenic understanding of bodily unity.

I.6 Scholarship

There are still many areas in this expansive corpus that have never been addressed in a long study, and the problem of the unity of Galenic physiology is one of them. However, such theme and focus would not be possible without building on the previous work on various aspects of Galen's physiology both in older monographs, such as C. R. S. Harris (1973) and E. Mendelsohn (1964), and in more recent works. In fact, Galenic scholarship has expanded significantly in recent years. The treatise *On the Doctrines of Hippocrates and Plato* in particular has received a lot of scholarly attention, including monographs devoted to it (e.g., Tieleman 1996). More recent monographs on various anatomical, physiological and psychological aspects of Galenic work include Stewart (2018), Rocca (2003), Salas (2020b) and Devinant (2020). In addition to these, some notable monographs investigated various literary and rhetorical aspects of Galen's work, including Mattern (2008) and Petit (2018) as well as Curtis (2010). In addition to full monographs, edited volumes, both dedicated to Galen specifically and those thematically broader, are important sources of Galenic scholarship, including Hankinson (2008c), Thumiger and Singer (2018), Petit (2019), Adamson, Hansberger and Wilberding (2014), Gill, Whitmarsh and Wilkins (2009), Horstmanshoff, King and Zittel (2012), and Bouras-Valliantos and Zipser (2019).

When it comes to works dedicated to Galenic physiology in particular, aside from the more dated and somewhat controversial study of Rudoph E. Siegel (1968–73), the important studies tend to focus on a specific area of physiology, for instance, the cardiac system and pneumatology in Debru (1996). Some of the most prominent examinations of Galen's thought in recent years have also been done in the article form, for example, van der Eijk (2014) or Hankinson (2003). Galen's understanding of human functioning overall is also often discussed in works not specifically dedicated to Galen, but to history of medicine more generally.[51] This monograph will complement the current scholarship by offering a book-length study of the unity of Galenic physiology in particular, focusing on its theorisation, coherence and significance for Galenic understanding of human identity.

The problem of how Galen conceptualises unity is also the main theme of Gill (2010), which focuses on psychology, presenting an innovative reading of what the author calls the 'high naturalism' of the Stoics and Galen.[52] The key argument is that Galen, despite his animosity to the Stoics in such works as *On the Doctrines of Hippocrates and Plato*, would have actually benefitted from adopting the Stoic understanding of the single *hēgemonikon* instead of the Platonic tripartition. Although this work does contain some physiological discussions (e.g., embryology in Chapters 2 and 3), its main focus is on psychology and related problems. The central topic of the present volume is also the question of unity, although it primarily focuses on those organs and systems that maintain vitality, such as nutrition, respiration, voluntary motion by means of nerves, muscles and bones, none of which feature prominently in Gill's discussion. Given its focus, this volume also does not address any significant problems in Galenic psychology, covered by Gill and others,[53] with one relatively small exception. The question on which psychology and physiology do overlap is the tripartition of the soul and organ systems. This question is briefly discussed in Chapter 5, but the overall discussion in the chapter puts an emphasis on the physiological aspects of the tripartition, concentrating on the interdependence of the organs rather than the psychological activities they underpin. Thus, my enquiry into the physiological unity runs parallel to Christopher Gill's investigation of the psychological unity, and, hopefully, complements it.

[51] For example, Cunningham (1997: 25–31). [52] Gill (2010: 66–77).
[53] For an overview of the Galenic psychology and pertinent problems, see Singer (2013a: 3–4, 18–30); Devinant (2020) is a major recent study of psychological illness in Galen. See also Trompeter (2018, 2025).

I.7 The Problem of the Substance of the Soul

There is one more significant problem that studying the unity of parts inevitably raises: the relationship between the psychic and the physical in Galen. He is committed to the traditional Platonising view that the body is an instrument of the soul,[54] which naturally raises the question of the nature of the interaction between these two. Is the soul a corporeal entity and this interaction is only a matter of a body affecting another body? If it is incorporeal, then how can it have an effect on the body, a corporeal and thus fundamentally different kind of entity?[55]

The problem of the substance of the soul and the potential reducibility of the psychic properties to the activities of the mixtures in the homoeomerous tissues is a well-known and widely discussed problem in Galenic scholarship. A number of recent studies explored what either could be called a kind of physicalism,[56] or the blurring of distinction between the body and the soul,[57] or the ways in which mixtures account for certain types of psychic content,[58] or how Galen makes no indication that pathologies of the 'soul' amount to more than the imbalances of the mixtures.[59] These studies, although concentrated on different topics, focus on the same broad question, that is, whether the Galenic stance somehow implies the conclusion that psychic capacities can be explained in terms of the properties of tissues, which are produced by the mixture of the four elements. Although, in many important ways, this volume builds on these arguments, by and large it adopts a modest approach, taking Galen's

[54] Galen makes this claim when contrasting the ape body and the human body. The former resembles the latter in the elements but not in the structure, because the structure is dictated by the soul (which implies instrumentality: certain kind of soul requires a certain kind of body), see *UP* 1.22 (1.59, 5–6 Helmreich=3.80–81K) and *UP* 3.16 (1.194, 9–11 Helmreich=3.264K); see also *QAM* 5 (54, 21–55, 7 Müller=5.795K). The ancient creationism that Galen is firmly committed to is distinctly anthropocentric; this point is discussed extensively throughout Sedley (2007), especially in the cases of Anaxagoras, Socrates, Aristotle and the Stoics.

[55] The Stoic physics puts a special emphasis on this problem, laying the ground for a materialist metaphysics that posits that all existing things are bodies; see, for example, Sextus Empiricus *M* 8.263=*SVF* 2.363=LS 45B.

[56] Gill (2010: 140–1, 145, 148), for example, suggests that Galen is leaning towards the Stoic style of physicalism. He further argues that embracing fully this kind of physicalism would have made Galen's own position stronger and more coherent (152–167). See also the discussion of this point in Chapter 3, note 165.

[57] Das (2020: 35–56).

[58] As in Havrda (2017), although it is worth noting that such an interpretation is only applied to those psychic properties that are underpinned by the activities of the vegetative and the spirited soul; Havrda concludes that Galen did not make the same claim about the rational soul. See also Vinkesteijn (2022).

[59] Singer (2018: 403–4).

claims that he does not commit himself to any theory of the substance of the soul at face value, just as the sources state. The reasons for this are twofold.

First, this approach is more consistent with Galen's ideas of what *phusiologia* ought to study. As his claim about the muscle movement in *On the Formation of the Embryo* indicates, the common philosophical problems ought not to overshadow the understanding of instruments. In fact, understanding instruments *qua* their instrumentality is no less important than the question of how the soul affects those instruments causally. Galen's position can be interpretated as follows: there is no doubt that the soul does affect the body and does use it as its instrument. Although the study of the mechanism by means of which it manages to do it is an important philosophical problem, there is a further, often overlooked but no less significant, problem: how are these instruments equipped to carry out the actions of the soul? It is all well and good to have opinions about the nature of causality between the body and the soul, but an account of *how* the body can enable the activities of the soul is equally necessary and no less philosophically interesting, according to Galen. This aspect of his understanding of the relationship between the body and the soul remains underexplored in the scholarship, and therefore this work prioritises it over the more standard philosophical question of causality.

Second, there is a potential methodological pitfall this approach aims to avoid. The key problem to looking for physicalist commitments in Galen is the interpretation of his explicit disavowal of the knowledge of the substance of the soul in various treatises.[60] It produces the following dilemma: on the one hand, if Galen was inclined to some form of physicalism, then the denial of the knowledge about the substance of the soul was disingenuous, and we ought to doubt the evidence of the text. If, on the other hand, Galen's denials were genuine, then we need an explanation of how the claim that psychic capacities follow the mixtures of the body is compatible with the lack of knowledge about the substance of the soul. This volume explores the second horn of this dilemma, because, arguably, it is a more productive way of approaching this issue. First, it does not require positing any extra-textual motivations for Galen's stance, so it survives the Occam's razor unscathed, unlike the first approach.

[60] For example, *Form. Foet.* 6, 32–4 Nickel (4.701–2K); *Prop. Plac.* 15.2 (136–8 Lami Garofalo); *PHP* 9.9.7 de Lacy (5.793K); in the context of the argument that even Plato himself went as far as to suggest that his account of the substance of the soul and the manner of the world generation is only a plausible and reasonable one (*PHP* 9.9.3 de Lacy (5.791–2K)).

Second, it is a more charitable reading; it is hard to motivate the view that someone who was micro-managing the spread of his work and attempting to guide his readers through his own corpus with treatises dedicated to that purpose would misdescribe his views in those treatises. It is not impossible, yet not very likely either.[61]

Finally, these two reasons also make it a more productive approach in the sense that, if answering the second horn of the dilemma succeeds, then the first horn dissipates. However, if we approach the problem as it is formulated in the first horn, then the second horn still remains a possible problem. In other words, in order to argue convincingly that Galen was leaning towards physicalism, it is necessary to establishing that there is no way of talking about mixture-mental capacity dependencies without physicalist commitments in the Galenic theoretical framework.

Taking into account all the recent arguments about the cases in which the psychic properties appear to share very close ties, if not identity, with the bodily mixtures, this volume explores how such dependencies can be explained in the physiological framework while maintaining that the substance of the soul is unknown. If there is such an explanation, it lies in Galen's conceptualisations of the scope of activities of each part of the body. Starting with the activities of the central governing parts, the brain, the heart and the liver, this volume also covers the significance of their interdependence and the role that the other, the so-called instrumental parts, play in the healthy functioning of the body. The discussion of what makes some parts vital and some instrumental culminates in the analysis of the Galenic claim that the body overall is an instrument of the soul, which leads to the key conclusions about the coherence and the unity of Galenic physiology.

[61] Salas (2020b: 17–27). *On My Own Books, The Order of My Own Books* and the late treatise *On My Own Opinions* could be arguably included in this list too. Although primarily dedicated to correcting the misinterpretation of his works (and thus defending Galen against criticism), it also provides an instruction for the reader on how to understand and interpret Galen's views, including the denial of ever claiming to know the substance of the soul.

CHAPTER 1

Galen on Parts
Taking the Body Apart

In contemporary English, the body parts are typically called organs. This term comes from the ancient Greek τό ὄργανον, but the primary meaning of the latter is an 'instrument' rather than a body part. The body parts can be, and often are, instruments in Galen's writing, but his conceptualisation of this term is more complex than it might seem at first sight.[1] For instance, in the description of the muscular motion, Galen states that the motor nerve is the demiurge and the bone is the instrument.[2] If the bone is broken, the motor nerves are completely hindered from exercising their activities – that is, walking. The instrument here is a crucial enabler of the activity. This is not true of all the instruments, however. In *On the Doctrines of Hippocrates and Plato*, while attacking Erasistratus' account of the veins as unclear, Galen notes that this Alexandrian doctor left their whole activity unexamined, despite the fact that they are more important than the stomach. He supports this by stating that, even if the stomach is no longer able to crush food, it is possible to stay alive by drinking fluids. The destruction of the generation of blood, meanwhile, results in inevitable death.[3] Presumably, it is not desirable to lose the activities of such an organ as a stomach,[4] yet it is, ultimately, an expendable part, owing to the fact that life is possible without it. The stomach is an instrumental organ in

1 In this work, I adopt both translations. In most cases, the translation 'organ' is suitable, with the caveat that Galen's definition of parts as organs is taken into account (discussed in this chapter, especially Section 1.1.4). When it comes to the topics pertaining to the soul, it is conventional to adopt the translation 'instrument'; for example, the question of whether the psychic pneuma is an instrument of the soul (Section 3.3.2), and I follow this practice here too.

2 *UP* 17.1 (2.437, 18–21 Helmreich=4.347K); see also the discussion in Chapter 4; for the notion of 'demiurge', see the discussion in Chapter 2. See also *UP* 17.2 (2.450, 6–16 Helmreich=4.363–4K), where knowledge of the bones is described as knowledge of the useful, not the same as knowledge of action (comprised of nerves and muscles), but also important.

3 *PHP* 6.6.26 de Lacy (5.554K) ff.

4 On the activities of the stomach, see *Nat. Fac.* 3.7 (217, 10 Helmreich=2.160K) ff.

the nutritive system governed by the liver,[5] just like bones are instrumental organs in the motor system governed by the brain, yet their instrumentality bears different significance; counter-intuitively, the bone seems to be a more significant instrument than the stomach!

Clearly, not all instruments are of equal value *qua* instruments; this point naturally raises the question of what kind of instruments there are and what determines their (relative or absolute) significance. In order to answer these questions, it is necessary to start from a simpler concept. The issue at stake here is the division of the body into parts. Starting with the examination of Galen's own critical account with the common terminology and presuppositions about parthood, this chapter explores two of the ways in which he divides the body into parts: homoeomerous and structured, and the four-fold division. In order to clarify the implications of the former, it also looks at the distinction Galen makes between parts and forms. Ultimately, I argue that Galen rejects the seemingly apt existing terminology (especially *meros/morion* distinction) and presents his own nomenclature for differentiating parts in order to put the activity or function at the forefront. The bodily parts, according to him, must be classified in reference to their activity more than their placement. The differentiation of activities that different parts have is further clarified in the four-fold division of parts, introducing a variety of relationships between the parts that self-manage and the principal parts that govern others, as well as those parts that are governed by the principal parts. Before concluding, the chapter addresses one further question that relates to the functionality of parts: the imperfect constitution of the body. The cases discussed here show that Galen understands activity in reference to vitality and, even while discussing normative imperfections of, for example, the female reproductive system, he praises its functional excellence in carrying and nourishing the embryo. Untangling Galen's preoccupation with activity ultimately leads to a better understanding of how parts make up the whole and why some of them seem to be more important than others.

1.1 What Is a Part?

When Galen talks about part divisions, he typically uses the term τό μέρος and its cognates. He defines the term at the beginning of *On the Usefulness*

[5] *PHP* 6.4.6 de Lacy (5.534K); *PHP* 6.3.7 de Lacy (5.521K). The distinction between necessary and subsidiary parts is already made in Aristotle *GA* 2.6 (744b11–27). The passage is discussed in Section 1.3, together with an argument concerning the differences between Aristotle and Galen.

of Parts in fairly simple terms. Every animal is *one* because it has its own circumscription; in the same way, the body parts have their own circumscriptions and by virtue of this, they are said to be one. They are not, however, circumscribed individually. They are also joined, and by virtue of sharing a connection with another entity, they are defined as parts. Galen concludes that 'all bodies that do not have their own circumscription at every point and are not everywhere joined to others are called parts'.[6] Mathematical terminology imbues this definition with authority, but the conceptualisation of parthood here is biological. The latter point becomes apparent if we consider the fact that this definition could have counter-examples. Once a piece of timber, for instance, is shaped into a plank of a ship, it can be used for one ship and then reused for another. It can be joined and rejoined to a number of different planks equally successfully, always acting as a part of a ship.[7] But what is true for parts of artefacts is not true of arms, hands and legs. From the point of their inception, body parts are physically connected in such a way as to form a closer unity that is never found among artefacts, no matter how well made. If body parts are separated, they are no longer proper body parts with their proper activities, and they cannot be reattached or attached to another body (not in the ancient world, at any rate). The condition of attachment implies inherent unity proper to living entities. Galen is, thus, implicitly preoccupied with this type of parthood that is distinct from artefact parthoods.[8] His preoccupation with a vitalist understanding of the body will be an important theme throughout this volume.

He is certainly not singular in his interest in vital parthood. In another set of passages, Galen reflects critically on the existing terminology of parts and expounds some of the principles that govern parthood, according to

[6] *UP* 1.1 (1.1, 8–10 Helmreich=3.2K), tr. May (1968: 67): ὥσθ' ὅσα σώματα μήτε πάντη περιγραφὴν ἰδίαν ἔχει μήτε πάντη συνῆπται πρὸς ἕτερα, μόρια ταῦτα κέκληται. See also the discussion in Barnes (1988: 243–4).

[7] A ship is a common example in the discussions of how wholes are constituted; the Stoics famously distinguished between the artificial unity of a ship and the proper unity of natural entities that possess a single tenor; see, for example, Sextus Empiricus *M* 9.78; 9.81; Simplicius *In Cat.* 214, 24–37=*SVF* 2.391=LS28M. This Stoic distinction has cosmological implications because it is often found in connection with the argument that the whole world is unified in the way that natural entities are; see Alexander of Aphrodisias *Mix.* 216.14–16=LS 48C. For the Stoic metaphysical commitments in this respect, see White (2003); Sauvé Meyer (2009: 78–80); Hensley (2020); Helle (2021).

[8] My reading differs from Barnes (1988: 243), who notes that 'the treatise is concerned with the parts of living things, but there is no reason to think that Galen's introductory discussion applies only to such parts'. While it is true that there is no explicit connection to the biological parthood in the text, I would argue that such a reading would be preferable not only because the context implies it but also because it is more charitable to Galen's conceptualisation, as I have argued.

him. The passage contains one of the more substantive discussions of parthood and can be found in his exposition of the correct therapeutic method in *On the Therapeutic Method*.[9] Having chosen the eye as an example for explaining his method, Galen writes the following:

> ὀνομαζέσθω τοίνυν ὀφθαλμὸς μὲν τὸ μόριον τοῦ σώματος, οὐδὲν οὐδ᾽ ἐνταῦθα διαφέρον εἴτε μέρος εἴτε μόριον εἴποι τις· ὅ τι γὰρ ἂν ᾖ τοῦ παντὸς συμπληρωτικόν, ἐκεῖνο μόριόν τε καὶ μέρος ὀνομάζεται, τοῦ ὅλου δηλονότι σώματος, οὗ συμπληρωτικὸν ὑπάρχει. ἐν γὰρ τῷ πρός τι τὸ μέρος· ὅλου γὰρ καὶ παντός ἐστι τὸ μέρος, ὥσπερ, οἶμαι, καὶ τὸ πᾶν καὶ τὸ ὅλον πρὸς τὴν τῶν οἰκείων μερῶν τε καὶ μορίων ἀναφορὰν ὀνομάζεται, καὶ ἔστιν ὥσπερ τὸ δεξιὸν πρὸς τὸ ἀριστερὸν καὶ τὸ ἀριστερὸν πρὸς τὸ δεξιόν, οὕτω καὶ τὸ πᾶν πρὸς τὸ μέρος καὶ τὸ μέρος πρὸς τὸ πᾶν. εἴ τις οὖν ταύτην φυλάττων τὴν ἔννοιαν αἱρεῖται μέρος λέγειν, οὐ μόριον, ἢ εἴ τις ἔμπαλιν οὐ μόριον, ἀλλὰ μέρος, ἐμοὶ μὲν οὐδὲν εἰς τὴν εὕρεσιν τῶν πραγμάτων ἐμποδίζει, δείκνυσι δ᾽ αὐτὸν ὀψιμαθῆ τῆς τῶν Ἑλλήνων φωνῆς· ὥσπέρ γε καὶ εἴ τις ὅλον καὶ τὸ πᾶν διορίζει, καὶ οὗτος ἀγνοεῖ τὴν τῶν Ἑλλήνων διάλεκτον.
>
> Let the eye, then, be called a part of the body, insofar as it makes no difference here if one says some component (*meros*) or part (*morion*). For whatever constitutes an essential part of the whole is called a part or a component, the whole, clearly, being the body of which it is an essential part. In this [body] the part is in relation to something because it is also the part of a totality and of a whole so that, in my view, the whole and the totality are so named with reference to its own parts or components. And just as the right is named with reference to the left, or the left to the right, so also the whole is named with reference to the part, or the part to the whole. If someone, while adhering to this concept, chooses to say 'component' (*meros*) and not 'part' (*morion*), or conversely 'part' (*morion*) and not 'component' (*meros*), as far as I'm concerned this presents no hindrance to the discovery of the matter but shows him to be laggard in learning the language of the Greeks. Similarly, if someone makes a distinction between the whole (*holos*) and the totality (*pan*), he, too, is ignorant of the Greek language.[10]

After an intermission dedicated to the criticism of the merely verbal disagreements, Galen continues as follows:

> ἡ μὲν οὖν ὄψις, αὖθις γὰρ ἐπὶ τὸν ὀφθαλμὸν ἰτέον, ἐνέργεια τοῦ μέρους ἐστίν· ὁ δ᾽ ὀφθαλμὸς αὐτὸς τὸ τοῦ ζώου μόριον, οὐδὲν γάρ, ὡς εἴρηται, διαφέρει μόριον εἰπεῖν, ἢ μέρος. ὄργανον δὲ ὀνομάζω μέρος ζώου τελείας ἐνεργείας ἀπεργαστικόν, οἷον ὀφθαλμὸν ὄψεως καὶ γλῶτταν διαλέκτου καὶ

9 He says this much at the end of his exposition at *MM* 1.7 (10.62K): ἐν τούτῳ δὲ τὸ πᾶν ἐστι, καὶ τοῦτο ἀρχὴ καὶ οἷον στοιχεῖόν τι πρῶτον ἁπάσης τῆς θεραπευτικῆς ὑπάρχει μεθόδου.

10 *MM* 1.5 (10.43–4K), tr. Johnston and Horsley (2011: 69).

σκέλη βαδίσεως· οὕτω δὲ καὶ ἀρτηρία καὶ φλὲψ καὶ νεῦρον, ὄργανά τε καὶ μόρια ζώων ἐστί. κατὰ ταύτην γοῦν τὴν χρῆσιν τῶν ὀνομάτων οὐ πρὸς ἡμῶν μόνον, ἀλλὰ καὶ πρὸς τῶν παλαιῶν Ἑλλήνων ὁρισθεῖσαν, ὁ μὲν οὖν ὀφθαλμὸς ὀνομασθήσεται καὶ μόριον ζώου καὶ μέρος καὶ ὄργανον· ὁ δὲ κερατοειδὴς χιτὼν μόριον μὲν καὶ μέρος, ὄργανον δ' οὔ· κατὰ ταὐτὰ δὲ καὶ ὁ ῥαγοειδὴς καὶ ὁ ἀραχνοειδὴς καὶ ὁ ἀμφιβληστροειδής· ἕκαστος γὰρ τούτων πρῶτον μὲν καὶ μάλιστα μόριόν ἐστιν ὀφθαλμοῦ, διότι δ' οὗτος προσώπου, διὰ τοῦτο κᾀκεῖνοι κατὰ δεύτερον ἤδη λόγον· οὕτω δὲ καὶ τοῦ σώματος ὅλου, διότι καὶ τὸ πρόσωπον ὅλου τοῦ σώματός ἐστι μόριον.

Sight then – for one must go back to the eyes once more – is an activity of the component (*meros*), while the eye itself is a part (*morion*) of the animal for, as has been said, it makes no difference to say part (*morion*) or component (*meros*). I call an organ a component (*meros*) of an animal which performs a complete activity: for example, the eye [effects] sight, the tongue speech, the legs walking, and in like manner, an artery, a vein and a nerve are both organs and also parts of animals. At all events, in accordance with this use of terms defined not only by us alone but also by the Greeks of old, the eye will be called a part (*morion*) of an animal, and a component (*meros*), and an organ, whereas the external 'tunic' (cornea, sclera) is a part (*morion*) and a component (*meros*) but not an organ, and it is the same for the choroid membrane, the arachnoid membrane and the retina, for each of these is primarily and particularly a part (*morion*) of the eye. But because the eye is part of the face, these are also parts of the face in a secondary sense, in the same way as they are also parts of the whole body because the face is a part of the whole body.[11]

A distinct terminology for portions of homoeomerous and structured parts would seem to be a desirable tool for Galen's conceptualisation of bodily constitution, but he is wary of adopting this nomenclature.[12] In vehemently rejecting such terminology, he also makes a number of pertinent remarks of how he thinks about parthood. One remarkable point in this passage is the description of parts and wholes as correlatives ('Just as the right is named with reference to the left, or the left to the right, so also the whole is named with reference to the part, or the part to the whole'). The passage also contains the identity conditions of an organ. It is a *meros* that 'performs a complete activity'.[13] The passage further states that the

[11] *MM* 1.6 (10.47–8K), tr. Johnston and Horsley (2011: 75), slightly altered.

[12] The *meros*/*morion* distinction under attack here is used to differentiate between a proper part and a part of that part, and both could be structured parts. This is not a distinction between homoeomerous and discrete parthood. At the same time, Galen's distaste for such terminological distinction sheds some light on his motivation to avoid a parallel distinction concerning homoeomerous and structured parts.

[13] See also *PHP* 1.8.11–15 de Lacy (5.203–4K).

parthood is transitive, that is, the parts of the eye are also part of the face in the secondary sense.[14] Each of these claims references some debates and views of the predecessors in a telling manner.

1.1.1 Meros *and* Morion

First, let's address the distinction between *meros* and *morion*. The diminutive *morion* is commonly found in physiological texts. A famous example would be the Greek title of Aristotle's *De Partibus Animalium* (Περὶ ζῴων μορίων). Galen's attack focuses on the use of the term when it is contrasted with *meros*, arguing that there is no ground for making a distinction between the terms. Galen's target here is a bit of a mystery, as the distinction is not at all common. Another source for it is a passage in Sextus Empiricus, and this text is a bit more generous with the detail. In his attack on the dogmatists and their accounts of parts and wholes, Sextus records the following:

> τὸ δὲ μόριον καὶ αὐτὸ λέγεται διχῶς, καὶ ὁτὲ μὲν ὡς διαφέρον τοῦ ἰδίως νοουμένου μέρους, καθά φασιν αὐτὸ μέρος μέρους εἶναι, καθάπερ δάκτυλον μὲν τῆς χειρός, οὖς δὲ τῆς κεφαλῆς, ὁτὲ δ' ὡς μὴ διαφέρον ἀλλὰ μέρος ὂν τοῦ ὅλου, καθό τινές φασι κοινῶς μέρος εἶναι τὸ συμπληρωτικὸν τοῦ ὅλου.
>
> And 'portion', too, is itself said in two ways, sometimes as different from the part properly conceived – as when they say that it is a part of a part, as a finger is of the hand, or an ear of the head – but at other times as not different, but as being a part of the whole, as when some say in general that a portion is what is such as to complete the whole.[15]

This short passage gives an account of two different ways of using the term *morion*. In the first case, it is used for referring to a part of a part only. In the second case, the term has no special reference. It is used to denote a part (*meros*) of the whole, so the two terms are interchangeable. The first use of the *morion* described by Sextus here is precisely the kind of position that Galen is criticising.[16] The scholars who commented on Sextus' passage

[14] Barnes (1988: 243) argues that Galen commits to the intransitivity of parts on the basis of the passage at the beginning of the *UP* (see note 6).

[15] Sextus Empiricus *M* 9.337–8, tr. Bett (2012: 63).

[16] There is a notable similarity between the second group of dogmatists and the way in which Galen describes a parthood in *MM* 1.5 cited above: τὸ συμπληρωτικὸν τοῦ ὅλου and ὅ τι γὰρ ἂν ᾖ τοῦ παντὸς συμπληρωτικόν, respectively. The key term here is συμπληρωτικός. In philosophy, this term is especially associated with Epicurus, who notably uses it in connection to health (*Ep. Men.* 128; Diogenes Laertius 10.131). By Galen's time, the term appears to be used fairly widely in metaphysics, without any distinctly Epicurean undertones, see Sextus Empiricus *PH* 3.100.

noted that the distinction between *meros* and *morion* is rare and puzzling, hardly adopted by any ancient philosopher.[17] Aristotle, for example, uses the terms interchangeably. One possible provenance of the distinction might be the Stoa. In very late antiquity, Ammonius employs it when arguing that logic is an instrument rather than a part of philosophy,[18] and his target is the Stoic conceptualisation of logic as a distinct *meros* of philosophy (rather than an instrument or a *morion* of physics or ethics). Jonathan Barnes notes that the Stoics clearly used the *meros/morion* distinction in order to delineate precisely the relationship between logic and philosophy, but there is hardly any evidence of the *meros/morion* distinction used in other contexts, and the terms are typically employed synonymously.[19]

The fact that both Galen and Sextus refer to the distinction hints at another possible source, namely, some scientific or medical text or texts. Sextus, after all, was a doctor just like Galen, and his work contains medical remarks and even anatomical examples.[20] The origin of the distinction, therefore, might be not purely philosophical. Indeed, something very similar to the *meros/morion* distinction shows up in Theophrastus' botanical work. The passage makes it clear that this terminology is used to describe human anatomy (as well as that of plants) as follows:

> Σχεδὸν δὲ καὶ τὰς ἄλλας μορφὰς ἑκάστων ταῦτα διασημαίνει. διαφέρουσι γὰρ πλήθει τῷ τούτων καὶ ὀλιγότητι καὶ πυκνότητι καὶ μανότητι καὶ τῷ ἐφ᾽ ἓν ἢ εἰς πλείω σχίζεσθαι καὶ τοῖς ἄλλοις τοῖς ὁμοίοις. ἔστι δὲ ἕκαστον τῶν εἰρημένων οὐχ ὁμοιομερές· λέγω δὲ οὐχ ὁμοιομερὲς ὅτι ἐκ τῶν αὐτῶν μὲν ὁτιοῦν μέρος σύγκειται τῆς ῥίζης καὶ τοῦ στελέχους, ἀλλ᾽ οὐ λέγεται στέλεχος τὸ ληφθὲν ἀλλὰ μόριον, ὡς ἐν τοῖς τῶν ζώων μέλεσίν ἐστιν. ἐκ τῶν αὐτῶν μὲν γὰρ ὁτιοῦν τῆς κνήμης ἢ τοῦ ἀγκῶνος, οὐχ ὁμώνυμον δὲ καθάπερ σὰρξ καὶ ὀστοῦν, ἀλλ᾽ ἀνώνυμον· οὐδὲ δὴ τῶν ἄλλων οὐδενὸς ὅσα μονοειδῆ τῶν ὀργανικῶν· ἁπάντων γὰρ τῶν τοιούτων ἀνώνυμα τὰ μέρη. τῶν δὲ πολυειδῶν ὠνομασμένα καθάπερ ποδὸς χειρὸς κεφαλῆς, οἷον δάκτυλος ῥὶς ὀφθαλμός. καὶ τὰ μὲν μέγιστα μέρη σχεδὸν ταῦτά ἐστιν.

> Trees moreover shew forth fairly well the other features also which distinguish plants; for they exhibit differences in the number or fewness of these which they possess, as to the closeness or openness of their growth, as to

[17] Barnes (1988); Bett (2012: 63n171); Ierodiakonou (2015).
[18] *in APr.* 8.34–6. It is worth noting that the commentary on *Prior Analytics* is not composed by Ammonius himself; it consists of notes written down by his students 'from the voice of Ammonius', see Blank (2000: 661). 'Ammonius' is not the only one of the late commentators using the terminology, he is the most explicit about the conceptual underpinning of the *meros/morion* distinction. As Barnes (1988: n.36) points out, Alexander of Aphrodisias, Olympiodorus and others use it too, only without explaining the distinction explicitly.
[19] See Barnes (1988: 241). [20] Sextus Empiricus *M* 9.339–40.

> their being single or divided, and in other like respects. Moreover, each of the characters mentioned is not 'composed of like parts'; by which I mean that though any given part of the root or trunk is composed of the same elements as the whole, yet the part so taken is not itself called 'trunk' but 'a portion of a trunk'. The case is the same with the members of an animal's body; to wit, any part of the leg or arm is composed of the same elements as the whole, yet it does not bear the same name (as it does in the case of flesh or bone); it has no special name. Nor again have subdivisions of any of those other organic parts that are uniform special names, subdivisions of all such being nameless. But the subdivisions of those parts that are compound have names, as have those of the foot, hand and head, for instance, toe, finger, nose or eye. Such then are the largest parts of the plant.[21]

Theophrastus reserves the term *morion* for portions of homoeomerous tissues and the term *meros* for structured parts. He states that the distinction he employs to differentiate between parts of plants is derived from the nomenclature used for human anatomy, which indicates that this distinction could come from a broader medical practice. This shows that the *meros*/*morion* distinction predates Galen's time significantly and possibly has a distinguished scientific pedigree.[22] At the same time, the fact that neither Galen nor Sextus attribute it to a specific school or figure but rather treat it as a generic kind of view indicates that the adoption of such terminology was either widespread or at least varied enough to be nondescript.

Galen also defines *meros* and *morion* in reference to the term 'organ' or 'instrument', *organon,* which is a species of parthood: all organs are parts but not all parts are organs. He defines the latter as a part that performs a complete activity or function (τελείας ἐνεργείας), such as the eye performing seeing. This definition is further clarified by the examples of the parts that are not 'organs' or 'instruments': various membranes and even the retina. In other words, the eye is an *organon* but none of the parts that make up the eye and enable the activity of seeing are. Here emerges a significant aspect of Galen's reasoning about body parts: the focus on activity and the attendant differentiation between the proper activity and supportive activities. At first glance, it might seem that his distinction between part and organ could very well be covered by the existing *meros*/

[21] *HP* 1.1, tr. A. Hort (2015: 15).

[22] There is some evidence of scientific discourse involving different terminology for different kinds of parthood in *An Outline of Empiricism* (*Subf. Emp.* 5). The topic in that case is the intradisciplinary divisions of medicine, however. Furthermore, the Greek text is not extant, and the fact that the treatise only survives in a Medieval Latin translation makes it difficult to draw any conclusions about the vocabulary used.

morion terminology. However, his emphasis on a complete activity makes it clear that, for him, it is not sufficient to divide the body into parts and their constituents; and in fact, the terminology focused on such divisions is not useful or reflective of ordinary uses of Greek language. Instead, it is more helpful to have terminology that differentiates the parts in accordance to distinctive activities they carry out, namely, organs. The importance of activity is a recurring theme in Galen's discussions of parthood, and we will come back to it in Section 1.2.

1.1.2 Pan *and* Holos

Galen also mentions another division, saying that those who distinguish between the whole (*holos*) and the totality (*pan*) are ignorant of the Greek language. Sextus' text presents a clear case where such a distinction is employed: 'But if all the parts are the whole, and the whole is nothing except the collection of the parts, neither will there be a whole nor will the parts turn out to be parts' (εἰ δὲ πάντα τὰ μέρη τὸ ὅλον ἐστίν, καὶ οὐδέν ἐστι τὸ ὅλον εἰ μὴ τὸ ἄθροισμα τῶν μερῶν, οὔτε ἔσται ὅλον οὔτε τὰ μέρη γενήσεται μέρη).[23] *Panta* seems to be used to denote all parts taken in totality *as parts*, distinct from *holos*, which is the unity (the whole) the parts constitute. This distinction comes from the Stoa,[24] where it is primarily employed in the cosmological context, and Sextus makes a note of this point earlier in the text.[25] Given how brief Galen's remarks on this distinction are, it is hard to determine what he is referring to here. It might be the Stoics themselves, although it is worth noting that Ps. Ocellus Lucanus' *On the Universe*, a pseudepigraphic Neopythagorean treatise, also employs such a distinction.[26] Furthermore, the terminology could have been adopted by contemporary doctors, perhaps some Stoicising doctors, such as the Pneumatists. Galen describes the latter as adopting Stoic doctrines,[27] and it is not impossible that, among other

[23] Sextus Empiricus *M* 9.343, tr. Bett (2012: 64).

[24] No surviving Stoic material points to a *meros*/*morion* distinction. The constituents of the blending are called *moria* in Galen's attack on the Stoics in *PHP* 5.3.8–9 de Lacy (5.447K) in which he reports the Stoic view that the *hēgemonikon* pneuma has two parts (*moria*), air and fire, blended through and through. Plutarch criticises the notion of blending with a reference *meros* in *Comm. not.* 1078B–D=*SVF* 2.465=LS 48E.

[25] Sextus Empiricus *M* 9.332. It is generally argued in the scholarship that they are likely to be the Stoics, and in that case, Sextus is misrepresenting their position; see Ierodiakonou (2015: 115–29).

[26] For example, in *Univ. Nat.* 1.11.4 Harder; the terms are used throughout the treatise.

[27] Galen *Diff. Puls.* 3.1 (8.642K); *CC* 2.1–6 Lyons; see also Ps. Galenic *Int.* 9.5 (21, 20 Petit=14.698K). See Petit (2009: xxxvi–li) regarding the question of authorship.

theoretical devices, these doctors embraced the cosmological terminology for discussing the body. At the same time, it is also possible that Galen's referent is yet another source, and we lack corroborating evidence to establish its provenance.

Cross-referencing Galen's claims with Sextus and other sources shows that he is writing in the context of a lively tradition of bio-mereology. Some of the views might have Hellenistic origins but the fact that we find the same or similar claims in Sextus or Ps. Ocellus Lucanus, Galen's near-contemporaries, shows that these questions were also very much current. Galen's stance is polemical, rejecting what must have been a popular practice, and his critical attitude naturally raises the question of what, according to him, is the correct way of thinking about parthood.

1.1.3 The Correlatives

One might very well wonder if the positive claims about parthood, interspersed with the critical, add up to a substantial and coherent position. The relationship between a part and a whole, Galen writes, is correlative, just like that between left and right hands. This claim indicates that the relationship between a part and a whole is relative. The manner in which something is a part is determined by the whole of which it is a part. Thus, there is only one way of being a part, viz. in relation to a certain whole.

The idea that parthood is relative did not originate with Galen. Sextus explicates this idea in his Pyrrhonian attack on dogmatist philosophers,[28] and Katerina Ierodiakonou has pointed out that his target are most likely Hellenistic philosophers; both Plato and Aristotle make somewhat similar claims,[29] but without the same language and explicit formulation that is found in Sextus.[30] However, there are two important differences. First, Galen applies it to the living body, and as we will see, this approach produces some innovative results. Second, Galen adopts the idea of the relativity of parthood with a clear polemical goal. The relative parthood is an alternative to the *meros*/*morion* distinction.

The distinction between *meros* and *morion* implies that there is more than one way of being a part. The parthood of a homoeomerous and a

[28] *M* 9.338–44; see also Ierodiakonou (2015: 109–10).

[29] Relativity also plays a role in the tripartition of the soul, to be precise, in accounting for the differentiation of desires; see Duncombe (2015). For psychology and physiology of tripartition, see the discussion in Chapter 5.

[30] Ierodiakonou (2015: 112–16).

structured part are entirely different. These part-whole relationships are non-transitive. The way in which, for example, all parts of a chair form the chair is different from the way in which portions of wood form a single leg of that chair. Thus, the terminology that Galen attacks conceptualises the parthood as coming in two different kinds. Galen's claims, meanwhile, implicitly argue for only a single kind of parthood. He explicitly subscribes to the transitivity of parts in this passage, saying that parts of the eye are also parts of the face and parts of the body as a whole.[31] Galen thinks that the relationship between a part and a whole is relative, and it is also transitive, so that the homoeomerous portions of, for example, a muscle are proper parts of an animal *qua* belonging to a structured part of that animal. In addition to these, Galen posits a definition of part: it is whatever forms a complete activity. The implications of this claim deserve a closer look, as they help to round out the Galenic understanding of parthood I have been sketching out so far.

1.1.4 The Priority of the Proper Activity

Galen defines an organ as a part (*meros*) of an animal that carries out a complete activity, such as the eye and sight, leg and walking. This also includes the vein, the artery and the nerve, which are both organs and parts of animals. It follows that:

(1) the eye is a full organ with a complete activity;
(2) the optic nerve is a full organ with a complete activity.

That would not be a problem if their activities were distinct, but this is not the case. The central part of the eye in regard to sight is the lens: 'The organ is the eye while sight is the activity. One of its parts is homoeomerous and is the primary organ of sight, which is the crystalline humour (lens), as has been demonstrated in my works on these, since this is what needs to be

[31] Although there is no direct reference to Hippocrates here, the same sentiment can be found in *Vict.* 1.6 (128, 25–130, 1 Joly–Byl=6.478 Littré) where the body is said to contain parts of parts and wholes of wholes. It is also worth noting that, in terms of activities, the parts are not entirely transitive. In *UP* 1.8 (1.13, 3–9 Helmreich=3.18K), Galen comments on the Hippocratic claim that, as a whole, all body parts are in sympathy, but taken separately, the parts of each body part cooperate for the effect of that part (*Alim.* 23 (81, 5–7 Heiberg=9.106 Littré)); see also Jouanna (2013: 306) for the argument that this 'Hippocratic' view has evident traces of Stoic influence, indicating that *Nutriment* was written after the rise of the Stoa in the Hellenistic period. Galen interprets this as claiming that large discrete parts act for the sake of an animal as a whole, while the parts of those parts, such as the eye, cooperate for the activity of their respective whole in order to bring about, in this case, vision.

altered by one of the colours externally for the animal to see.'[32] However, the eye is dependent on the nerve for sight too. Galen spells this point out quite explicitly when discussing a pathology of the eye as follows: 'if you ever see a person with one eye as a whole more prominent, you may know that if he can still see and the condition is not the result of a blow, that soft nerve has been stretched because of the paralysis of the muscle which is no longer able to hold, control, or bind it. And if he cannot see any longer, the nerve too is already affected.'[33] There is a seeming overlap of activity, with the result that the eye is an organ containing another organ. The sight is dependent on the lens; if it is damaged, the animal cannot see. At the same time, the vision also depends on the optic nerve. If the nerve is severed, the animal does not see either. The activities of the lens and the optic nerve, then, appear to coincide! Such overlap is a problem for Galen's own theoretical commitments. He states explicitly in *On the Usefulness of Parts* that each activity has its distinct proper part as follows:

> χρῆναι γὰρ δή φαμεν ἐν τοῖς συνθέτοις τοῦ σώματος μορίοις τοῖς ἐνέργειάν τινα πεπιστευμένοις, ἃ δὴ καὶ ὄργανα καλοῦμεν, ἐπισκοπεῖσθαί τι διὰ τῶν ἀνατομῶν τοιοῦτον μόριον, οἷον μηδαμόθι τοῦ σώματός ἐστιν ἑτέρωθι, καὶ τοῦτο μὲν τῆς ἰδίας κατὰ τὸ πᾶν ὄργανον ἐνεργείας αἴτιον εἶναι νομίζειν, τὰ δ' ἄλλα τῶν κοινῶν.
>
> I have said that in studying a composite part of the body to which some one activity has been entrusted and which we call an instrument, it is necessary to find by dissection a certain part of it that resembles nothing else anywhere in the body and to regard this as the cause of the special activity of the whole instrument, whereas its other parts are the causes of activities common [to all instruments].[34]

The passage begins with the definition of the term τό ὄργανον: it is used to refer to a structured part when talking about its proper activity. The rest of the passage explains that such a part is found via dissection, by identifying its properties not shared with any other parts. As shown in the recent scholarship, this is a key methodological principle guiding

[32] *MM* 1.6 (10.48–9K), Johnston and Horsley (2011: 77), slightly altered: τὸ μὲν γὰρ ὄργανον ὀφθαλμός, ἐνέργεια δ' ἡ ὄψις· ἓν δ' αὐτοῦ τῶν μορίων ὁμοιομερές τε καὶ πρῶτον ὄργανον ὄψεως, τὸ κρυσταλλοειδὲς ὑγρόν, ὡς ἐν τοῖς περὶ αὐτῶν λόγοις ἀποδέδεικται· τοῦτο γάρ ἐστι τὸ δεόμενον ἀλλοιωθῆναι πρός τινος τῶν ἔξωθεν χρωμάτων, ἵν' ἴδῃ τὸ ζῷον.

[33] *UP* 10.8 (2.82, 20–26 Helmreich=3.798K), tr. May (1968: 483–4): καὶ εἴ τινος ἐθεάσω ποτὲ προπετέστερον ὅλον τὸν ἕτερον ὀφθαλμόν, εἰ μὲν ἔτι βλέποι καὶ χωρὶς πληγῆς εἴη τὸ πάθημα γεγονός, ἐκτεταμένον ἴσθι τούτῳ τὸ μαλακὸν ἐκεῖνο νεῦρον ἐπὶ παραλύσει τοῦ μυὸς οὐκέτ' ἀντέχειν οὐδὲ κρατεῖν οὐδὲ σφίγγειν αὐτὸ δυναμένου· εἰ δὲ μηκέτι βλέποι, καὶ αὐτὸ τὸ νεῦρον ἤδη πέπονθεν.

[34] *UP* 4.12 (1.217, 17–23 Helmreich=3.296K), tr. May (1968: 221, slightly altered).

Galenic anatomical practice and theory.[35] For the current purposes, the most relevant aspect is the implications of this principle to physiology: if the activities of parts cannot duplicate, how can we explain the seemingly identical role of both the optic nerve and the lens? The answer is suggested by terminology. Galen explains that he uses the term τό ὄργανον to talk about the part in its proper activity. In the passages describing the dependence of sight on both the lens and the optic nerve, he only uses this term to describe the lens, noting that its mixture is peculiarly suitable to process sight.[36] Elsewhere, he describes the lens as having a light-like property that allows it to act as a communicator between the outside air and the pneuma inside the optic nerve.[37] Thus, the language makes it clear enough that only the lens is the proper part, the instrument, of sight. But how can sight be dependent on a non-proper part too, that is, the nerve?

The role of the (optic) nerve deserves a closer analysis. Throughout *On the Usefulness of Parts*, nerves are mentioned constantly as parts of other organs, but at the same time, a distinct set of chapters is dedicated to nerves themselves. They are and are not parts of other organs, mainly due to the fact that they are distributed throughout the body and often share physical connection with the proper parts.[38] For example, in the eye, the sensory nerves are inserted into the most important instrument of sight, the lens, while the hard nerves are to be found in the muscles.[39] The placement of the optic nerve hints at the reason the sight is dependent on it (even though it is not the proper organ of sight): the activity of the nervous system (and thus the optic nerve) is not to 'see' but to pass on the sensation of sight.[40]

One of the primary activities of the nervous system, according to Galen, is sensation (the other being voluntary motion and, sometimes, sensitivity to pain).[41] Yet, nerves themselves are not inherently capable of sensation; rather, they attain this ability by virtue of being connected to the brain, the latter being the proper sensory part.[42] When it comes to the eye, the optic

[35] See the discussion in Salas (2020b: 158–68).

[36] See also *MM* 2.6 (10.118–9K). The organ of sight is the crystalline humour (the lens) while each of the other parts exists for the sake of that (τὸ μὲν τῆς ὄψεως ὄργανόν ἐστι τὸ κρυσταλλοειδὲς ὑγρόν, ἕκαστον δὲ τῶν ἄλλων μορίων ἐκείνου χάριν ἐγένετο).

[37] *PHP* 7.5.22–6 de Lacy (5.623–4K). [38] *UP* 2.19 (1.122, 20–21 Helmreich=3.166K).

[39] *UP* 8.5 (1.460, 3–6 Helmreich=3.635K). The distinction between the two types of nerves is discussed in more detail in Chapter 4.

[40] See Chapter 4 on the nervous system for the full argument.

[41] The tripartite purpose of the nervous system is elaborated at the beginning of Chapter 4.

[42] *MM* 6.4 (10.409K); there is a lot at stake in the discussion of the sensitivity of the nervous tissue; see the discussion in Chapter 4 for details.

nerve and the lens have different roles. Although seeing depends on this nerve, it does not 'do' the seeing, it merely passes on the sensation to the brain. Given that the nerve is necessary for sight, one might wonder whether Galen envisioned the eye as just a supporting part of the brain responsible for seeing. The eye, in other words, would be in that case just a section of the extended brain complex. Yet Galen explicitly warns against drawing such conclusions. In the same treatise, *On the Affected Parts*, he writes that 'one could assume that it [i.e., the organ containing the soul] can see or hear, whereas only the eye sees and the ear hears. However, our thought, memory, reason and voluntary movement avail themselves neither of the eyes nor of the ears nor even of the tongue or any other part.'[43] The brain does not 'see', even if this activity cannot be accomplished without it.

This leads to the conclusion that the body parts can be co-dependent in complex ways; the knowledge of the proper organ is only one part of understanding how its activity takes place and how ailments ought to be treated. Furthermore, such a conclusion indicates that the boundaries of a bodily part, such as the eye, are in a certain sense, relative. The claims Galen makes in the aforementioned passage from *On the Therapeutic Method* helps to make sense of this. In the case of the eye, for example, the optic nerve is an anatomical part of the eye. Functionally speaking, however, the nerve is a part not of the eye but of the brain/nervous system. The proper activity of the nerve is to pass on the sensation. The nerve then is not a proper part of the vision. Thus, the optic nerve is both the part of the brain/nervous system and the part of the eye. To the extent that it participates in 'seeing', it is a correlative part of the eye. To the extent that it passes the sensation, it is a correlative part of the brain/nervous system.[44]

Sight, the activity of seeing, involves a series of actions carried out by different organs. First, an external impression travelling through the air has to be 'taken in' and passed on to the psychic pneuma. This is the activity of the lens. Seeing, however, also has a cognitive element. An animal can recognise or identify an external object as, for example, another animal (this act does not require rationality). For this, the brain is necessary. Overall, the sight can be described as a series of reactions, from light and

[43] *Loc. Aff.* 2.10.14 Gärtner (8.127K) , tr. Siegel (1976: 67): κατὰ μὲν γὰρ τὸν ἀληθῆ λόγον καὶ βλέπειν αὐτὸ τοῦτο καὶ ἀκούειν ὑποληπτέον, ἀλλὰ δι᾽ ὀφθαλμῶν μὲν βλέπειν, δι᾽ ὤτων δ᾽ ἀκούειν. ἐννοεῖν μέντοι καὶ μεμνῆσθαι καὶ λογίζεσθαι καὶ προαιρεῖσθαι μήτ᾽ ὀφθαλμοῖς ἔτι μήτ᾽ ὠσὶ μήτε γλώττῃ μήτ᾽ ἄλλῳ τινὶ προσχρώμενον.

[44] There is, then, some symmetry in this scheme: because the eye as an organ and the nerve as an organ depend on each other.

external air to the lens, from the lens to the psychic pneuma in the optic nerve, and from the psychic pneuma in this nerve to the psychic pneuma in the ventricles of the brain.[45] This means that the functioning of an animal is highly systematic and, as a result, the boundaries of organs can be relative from a functional point of view.

Galen's approach is presumably motivated by its therapeutic use. The first step in establishing the origin of an ailment of the eye – the example he uses in *On the Therapeutic Method* – is determining what aspect of the anatomical compound of the eye is injured. Corroborating cases can be found in other treatises too. In *On the Affected Parts*, for example, he argues that, when cognitive activities are damaged, a well-trained doctor knows that the *hēgemonikon* has suffered damage. Even when this happens in a patient with pleurisy and pneumonia, no one assumes that the damage was caused by the lungs. Instead, they invoke sympathy, in the manner of their particular doctrine.[46] The *hēgemonikon* is said to be liable to be affected where one of its specific activities are damaged, viz. those that cannot be done by means of any other part *qua* an instrument.[47] Knowing what exact role each bodily part plays in a healthy activity allows for proper diagnosis and treatment in the case of injury or pathology.

The passage in *On the Therapeutic Method* reveals that Galen's attempts to define parts are more complex than one might suspect from reading the opening of *On the Usefulness of Parts*. He does not simply define vital parts as more unified with the whole than artefactual parts, he also engages in polemics. His project in these passages is primarily critical: he attacks the inflated technical terminology that must have been present in medical and philosophical discourses and instead proposes a 'common-sense' understanding of terminology grounded in the ordinary use of the Greek language. However, the passage also contains some reflections on the relationships that govern part-whole relationships: transitivity, correlativity and so on. If we turn to the passages in which he expounds his own views, we find him using complex and less-than-crystal-clear distinctions, as well as at least two distinctive classifications of parts that are, strictly speaking, no less theoretically laden than the terminology he criticises in *On the Therapeutic Method*. In the following two sections, I examine two broad divisions of parts that represent Galen's own attempts to theorise parthood: the division of parts into homoeomerous and structured and the

45 For Galen's account of sight, see Boudon-Millot (2012) and Ierodiakonou (1999, 2014, 2022).
46 For Galen's own 'hippocratising' of *sumpatheia*, see Holmes (2012, 2015, 2020).
47 *Loc. Aff.* 2.10.14 Gärtner (8.127K): ἃς δι᾽ οὐδενὸς ἄλλου μορίου ποιεῖται καθάπερ δι᾽ ὀργάνου.

four-fold division of parts. The former is, in many respects, straightforward, but Galen employs it in an argument about the tripartition of the soul as an explanatory reference. His analogy that is more nebulous than lucid. I argue that untangling the implications of the comparison reveals much not only about tripartition but also the significance of the division of parts into homoeomerous and structured.

1.2 Homoeomeries, Structured Parts and Forms

The division into the homoeomerous and the structured parts is possibly the most common part-division in Galenic texts.[48] He rarely dwells on it, but if the frequency with which he uses this division is indicative of its importance (which seems reasonable enough), then it must be a key building block in his physiology. Homoeomerous parts are tissues, constituted of the mixtures of four elements but lacking discrete parts. Structured parts, meanwhile, have discrete parts. The activities of the former are explained in reference to mixtures, whereas the activities of the latter in reference to the actions of discrete parts. It has been pointed out that this terminology has a clear Peripatetic pedigree,[49] but arguably, Galen is also influenced by the medical tradition. It has also been noted that the Peripatetic concepts were already adopted by the Alexandrian doctors,[50] but there is a striking similarity in broad conceptualisation of this division in Hippocratic works that served as the definitive authority for Galen. The author of the Hippocratic *On Ancient Medicine* claims that affections (παθήματα) arise either from capacities (δυνάμεις) or from structures (σχήματα), explaining that the latter is the strength of the fluids and the structure are the shapes and textures of the parts.[51] The main

[48] *MM* 2.6 (10.118K); 2.6 (10.125–6K); 3.3 (10.184K); 3.10 (10.229K); 7.2 (10.458K); 9.14 (10.646K); 13.10 (10.900K); *Symp. Caus.* 1.2.1 (7.87K); 1.2.4 (7.93–4K); 1.2.9 (7.99K); 3.8.1 (7.249K); 11.1 (7.262K); *Opt. Corp. Const.* 1.2 (10, 8–13 Helmreich=4.742K); 1.3 (13, 10 Helmreich=4.745K); 1.4 (16, 10–11 Helmreich=4.749K); *San. Tu.* 1.1.3 Koch (6.2K); 1.5.48 Koch (6.25K); 6.15.11–12 Koch (6.452K); *Ars. Med.* 2.1 (279, 5–6 Boudon=1.310K); 27.1 (359, 9–10 Boudon=1.379K); *Loc. Aff.* 6.2.2 Brunschön (8.381K); 4.4 (8.235K); *Praes. Puls.* 3.1 (9.331K); *Morb. Diff.* 13 (6.876K); *CAM* 11, 1–2 Fortuna (1.260–1K); *PHP* 9.6.63 de Lacy (5.777K); *Comp. Med. Loc.* 2.1 (12.499K). See also *Morb. Diff.* 3 (6.841K) cited later.

[49] See, for example, *GC* 1.1, 314a19–20; *HA* 1.1 (486a5–8); *Mete.* 4.12, 390b5–8. Guthrie (1965: 325–6) argued that the term is an Aristotelian neologism. Galen describes it as an Aristotelian term in *San. Tu.* 6.2.2 Koch (6.384K). See Berman (2015) for a conceptual study of Aristotle's notion of a homoeomery.

[50] Leith (2015).

[51] Hippocrates *VM* 22 (149, 1–3 Jouanna=1.626, 6–13 Littré); see also Gundert (1992: 459–62) for a more detailed discussion.

difference from the Galenic division of the body into homoeomerous and structured parts is the complete distinction of capacities as fluids and structures as more or less solid parts. Galen does not make such a sharp cut: solid tissues are imbued with capacities owing to their mixtures too. But the idea that some parts of the body act via their structure and some via their elemental composition is present in Galen as well.

In general, the division of parts into homoeomerous and structured is presented as a simple and straightforward matter by Galen: there are hardly any problems relating to the division itself. However, the seemingly straightforward distinction between the two kinds of parts is invoked in a complicated passage that juxtaposes 'parts' with 'forms', and his argument reveals some significant aspects of his reflection on not only homoeomerous and structured parts but also parthood in general. The somewhat convoluted passage comes from *On the Doctrines of Hippocrates and Plato*. At the beginning of Book 6, Galen outlines his plan to inquire whether the powers governing humans are singular and placed in the heart, or three in number. He adds that he was distracted by Chrysippus' position that denies not only the trilocation but also the three types of capacities.[52] Having covered the criticism of Chrysippus in the previous books, he now comes back to the question of the trilocation. He starts, in his customary manner, by explaining the terms, in this case, the difference between activity or function (ἐνέργεια) and affection (πάθος).[53] Then he launches into an exegesis of a passage from Plato's *Republic*, in order to address the problem of seeming inconsistency: Plato refers to the souls as both parts and forms (εἴδη).[54] Galen explains away the inconsistency as follows:

> καὶ γὰρ εἴδη καὶ μέρη ψυχῆς ὀρθῶς ἄν τις ὀνομάζοι τὸ λογιστικὸν καὶ τὸ θυμοειδὲς καὶ τὸ ἐπιθυμητικόν, ὥσπερ εἰ καὶ σώματος εἴδη τις εἰπὼν εἶναι φλέβα καὶ ἀρτηρίαν καὶ νεῦρον ὀστοῦν τε καὶ χόνδρον καὶ σάρκα καὶ τἆλλα ὅσα τοιαῦτα, μετὰ ταῦθ' ὡς περὶ μερῶν αὐτῶν διαλέγοιτο. καὶ γὰρ καὶ μέρη τοῦ σώματος ἡμῶν ἀληθῶς ἄν τις εἶναι λέγοι τὰ τοιαῦτα– συμπληροῦται γὰρ τὸ ὅλον ἐξ αὐτῶν–, καὶ μέντοι καὶ εἴδη τοῦ σώματος οὐδὲν ἧττον· ἐν μόνοις γὰρ τοῖς ὁμοιομερέσι τὸ διαφέρον εἶδος οὐκ ἔστιν, οἷον τὸ τῆς σαρκὸς μέρος ἢ τὸ τῆς φλεβὸς ἢ τὸ τῆς πιμελῆς, οὐδὲ ἀληθὲς εἰπεῖν ἐπὶ τῶν τοιούτων ὡς ἐκ τοσῶνδέ τινων εἰδῶν σύγκειται τὸ ὅλον· ἐν δὲ τοῖς ἀνομοιομερέσιν ἡ τῶν εἰδῶν διαφορὰ τὸν ἀριθμὸν ὁρίζει τοῖς

52 *PHP* 6.1.2 de Lacy (5.505–6K); for the extensive studies of this disagreement, see Gill (2010) and Tieleman (1996).

53 *PHP* 6.1.4–27 de Lacy (5.506–513K).

54 *PHP* 6.2.1 de Lacy (5.514K).

μορίοις. τοιοῦτον δέ τι χρῆμα καὶ ἡμῶν τὴν ψυχὴν ὁ Πλάτων εἶναί φησιν ἐκ τριῶν μερῶν συγκειμένην.

It would be correct to term the rational, the spirited and the desiderative both 'forms' and 'parts' of the soul, just as one might say that vein, artery, nerve, bone, cartilage, flesh and the like are forms of body, and then speak of them as parts. Indeed, one could say of such things both that they are truly 'parts' of our body – for the whole is made up of them – and again that they are no less truly 'forms' of the body. For it is only in homoeomerous structures that differences are not forms, for example, different parts of flesh or of a vein or of fat; and it is not correct to say of such things that the whole is composed of such and such forms. But in things that have unlike parts the difference in the forms determines the number of parts. Plato says that our soul is this kind of thing, being composed of three parts.[55]

Galen ultimately argues that there is no inconsistency in Plato's terminology, because referring to the souls as 'forms' is equivalent to saying that they are the kind of parts that have forms. This point is important for supporting his views about the tripartition of the soul, but it is equally pertinent for the distinctions that Galen makes in regard to parthood. He brings in the description of the structured and the homoeomerous parts to support this argument, arguing that the souls are not divided like the latter. Ultimately, this comparison suggests that the soul is more like a structured part than a homoeomery, but does this point mean that the soul is like a structured part because it is a form, whereas homoeomerous parts do not have forms?

This question must surely be answered in the negative. In other contexts, Galen clearly talks about the forms of the homoeomerous bodies too, and, furthermore, he tends to use the term μορφή, typically referring to mere shape, for structured parts. One notable example is his reference to the mixtures of homoeomerous parts in *That Capacities of the Soul Follow the Mixtures of the Body* while commenting on Aristotle.[56] Here he discusses two concepts of the 'form': the form as a mixture and the form as a shape (μορφή), as found in the structured parts (ὥσπερ ἐν τοῖς ὀργανικοῖς σώμασιν). The shape of the structured parts is denoted by the word that refers to artificial appearance,[57] while the term for the substantial form is εἶδος, the one used in the *On the Doctrines of*

[55] *PHP* 6.2.1–3 de Lacy (5.513–515K), tr. de Lacy (1978–84: 369). See also Schiefsky (2012). Galen's reception of Plato, and especially the problematic adoptions of views from both the *Republic* and the *Timaeus* is discussed extensively in Gill (2006: 296–9).

[56] *QAM* 3 (37, 6 Müller=4.773–4 K); see also Vinkesteijn (2022: 14–25).

[57] See, for example, Plato *Phd.* 103E.

Hippocrates and Plato passage. Furthermore, in *Differences of Diseases*, Galen divides the composition and construction of the body into three kinds: of homoeomeries (arteries, veins, nerves, etc.), of structured parts (the brain, the heart, the lungs, etc.) and of the body as a whole. He notes that the *differentiae* of flesh *qua* flesh arise from only the combination of primary elements; but when flesh is a part of a structured part, the *differentiae* arise from construction and size (παρά τε τὴν διάπλασιν καὶ τὸ μέγεθος).[58] Thus, he consistently describes the distinguishing features of the structured parts as grounded in size and construction, nothing more than μορφή. Galen appears to claim that the structured parts have εἶδος in this text, while in others that they are described as having μορφή.

Is there inconsistency in Galen's use of the term εἶδος in reference to parts? Arguably, no. The comparison between homoeomerous/structured parts to the soul can, and perhaps ought to, be read as referring not to the differentiation of parts but to the differentiation of the ways in which parts constitute wholes. In the passage, he is making a subtle distinction between a part *qua* part and *qua* form. The souls according to him are both parts and forms. They are parts, because they constitute the whole person. Thus, a part denotes the simplest constitutive relationship: if A is made up of B, C, D, then these are the parts of A. But it is not always enough to know what parts there are. Sometimes, it is also necessary to know *how* the parts constitute the whole,[59] and this is where the notion of the form comes in. Although the term εἶδος has significant metaphysical baggage, Galen uses it here in a rather specific sense, as the foundation of distinctive kind-identity. It grounds the difference between two *kinds* of homoeomerous tissues. The description of some tissue as a part tells us that it forms part-whole relationship with the body and the description of the same tissue as a form tells us *how* it forms that relationship, that is, as a distinctively identifiable part.

The comparison to the division of parts into homoeomerous and structured illustrates this point and serves to introduce different relationships of constitution. Homoeomerous tissues can be divided endlessly, with each new division sharing the same properties with all the others.[60]

[58] *Morb. Diff.* 3 (6.841K).

[59] For current purposes, I focus on the metaphysical aspect of Galen's claim, but it certainly has a psychological implication too, for which see Hankinson (1991a); Mansfeld (1991: 138–45); Schiefsky (2012); Tieleman (2003a: 34–9).

[60] Galen says this explicitly later in the text, after supplying a number of passages from Plato's *Republic* and *Timaeus* supporting this interpretation. *PHP* 6.2.16–17 de Lacy (5.518–9K) ὅτι μηδ' ἐγχωρεῖ λέγειν μηδὲν σύνθετον ὁμοιομερές, ἑαυτῷ γε <μὴ> συνεχὲς ὅλον ὑπάρχον· ἐξ ὡρισμένων γὰρ τὸν

Furthermore, two numerically distinct portions of homoeomerous matter constitute the whole in the same way. Their status as parts is exactly the same. The sub-parts of a structured part are different in *form*. The vein and the bone (or the spirited and the rational soul, for that matter) are parts in a different sense, they play different roles *qua* parts of the same whole, owing to their difference in form.[61]

This distinction is significant for Galen's argument that the soul is tripartite: there are three entities that constitute the human soul *qua* parts and they are three in kind *qua* forms. The soul is like a structured part, it is divisible into parts with discrete identities, and this fact grounds the tripartition. If the soul were like a homoeomerous part, its parts would have no distinct discrete identity: it could, in principle, be divisible into three, five or ten parts, but this division would not be meaningful since nothing would separate them from each other substantially. For all intents and purposes, the soul would be unitary.[62]

The distinction between forms and parts and, less directly, the division into homoeomerous and structured parts play a significant role in theorising the tripartition, one of the major preoccupations of Galen's. I will come back to the notion of form in the final chapter of this work, where I look at the ways in which it plays the role of unifying bodily activities. In this context, however, it is a tool for dividing the soul in a very particular way, that is, into distinctive parts or kinds. In this way, the division of parts into structured and homoeomerous, despite its apparent simplicity, serves as a crucial conceptual tool for motivating other theoretical divisions of the body.

There is another significant aspect to this bipartite division that renders it, in a certain sense, fundamental to thinking about the body: it is non-reductive. Given his choice to describe structured parts as differentiated by size and structure in *Differences of Diseases*, one might wonder if ascribing διάπλασις and size, rather than form, to these parts suggests that they are

ἀριθμὸν σύγκειται μορίων· οὐδενὸς δὲ/ὁμοιομεροῦς ἀριθμῷ περιλαβεῖν ἐγχωρεῖ τὸ πλῆθος τῶν μορίων.

61 Galen also shows some affinity to the Aristotelian approach to homoeomerous parts, cf. Aristotle *PA* 2.1–4, especially 2.2 (647b29–648a20), where he discusses how homoeomerous tissues differ in kind with an example of blood. See also *GC* 1.1 (314a19–20), which describes homoeomerous tissues (bone, flesh, etc.) as entities in which whole and part are synonymous.

62 This would also mean that such souls do not have activities that are distinct from each other; the notion of the form, therefore, must be closely related to activity. Galen could, in principle, introduce the notion of instrument in the context of this discussion, because each of the souls performs a complete activity, and so they have both distinctive forms and activities. However, given that he is commenting on Plato's use of the terms 'part' and 'form' in reference to the souls, it is not surprising that he does not address the question of souls as instruments as well.

derivative. After all, the form is notably associated with substantial identity in ancient philosophy. But when he talks about the *differentiae* of parts, he seems to emphasise a difference in activity, not in fundamentality. In fact, the prominence of this division precisely indicates that it is, in some way, pinpointing important non-reducible differences. Ultimately, in Galen we find the idea that the activities of the structured organs cannot be reduced to homoeomerous parts and these parts cannot account for the activities of the structured organs. The differences between the two types have significant consequences for medical practice. In order to understand human physiology, a Galenic doctor needs to understand two types of 'behaviour': the 'behaviour' of homoeomerous tissues *qua* their mixtures and the 'behaviour' of structured organs *qua* their shape and structure.[63] The latter parts are designed to perform certain activities in a set way. The size of the offshoots from the stomach, for example, is directly dependent on whether it is useful to permit a passage of coarse food or whether only digested matter ought to be allowed.[64] The homoeomerous tissues, which constitute the structured organs, are designed to perform a range of activities deriving from the four natural capacities that underpin such functions as nutrition and growth of all living beings. They will be discussed in more detail in the following chapter.

It is surprising that Galen did not adopt the terminology for distinguishing the portions of homoeomeries and the sub-parts of discrete parts, denoted by *morion* and *meros*, respectively, and instead chose to criticise it as superfluous.[65] After all, it could be utilised very effectively together with his own distinction between parts *qua* parts and parts *qua* forms. Presumably, his interest in distinguishing proper activities from other types, quite evident in his critique of the terminology, motivates the rejection of this terminology. And, in fact, his four-fold division of parts, much less known than the distinction between homoeomerous and structured parts, shows quite explicitly that he envisions the hierarchical divisions of the body according to their proper activities.

1.3 The Four-fold Division

This little-discussed classification can be found in a short treatise *Art of Medicine*. Having stated the signs of the best constitution, Galen starts the

[63] The most extensive discussion is in *On Mixtures*, which begins with the claim that mixtures of hot, cold, wet and dry are not the same in every case, see *Temp.* 1.1 (1–3 Helmreich=1.509K).

[64] *UP* 4.7 (1.205–6 Helmreich= 3.280–1K) .

[65] *MM* 1.6 (10.47–8K). This passage is cited and discussed in Section 1.1.

discussion of the constitutions that fall short of the ideal. He notes that he has already written about the signs of a diseased body in *On the Best Constitution of Our Bodies* in regard to genus,[66] and in *Art of Medicine* he is going to write about them in terms of species (κατ' εἶδος). Before doing so, he sets out the division of parts as follows:

> τέσσαρες δ' αὐτῶν εἰσιν αἱ πᾶσαι διαφοραί· τὰ μὲν γὰρ αὐτῶν ἀρχαί τινές εἰσι· τὰ δὲ ἀπ' ἐκείνων ἐκπέφυκε· τὰ δὲ οὔτ' ἄλλων ἄρχει τῆς διοικήσεως, οὔθ' ὑπ' ἄλλων ἄρχεται, συμφύτους ἔχοντα τὰς διοικούσας αὐτὰ δυνάμεις· ἔνια δὲ συμφύτους τε ἅμα καὶ ἐπιρρύτους ἔχει· ἀρχαὶ μὲν οὖν εἰσιν ἐγκέφαλος, καρδία, ἧπαρ, καὶ ὄρχεις· ἀπ' ἐκείνων δ' ἐκπέφυκε, κἀκείνοις ὑπηρετεῖ, νεῦρα μὲν καὶ νωτιαῖος μυελὸς ἐγκεφάλῳ, τῇ καρδίᾳ δὲ ἀρτηρίαι, φλέβες δὲ ἥπατι, τὰ σπερματικὰ δὲ ἀγγεῖα τοῖς ὄρχεσιν· αὐτὰ δὲ αὐτὰ διοικεῖ χόνδρος, ὀστοῦν, σύνδεσμος, ὑμήν, ἀδήν, πιμελή, σὰρξ ἁπλῆ· τὰ δ' ἄλλα πάντα μόρια κοινὴν τούτοις ἔχοντα τὴν ἐξ αὐτῶν διοίκησιν, ἀρτηριῶν τε καὶ φλεβῶν καὶ νεύρων προσδεῖται· τριχῶν δὲ καὶ ὀνύχων οὐδὲ διοίκησίς τίς ἐστιν, ἀλλὰ γένεσις μόνη· αὗται μὲν οὖν αἱ τῶν μορίων διαφοραί.
>
> The differentiae of these parts are four in all. Some of them are principles; some grow out of those; some neither control the governance of others nor are controlled by others, having innate powers that [allow them to] administer themselves; and some have both innate and inflowing capacities. The principles are brain, heart, liver and testicles. Growing out of those and serving them are nerves and spinal cord for the brain, arteries for the heart, veins for the liver and spermatic ducts for the testicles. Those parts that govern themselves are cartilage, bones, ligaments, membranes, glands, fat and simple flesh. All the other parts which have in common with these the governance of themselves need arteries, veins and nerves as well. There is no governance of hair and nails, only genesis. These, then, are the differentiae of the parts.[67]

All the parts named in this passage are instruments, in the sense of being parts that carry out complete activities. However, not all instruments are made equal, and this classification reveals the grounds on which these parts can be differentiated in their relationship with other parts. Only the principles (the brain, the heart, the liver and, interestingly, the testicles) are able to exercise influence on other parts (ἄρχειν).[68] They do this by

[66] *Opt. Corp. Const.* 3–4 (12–16 Helmreich=4.744–748K).

[67] *Ars. Med.* 5.1–3 (286, 13–287, 10 Boudon=1.318–19K), Johnston (2016: 177–9), slightly altered.

[68] Two points are worth noting in reference to the last principle. First, this organ can be found in both male and female animals (this is made explicit in Book 14 of *On the Usefulness of Parts*, where the anatomy of the reproductive system is discussed – the most pertinent passages are discussed in the following section). Second, one might wonder why testicles are classified with principles here but not in many other cases. An argument explaining this point will be presented in Section 5.4.

means of their offshoots (nerves, arteries, veins and spermatic ducts). Galen does not say it explicitly, but the rest of the passage implies that the offshoots are fully governed by the principles from which they spring. The third group, by contrast, is comprised of the parts that are completely self-sufficient. These are discrete parts, each with its own form, composed of just homoeomerous tissues. The fourth category is comprised of parts that are both self-managed and connected to the principles by means of their offshoots. Galen does not give examples of such parts, but, presumably, many of the organs would fall into this category, as they are made up of homoeomerous tissues and connected by means of some of the offshoots.

The last category, not mentioned in the four-fold division at the beginning of the passage, differs significantly from the rest by virtue of containing organs that have no self-management (διοίκησις), only genesis. The genesis must refer to growth,[69] and the absence of the ability to self-manage (διοικεῖν) presumably amounts to the absence of peculiar vital action. The hair and nails simply increase in size, but do not attract what benefits, reject what harms and so on. These parts 'grow' in a way that resembles more closely inanimate objects rather than other animate tissues.[70]

At first glance, the passage echoes Aristotle's hierarchy of body parts outlined in *The Generation of Animals*. Here, Aristotle also distinguishes between necessary and subsidiary parts, dividing the latter into two further categories. Unlike Galen, he associates functional priority with earlier generation and better material constitution. Comparing nature to a good housekeeper (οἰκονόμος), he notes that the purest nutriment is concocted first and forms the noblest, the necessary organs: the flesh and the sense organs. In an *oikos*, this nutriment is comparable to food set aside for the free people. Meanwhile, the leftover food is divided hierarchically further into the food for the enslaved people and for animals. In the body, the

In short, when discussing the governing organs, Galen is typically concerned with vitality (*MM* 9.10 (10.635–7K)). The removal or malfunction of the testicles obviously does not result in the loss of life. Thus, it is a principle insofar as it is the epicentre of a reproductive system but it is not a vital organ, and the testicles do not belong to the list of the overall principal parts on which vitality depends.

69 Confusingly, given that in *On the Natural Capacities* Galen accuses his rivals of not keeping this distinction clear.

70 In fact, in *Natural Faculties*, he distinguishes between animate 'growth' and 'inanimate' genesis, see Section 5.2.1 for the discussion of the passage. See also Nussbaum (1978: 76–7), who argues that the self-nourishment is a condition for animate life in Aristotle, notes the following: 'An icicle grows by absorbing material from the environment; a fire "nourishes" itself by consuming surrounding matter. Yet we do not call these living, because there appears to be no selectivity.'

residual nutriment is given first to bones and sinews and only then to hair, nails and so on.[71]

Aristotle has three categories rather than four, but Galenic and Aristotelian bodily hierarchies appear to be similar, starting from organs responsible for perception and ending with hair, nails and so on. However, there are also several significant differences. Galen emphasizes offshoots (undoubtedly an influence of Hellenistic medical discoveries) and makes no mention of the generation of parts or their nutrition. Most notably, the hierarchies are organised differently: while Aristotle ties the significance of parts proportionally to their place in line of generation and nutrition, Galen divides them according to the way in which they are governed. In Aristotle, the nature is a metaphorical οἰκονόμος, but, in Galen, the capacity of parts to ἄρχειν others and to διοικεῖν themselves becomes the central preoccupation, and the terms are used not as metaphors but as technical vocabulary.[72]

Principles govern themselves and other organs. Their offshoots depend on them. The rest of the structured parts have their own distinct self-managements owing to their innate natural capacities, but they can be also governed by principles or not, depending on whether they are connected via offshoots. The fact that Galen adds the fifth category to his four-fold division is revealing: it shows that he thinks of body parts as divided (and connected!) primarily in reference to their activities, and the parts that merely grow serve as a useful contrast to the parts that do possess capacity for the internal διοίκησις.

Apart from the final category containing nails and hair, all the parts are described in relation to other parts. All of them require each other in order to carry out their peculiar activities, even those with the capacity to ἄρχειν. In another treatise, Galen poignantly points out that 'neither the brain alone without the foot nor the foot without the brain would be very useful, for one of them, of course, needs something to support it and the other needs sensation'.[73] The degree of co-dependence of the parts can vary. They are especially tightly connected when some parts of one organ appear

[71] *GA* 2.6 (744b11–27); for a further discussion, including the differentiation of formal and material causes, see Leunissen (2010: 83–4, 129).

[72] The comparison between the *oikos* and its management to the body is not uncommon, it can be used both to explain the body (as we see here) and the management of the *oikos*, see, for example, Čelkytė (2023). On the language of household management and its connection to Galen's concept of nature, see Jouanna (2013: 290–1).

[73] *UP* 3.11 (1.178, 7–9 Helmreich=3.243K), tr. May (1968: 192, slightly altered): οὔτ᾽ ἐγκέφαλος ἄνευ ποδὸς ἦν ἄν ποτε καλὸς μόνος οὔτε πoὺς ἐγκεφάλου χωρίς. δεῖ γὰρ οἶμαι τῷ μὲν ὀχήματός τινος, τῷ δ᾽ αἰσθήσεως.

to also be parts of another one. This problem was already raised in Section 1.1, on the basis of the passage from *On the Therapeutic Method*, with the conclusion that parthood is relative, or properly speaking, correlative to the activity it contributes to the body. This passage from *Art of Medicine* further explains how the correlative status of parts ought to be understood: some parts both self-manage (διοικεῖν) and are subject to the principles that govern them (ἄρχειν), which renders their activities correlative. The eye, for example, is capable of sight both in virtue of parts that are self-managing (the lens) and parts that are offshoots of the governing part, the brain (the optic nerve).

Just like Aristotle, Galen sees body parts as hierarchically arranged: some necessary, others subordinate. But unlike Aristotle, he sees them as (1) varying in their degree of independence *qua* governance and self-management and (2) extensively interconnected. His interest in differentiating parts in reference to their activities seems justified, given that he presents the body parts as physically intertwined in multiple complex ways, and activities help to 'untangle' the connections and to identify their relevant aspects for diagnostic and therapeutic purposes.

These purposes are, of course, of primary interest to someone identifying as a doctor. Medicine, in essence, is the domain of knowledge that becomes relevant when things go wrong and when it is necessary to restore the healthy functions of the body. But bodies can veer off the ideal in different ways: by means of injury, illness or even innate constitution. In the division of the body that prioritises activities, the innate imperfections present a theoretical challenge.

1.4 The Imperfection of Parts

Apart from health and injury, there is the third kind of physiological state that Galen addresses: the imperfect functioning. An example of such a state could be the loss of stomach described at the beginning of the chapter. In such cases as these, the loss of a part can be compensated by the activities of other parts. What do such cases tell us about the relationship between the body as a whole and its parts? In order to understand Galen's approach, it is worth turning to the passages concerned with the loss of parts and the inherent deformity of body parts.

In *On the Therapeutic Method*, Galen argues that it is important to make a careful distinction between how the notion of 'in accordance with nature' ought to be understood. He argues that, for example, when a person has the sixth finger or is missing the fifth finger, there is no need to try to 'fix' this as if it was 'against nature'. He adds that the term 'against nature' ought to be applied only to those things that cause injury to activities.[74] As Galen warns against attempting to 'fix' people in accordance to what would be the perfect shape, he makes it clear that activities ought to be prioritised over the 'typical' number or arrangement of parts. His concern here is that the claim 'everything against the nature ought to be eliminated/fixed' could be misunderstood as referring to everything *tout court*. Yet this is certainly not the case. The medical intervention has clear limits: it ought to be only concerned with the activities. Similarly, the beginning of the treatise *To Thrasybolous* contains a rhetorically charged claim that it is for the activity, not the constitution, that we need parts; the parts, therefore, are judged to be useful simply in regard to their actual action.[75]

Thus, Galen suggests that the focus of medicine is activities that take place within the body, especially those that maintain its vitality. The theoretical perfection and medicine, as a result, are completely divorced notions. In addition to this, it is notable that Galen does not speak of the 'perfection' of parts as common. In fact, quite the opposite is the case. In *On the Best Constitution of Our Bodies*, Galen discusses the perfection in a human body as exceptional as follows:

> εἰ μέλλει χρήσιμος ὁ λόγος ἔσεσθαι τοῖς ἐργαζομένοις τὴν τέχνην, μὴ μόνον τὸ σπάνιον ἐν αὐτῇ σῶμα καὶ οἷον παράδειγμά τι τοῦ Πολυκλείτου κανόνος ἐν τῷ λόγῳ πλάττειν ἀλλὰ καὶ τῶν ἀπολειπομένων μὲν αὐτῆς κατά τι, μὴ μέντοι κατάφωρον ἤδη καὶ μέγα τὸ σφάλμα κεκτημένων ἀναμνησθῆναι.
>
> If, then, our discussion is to be of any value to practitioners of the art, it would appear sensible not to confine ourselves to the construction, in our argument, of that rare body which might be called the exemplification of the Canon of Polycleitus, but to include also bodies which fall short of it in some small respect, without, however, manifesting any large defect.[76]

The contrast with the famous perfectly proportioned statue of Polycleitus shows that the deviation from the perfect norm can be assumed in the vast majority of people, because the perfect constitution is exceptionally rare. And it is worth remembering that even if one is lucky enough to be born

[74] *MM* 14.14 (10.991–2K). See also *MM* 14.15 (10.993K). There is a difference between nature and medicine, and the case of the extra finger is in the domain of nature.

[75] *Thras.* 11 (45, 13–46, 4 Helmreich=5.823K).

[76] *Opt. Corp. Const.* 3 (12, 23–13, 5 Helmreich=4.744–5K) tr. Singer (1997: 293). See also *Ars. Med.* 25.3–4 (353, 7–15 Boudon=1.373K) for the argument regarding the existence of the many classes of bodies that are only slightly short of the best constitution; a doctor ought to adapt the causes that preserve health to them proportionally.

with it, the state would only be temporary, because with age, the mixtures of the animal body inevitably dry out, as it is stated in the passage from *On Hygiene*.[77] In that case, the issue at stake is homoeomerous tissues, but Galen does not distinguish between homoeomerous and discrete parthood, so a person lacking, for example, moistness in her mixture is still lacking a part, just like she would be lacking a part if she lost a limb. Ultimately, some imperfection of parts is a given at least at some point in human life and very likely present throughout lifetime.

It is quite clear that, according to Galen, every constitution is full of shortcomings. At the same time, he also adopts a notorious piece of Aristotelian biology concerning deformed animals.[78] This notion theorises imperfections of certain species and kinds, with profound implications for how the nature of such animals ought to be understood. There are some debates going on in the current Aristotelian scholarship on how one ought to interpret the notion of an incomplete animal that encompasses a staggering number of species, from frogs to hippopotami.[79] Most relevant for Galen is the inclusion of female mammals in this category. He takes it upon himself to comment on this following Aristotle and to finish the work that Aristotle left undone in Book 14 of *On the Usefulness of Parts*.[80] As Sophia Connell has shown, Galen's attack on Peripatetic views is not entirely justified, and his own view, often lauded as more egalitarian, is not substantially less sexist than Aristotle's.[81] However, given that Galen makes the female reproductive system inferior to male, the former presents an important case study for understanding how he reconciles the supposed imperfection of parts with his interest in the functionalist approach to parthood. The remainder of this section is dedicated to this question, and, having briefly outlined Galen's account of female reproduction, I argue that his view shows a strong commitment to functional understanding of the body parts in this case too.

There are, according to Galen, two points on which female is inferior to male: (1) the colder constitution and (2) the internal construction of the organs that can be seen in the dissection.[82] These two claims turn out to be

[77] *San. Tu.* 1.2.6–7 Koch (6.4–5K); see also Chapter 5.

[78] See the discussions in Boylan (1984, 1986).

[79] See, for example Witt (2012) and major studies in Connell (2016) and Mayhew (2010).

[80] *UP* 14.5 (2.296, 1–7 Helmreich=4.157–8K). Galen's conceptualisation of the woman is explored extensively in Flemming (2000: 306–29).

[81] Connell (2016: 109–120).

[82] Such claims regarding the 'colder constitution' can be found in Hippocratic texts as well, which was undoubtedly important for Galen. See, for example, *Aër.* 10, 3 Diller (2.44 Littré). See King (1998: 28–33) for a further discussion of the 'wet' constitution of women and its implications for medical

connected once he sets out his point (2), which he describes as not easy to explain. Ultimately, the anatomical inferiority amounts to the internal/external distinction of the female and male reproductive systems. In respect to (1), Galen is reiterating the Aristotelian view, although he is critical of the Peripatetic for the claim that the female form fails by virtue of not being hot enough to produce seed.[83] In Galenic biology, females do produce seed,[84] while nonetheless possessing colder constitutions.

The colder constitution is causally connected to the anatomical inferiority of the female reproductive system. This argument is grounded on the assumption that female and male reproductive systems are, in a certain sense, not two but one kind of system. According to Galen, females have the same reproductive parts as males, except in the former they are internal, and in the latter they are external. A lengthy exposition follows arguing that the female reproductive organs would overlap exactly with the male if they were turned inside out.[85] Galen illustrates this claim with a comparison to the eyes of a mole, possibly the best-known example of the Aristotelian deformed animal.[86] He notes that, according to Aristotle, there are animals with varied natures, and they can be arranged hierarchically depending on how many senses they have. Then he explains the inferiority of the female reproductive system by combining points (1) and (2). He states that the colder constitution of the female embryo is unable to push the reproductive organs outside.[87] This accounts for the analogy between the mole's eyes and the female reproductive system: both are incomplete (by being internal) owing to their cold constitutions.

One might wonder if this is perhaps an unfortunate analogy. The eyes of moles are incomplete because, despite having all the required organs, the

practice. This discussion also highlights a controversy concerning another elemental property, 'heat'/'cold', of a female body both in Hippocratic texts and in broader medical tradition (King 1998: 32–33).

83 *GA* 1.20 (728a17–20); 2.3 (737a28). Galen's reading is not entirely correct, as Connell (2016) shows, see especially Chapter 3 on this issue. Connell demonstrates that the female side of reproduction does offer an important generative contribution, including a seed-like material that complement the paternal seed and is capable of producing maternal resemblance in an offspring.

84 See, for example, *Sem.* 2.5.4–5 de Lacy (4.627–8K), where the two types of semen are used for explaining the maternal resemblance in some parts and the paternal resemblance in others. A similar argument, although in a very different context, can be found in Galen's near-contemporary Plotinus, see *En.* 5.7.2.

85 *UP* 14.6 (2.296, 7–297, 3 Helmreich=4.159K).

86 *UP* 14.6 (2.297, 26–298, 9 Helmreich=4.160K). See also Aristotle *HA* 4.8 (532b4–533a12); *de An.* 3.1 (425a9–10); *PA* 4.8 (684a32–b1). See also Witt (2012: 95).

87 *UP* 14.6 (2.299, 14–19 Helmreich=4.162K). See also Connell (2016: 117–18) for an argument that, in this respect, Galen has a more sexist conception of gender than Aristotle.

mole lacks good sight.[88] This is not the case in female animals. In fact, Galen immediately follows with an extensive discussion of how the internal reproductive system – which is supposed to be falling short – is of great usefulness,[89] especially because a colder constitution can retain nutriment better, which enables gestation. Galen's exposition of the excellence in the design of the female reproductive system has an odd result. The female reproductive system does not fail in any way *qua* a reproductive system, and in this way, it is nothing like the eyes of moles. It exhibits functional excellence, just like all the other systems. The only respect in which the female reproductive system fails is by not being male. This is a normative failure, not a functional one. It has been pointed out by Rebecca Flemming that Galen's (mis)treatments of women as epistemic agents is not necessarily a result of making judgements about the gender but rather a reference to the dominant cultural norms.[90] Presumably, cultural assumptions about gender roles can explain the somewhat incoherent approach to reproduction too.[91]

Despite not being an outstanding example of Galen's analytical prowess, this argument proves to be revealing when put against the background of his theoretical understanding of parthood. A female animal, according to him, lacks a part normatively. At the same time, the lack of this part not only does not interrupt activities but, in fact, aids them. The gestation could not take place successfully if the female constitution were not imperfectly cold. When this point is combined with the claims in therapeutic treatises – much less culturally and politically charged – Galen appears to acknowledge the normative failure while warning very explicitly against prioritising it above activity or function. This sentiment is echoed in other treatises too. He writes about the shape of the organ as the structure that enables the activity of that organ numerous times.[92] In *On the Doctrines of Hippocrates and Plato*, for example, Galen prioritises functionality over shape, writing that the essence is not tissues and

88 Aristotle *de An. 3.1* (425a11–13); *Metaph.* 5.22 (1022b26). It is also surprising not to find Galen adding that the construction of the eyes in moles is, in fact, a greatly beneficial design for an animal that lives underground. This argumentative strategy is so consistently reiterated throughout the treatise, that its absence is noticeable. Perhaps the distinctly anthropocentric focus could account for that; *UP* 1.22 (1.59 Helmreich=3.80K) is a notable example of Galen portraying the constitution of apes as inferior in principle.

89 *UP* 14.6 (2.299–300 Helmreich=4.162–3K).

90 Flemming (2000: 286–7).

91 Although it is worth bearing in mind that, as Flemming (2000: 322) notes, 'in none of these cases, however, is the concern to naturalise the conventions of the Roman sexual order, but rather to bring these conventions to bear on nature'.

92 For example, *UP* 1.9 (1.17 Helmreich=3.23–4K), see esp. the conclusion in lines 19–22; *Loc. Aff.* 1.1.25 Gärtner (8.16K); see also the case of the brain in *Cur. Rat. Ven. Sect.* 8 (11.275–6K).

arrangements, but actions and uses; in effect, he emphasises the functional aspect over the normative.[93]

Thus, Galen fully commits to the view that nature's design is nothing but excellent, and even when it seems to fall short, it is, in fact, accomplishing significant tasks. His commitment to design theory has been thoroughly explored in the scholarship,[94] and his views on the imperfect reproductive system are a reflection of those beliefs. However, the strong emphasis on the functional excellence could also be influenced by his immediate medical context. As Soranus reports in his *Gynaecology*, the claim that women have different natures (e.g., colder *kraseis*) became contested by various fashionable doctors in the Hellenistic period. Herophilus, for instance, claimed that the only women-specific medical facts are the ones concerning the reproductive system. Asclepiades of Bithynia appears to reject any difference as well, and Soranus explicitly contrasts their position with the Aristotelian view.[95] It is significant that Soranus mentions Herophilus and Asclepiades specifically. These two doctors have hardly anything in common otherwise,[96] so naming these two figures shows that the view was held by a wide range of doctors, not just members of one specific school.

It seems likely that, by the time Galen was active, Aristotle was, deservedly or not, associated with the view that the female gender necessitates a certain physiological constitution, inferior to the male one. This view was, furthermore, understood to contrast with the views of celebrated Hellenistic doctors. Galen is polemically engaged with both Aristotle and some of these doctors. In fact, *On the Usefulness of Parts* not only presents a criticism of Aristotle's understanding of the reproductive system but also critiques of such figures as Anaxagoras and Asclepiades.[97] However, it is

[93] *PHP* 1.8.11–15 de Lacy (5.202–3K). There is a similar concept of 'functional' parthood in modern mereology. However, given that modern mereology is committed to principles and methods that are very different from ancient preoccupations, my use of this term only refers to Galen's conceptualisation.

[94] See, for example, van der Eijk (2017) and Hankinson (1989).

[95] Soranus *Gyn.* 3.3.5 Ilberg.

[96] Asclepiades notoriously denied the existence of the *hēgemonikon*, see Sextus Empiricus *M* 7.1.202; Caelius Aurelianus 1.14.115. See Tertullian, *De anim.* 15.2 (Waszink) for the anatomically motivated argument against its existence that clearly targets both the cardiocentrists and the encephalocentrists, Herophilus being the most prominent of them (as discussed in the chapter on the nervous system). For Herophilus' encephalocentrism, see von Staden (1989: 155–60). The most substantial work on Asclepiades is Vallance (1990), although see also Leith (2012) and Polito (2006).

[97] Anaxagoras (*UP* 1.3 (1.4, 3 Helmreich=3.5K)), Asclepiades and the Epicureans (*UP* 1.21 (1.54, 12–13 Helmreich=3.74K)) are all mentioned in the very first book of the *UP*. See also Galen's attack of Asclepiades regarding the explanation of why the vein is arterial, and the artery is veinous discussed in Chapter 5.

quite clear that the two positions are not equally faulty: the former is much less so than the latter. Galen positions himself against the atomistic understanding of the body and often assigns a respectable Peripatetic pedigree to his own views. The treatise itself, after all, is dedicated to a Peripatetic Boethius.[98] At the same time, the 'traditional' view associated with Aristotle comes with a possible risk of being perceived as too old-fashioned, given the progress of medical tradition in the Hellenistic period. Galen's strong emphasis on the high functional value of the female reproductive system allows him to navigate this rhetorical Scylla and Charybdis. He commits to the Peripatetic view on the female constitution (female animals do have different mixtures) but adds a claim about its high functionality, which puts him in more direct conversation with the doctors knowledgeable of and invested in the Hellenistic medical discoveries and theoretical preoccupations. Galen both distances himself from certain Aristotelian views (most notably, regarding the existence of the female seed) and reinvents others (the female *krasis*) for his own purposes in his contemporary debates. The interesting consequences of such polemic manoeuvring is that Galen is no less influenced by the Hellenistic doctors, including such figures as Asclepiades, than by Aristotle.

1.5 Functional and Normative Parthood

There is a notable consistency between Galen's approach to the imperfections of the body, whether they are imperfections of the innate constitution or imperfections of shape. Neither the sixth finger nor the inherently cold mixture of the female body is something that needs to be fixed; they are not 'against nature' *per se* and, therefore, not a concern to medicine. What medicine does concern itself with is activity, and imperfections are only important when they affect the functioning of the body. Therefore, the Galenic understanding of human nature puts a strong emphasis on functionality of the activities.[99]

This point helps to explain why certain parts are expendable while others are not. The chapter started with the curious claim that the loss of bone is, effectively, more disruptive to the body than the loss of the stomach, because it destroys the activity. Key to explaining this

[98] *Lib. Prop.* 1.17 (139, 27–140, 5 Boudon-Millot=19.15–16K), for further discussion, see Hankinson (2022b).

[99] Galen's inspiration here could very well be Aristotelian. The activity bears ontological significance in the works of the latter too, for example, in *de An.* 2.1 (412b18–23), which famously argues that the eye that no longer sees is an eye only homonymously, not properly.

surprising claim is Galen's prioritisation of functional over normative parthood. The key question in determining the results of a loss of a part is whether the part has a unique activity or if it shares the type of activity it performs with another part. The difference can now be explained by the roles each of these parts play in their respective anatomical location, and the four-fold division of body parts in the *Art of Medicine* is useful for clarification. Some discrete parts are self-sufficient in their activities, while others are not. The bone belongs to the group that Galen describes as the organs with innate capacities that are neither governed by nor govern any other parts. This means that it functions by virtue of properties that are entirely self-contained. The stomach, meanwhile, is a structured organ. It means that its activity relies both on its homoeomerous tissues and on the veins, nerves and arteries.

Veins especially are crucial, as they connect the stomach to the liver, which is the actual overseer of nutrition. The nutritive system, as Galen notes in *On the Natural Capacities*, is comprised of many organs because food has to be converted into blood by stages. The stomach, thus is not simply a part of the body like a bone is; it is also a sub-part of the nutritive activity. As nutrition is taken care of by multiple organs, the loss of a stomach can be compensated by the fact that the other organs keep on performing related activities. Whereas the 'activity' of a bone is lost when that bone is damaged, the activity of nutrition can be compensated by other parts.[100]

The compensation mechanism can also take place via the doubling of the parts, as Galen notes in Book 8 of *On the Usefulness of Parts*, when discussing the head anatomy. Having noted that it is better that there are two lateral ventricles because there are two downwards-leading channels and sense instruments are paired, he explains that the main usefulness of paired instruments is the possibility to maintain activity through one if another one if injured.[101] The first priority of the design of the human body is, after all, the maintenance of the activity, and the significance of parts is determined in reference to the activity.

Consequently, by identifying an organ with one of the four categories of parts, it is possible to calculate how much damage to life and health the loss of that organ will cause. The principles are most important when it

[100] As long as the liver is active; but the liver has a special status as the seat of one of the principles, so *qua* a body part, it is different from simple structured organs such as the stomach.

[101] *UP* 8.10 (1.481, 14–22 Helmreich=3.663–4K), esp.: ἀλλ' ἥ γε πρώτη τε καὶ κοινοτάτη πάντων τῶν διφυῶν ὀργάνων ἥδ' ἐστίν, ἵν', εἰ καὶ θάτερον αὐτῶν πάθοι, τὸ λοιπὸν ὑπηρετοῖ.

comes to vitality.[102] The loss of them will undercut any functioning of all the other parts.[103] The capacities of the self-sufficient tissues, although simple, are irreplaceable. The structured organs (the ones that are not principles), meanwhile, are somewhat replaceable, to the extent that similar organs in the same system can compensate for their activity. Finally, there are body parts that have no capacities, only reproduction. As these do not perform any action as such, they are quite expendable. The regular loss of hair and nails illustrated this well.

Galen's four-fold division of parts, thus, illuminates an interesting equilibrium. The systematic constitution of human animals renders them, on the one hand fragile, because a loss of one part can be highly dangerous, (and they have very many parts that can be damaged). On the other hand, human animals are also reasonably sturdy, because the systematicity of some of their organs allows the activities of that system to continue while a part is lost. This means that, although human beings have a multitude of parts, it is only in a few cases that damage to a part results in the loss of life.

1.6 Concluding Remarks: The Problem of Unity

The emerging picture shows Galen's interest in approaching the human body not just as a static combination of parts but also as a hierarchy of activities carried out by those parts. In Galenic physiology, it is important to know not only that certain parts make up certain organs but also *how* those parts are connected both to each other and to other organs, as well as how these connections enable them to fulfil their activities. The notion of governance plays a key role in determining the relationship that one part has with another. Whether a part only self-manages, both self-manages and is governed or governs determines how irreplaceable its activity is. The application of these notions is wide-ranging, and they will continue

102 In yet another kind of division of parts, Galen explains that while some parts are crucial for life itself (the brain, the heart and the liver), others are created simply for improving life; see *UP* 14.1 (2.284–5, 23 Helmreich=4.142K); 6.7 (1.318, 10 Helmreich=3.435K); see also *AA* 7.1 (622 Garofalo=2.590K). He classifies all the organs into three categories according to their purpose: those for the sake of living, those for the sake of living well and those for the sake of reproduction. Galen takes the sensory organs (the eyes, the ears and the nostrils, to be precise) to be a condition for living well, not just living.

103 The notion of a vital part (in the sense that damage to it results in death) is also present in the Hippocratic corpus, but the lists of vital parts are different, see *Morb.* 1.3 (6.144, 1–2 Littré) for the list that includes the brain, the spinal medulla, the cavity, the liver, the diaphragm, the blood vessel, the heart; and *Aph.* 6.18 (4.566–8 Littré) for the bladder, the brain, the heart, the diaphragm, intestines, the cavity, the liver. See Singer (1996) for a study of Galen's dubious claim in *PHP* that the notion of the three governing parts is Hippocratic.

reappearing in the remainder of this study. The importance of this division of parts can hardly be overstressed: it explains how life can continue when some parts of a body are damaged (or missing altogether) and why the loss of some parts is much more harmful than the loss of others. Ultimately, it is a very helpful tool for understanding what makes a body *one*.

There is a strong emphasis on the activities of parts in reference to vitality in particular. The case of (im)perfect parts and constitutions illustrates this point well: the normative imperfection does not necessarily need to be fixed, as long as it does not threaten life, and other types of imperfections, such as the constitution of the female reproductive system, is even desirable, as its flaws are in fact useful features, enabling reproduction.

Understanding how Galen theorises human nature, it follows, requires centring the discussion around the question of how parts come together to perform vital functions, such as nutrition or respiration. These functions are underpinned by the activities not of single parts but of the entire physiological systems ruled by their respective governing parts: the liver, the heart and the brain. The following three chapters are dedicated to the systems that these organs govern: the parts that they consist of, the activities they carry out and their overall significance. Special attention will be paid to the question of how each system renders a living being unified and how the two animal-only systems (the nervous and the cardiac) built on the vegetative system, with profound mutual effects. In Chapter 5, the discussion turns to the question of how these three governing parts and their respective systems that seemingly have an equal status form a single coherent physiological system. In other words, having discussed how Galen 'takes the body apart' by dividing it conceptually into various parts, the rest of the work is the study of how he puts it back together, one vital process at a time, with the emerging Galenic account of human nature and vitality.

CHAPTER 2

Nutrition, Growth and Vegetative Capacities

In most contexts, the distinction between living and non-living things is easily made and so obvious that it hardly bears thinking about it. However, there are cases that blur the line, for example, very complex automata or single-cell living organisms. In antiquity, it is not the latter but ordinary plants that are taken to be the simplest entities that pass the threshold of vitality. At the beginning of *On the Natural Capacities*, Galen states that sensation and voluntary motion are specific to animals, while growth and nutrition are also observable in plants. The former are the effects of the soul, while the latter are the effects of nature.[1] He goes on to claim that animals are governed both by nature and the soul.[2] This treatise focuses on the effects of nature, examining how growth and nutrition take place. In Galenic physiology, these activities are treated as fundamentally vital, and they represent the distinguishing features of living beings.[3]

These processes, common to humans, animals and plants, are governed by the vegetative soul.[4] In this respect, Galen adopts elements of the prominent philosophical traditions without making very nuanced

[1] *Nat. Fac.* 1.1 (101, 3–4 Helmreich=2.1K); see also *Loc. Aff.* 1.6.27–1.7.3 Gärtner (8.66–7K), spelling out the difference between the natural capacities as being innate to the organs and the psychic capacity as flowing from elsewhere, like sunlight; see Hankinson (2014: 92–3). This passage, as well as the other texts discussed in this section, might pose a problem for the interpretation of Galen as a Stoically leaning physicalist, discussed in the Introduction. The similarity between the Stoics and Galen lies in Galen's 'belief that matter can be analysed, ultimately, in terms of a complete fusion or mixture of elements and that this mixture provides the basis for the inbuilt vitality of natural entities. This postulate of inbuilt vitality underlies, in turn, Galen's conception of living things as coherent complexes of natural faculties or capacities' (Gill 2010: 145). While Gill's emphasis on the connection between natural capacities and vitality must be correct (the discussion in Chapters 3 and 4 will also lead to similar conclusions), this passage shows Galen distinguishes between the natural capacities and the soul capacities, so the former do not account for all the capacities a human body has. The so-called higher-order capacities of the brain cannot be accounted for by the natural capacities, as I later argue.

[2] *Nat. Fac.* 1.1 (101, 12–13 Helmreich=2.2K).

[3] See Holmes (2017: 379–80).

[4] It also could be called 'nutritive soul' and 'nature'; for the sake of clarity and consistency, I mostly use this term.

differentiations, and his tendency to present certain differences in terminology (and even concepts) as merely verbal disagreement is well-known, even if puzzling.[5] For example, he often conflates the Platonic notions of the desiderative soul and the Aristotelian nutritive soul without referring to the crucial difference, viz. the acts of desire.[6] Similarly, at the beginning of *On the Natural Capacities*, he writes that it does not matter whether one calls the entity in question 'nature' (φύσις) or 'nutritive soul' (θρεπτική ψυχή) because neither of the terms is revealing enough of what is at stake, which reduces the difference between the Stoics and Peripatetics to a verbal dispute.[7] Despite a convoluted approach to the preceding tradition, Galen's own focus is clear enough: the two fundamental activities that separate the living from the non-living are nutrition and growth.

In highlighting nutrition and growth as the threshold for vitality, Galen is in line with Aristotle's account of lower and higher soul-activities. In Book 2 of *On the Soul*, Aristotle clearly delineates nutrition as the basic capacity of living things, noting that it can be separated from more advanced capacities, such as thinking, perception, movement, rest and so on, but the latter cannot be separated from it. It indicates that these capacities are common and necessary for something to be considered living; but for an entity to be considered a living *animal*, it must possess the capacity for sensation too.[8] Furthermore, nutrition also allows plants to grow, that is, to expand spatially.[9] Galen names these two activities as basic attributes of the vegetative life too, presumably following Aristotle's analysis of the basic vitality.[10]

[5] See Hankinson (1991b). [6] see Holmes (2017: n43).

[7] *UP* 4.13 (1.226, 21–25 Helmreich=3.309K). The ones identifying this entity with nature are the Stoics, *PHP* 6.3.7 de Lacy (5.521K); *Form. Foet.* 6, 31 Nickel (4.700K). See also Ps. Galen *Int.* 13.1 (45, 13–19 Petit=14.726K=*SVF* 2.716=LS 47N). The nutritive soul is an Aristotelian term (*de An. 2.3* (413a23)). Hankinson (1991a: n8) points out that Galen sides with the Stoics in allocating the vegetative capacities to nature rather than the soul, as Peripatetics do. See also von Staden (2000: 102): 'it is historically plausible that Chrysippus' radical distinction between nature and soul, between *physis* and *psyche*, was prompted by Herophilus' distinction between "physic and natural" capacities within a living being'; Galen may have known this distinction from Herophilus too. However, see Leith (2020) for the argument that Herophilus most likely posited four capacities of the body. Regardless of the provenance of nomenclature, I argue later in this chapter that the conceptual apparatus that Galen employs to account for the generative power of these capacities is, predominantly, Peripatetic.

[8] *de An.* 2.2 (413a32–b5). [9] *de An.* 2.2 (413a25–30).

[10] Although Plato *Ti.* 77A is probably a relevant background too. Furthermore, Galen also takes it that sense perception and voluntary motion are higher, animal-level activities. The exact nature of this distinction as made by Galen is a matter of debate in the scholarship; see note 58.

However, Aristotle also takes reproduction and nutrition to originate from the same psychic power.[11] Galen does not identify reproduction as an activity of the vegetative soul at the beginning of *On the Natural Capacities*, although the vegetative soul does oversee the regeneration of tissues and the generation of an embryo.[12] On one occasion, he even claims the vegetative soul, not the pneuma in the seed, is the demiurge of an embryo.[13] Section 2.7 will address the problem of the generative power of the vegetative soul by outlining the cases in which it manifests itself and in which it does not arguing that, ultimately, Galen assigns a minor generative role to these capacities. Before turning to this problem, the chapter will discuss another divergence from Aristotle: the very Platonic emphasis on the liver as the seat of the vegetative soul. A careful outline of its activities as a governing part, as well as the parts that it governs, shows that Galen reflects on vitality in a coherent and nuanced way, even if he does not always provide all the answers one might wish. This chapter starts with the anatomy that underpins the physiological domain of the vegetative soul and its activity, nutrition. Then the discussion delves into a more minute analysis of natural capacities that enable these activities on both self-managing parts and the governing principal part, before turning to the discussion of generative aspects of these capacities and the Galenic notion of nature as a demiurge. The conclusion draws the insights together, explaining how the presence of the vegetative capacities unifies a living being in a fundamental way.

2.1 The Seat of the Vegetative Soul and Its Anatomy

Chapter 1 covered the odd case of Galen arguing that the loss of a bone is more damaging than the loss of a stomach. The explanation for this claim turned out to be the fact that the stomach is subordinate to the liver. The liver, furthermore, is one of the principal organs with the capacity to govern (ἄρχειν) other parts, according to the four-fold division of parts discussed in Chapter 1. He assigns a Platonic pedigree to this understanding of the liver's significance, although Plato's *Timaeus* is, in fact, more vague and only talks about the region in which the vegetative soul is

11 *de An.* 2.4 (416a19).

12 See, for example, *Sem.* 1.13.16–18 de Lacy (4.560–1K), which will be discussed later.

13 *Sem.* 1.9.17 de Lacy (4.546K) and 1.10.1 de Lacy (4.546–7K).

located.[14] Galen's main argument that it is the liver specifically can be found in Book 6 of *On the Doctrines of Hippocrates and Plato*. At the beginning of this book, he states that, having proven that the spirited soul is located in the heart and the rational one in the brain, he is setting out to prove the location of the third, the vegetative soul. It is much harder, however, to demonstrate this point than the previous two. This proof follows not from the nature of the things investigated but from the properties peculiar to them. He illustrates the difficulty by reminding his readers that when the nerves are cut, the parts connected to the brain retain their capacities (*dunameis*), while the parts below the ligature lose them. The same is the case with arteries. They lose pulse once they are separated from the heart by ligature.[15] It is not possible, however, to perform the same type of demonstration by cutting veins, the offshoots of the liver. This governing part is not a source of clearly perceivable motion, and its injury produces harm very slowly, as it takes time to affect nutrition and colouring.[16]

Galen's project also has a polemical aspect: he is attacking the accounts that attribute the activities of the liver, such as blood production, to the heart. In order to show that the liver is the *hēgemon*, he develops a multi-step argumentative strategy, with the key claim that the liver is a source of the same kind of capacity that is also present in plants.[17] A comparison to plants turns out to be a significant explanatory device, and it plays an important role in the first step, that is, showing that the liver – and not the heart – is the source of veins.[18] He describes the growth of a tree from a seed to a large plant and points out that its roots are always the 'mouths' through which the plant feeds.[19] Then he describes the animal body using this very same pattern. He first compares arteries, the offshoots from the heart, to the branches growing from the trunk of a tree. The arteries drawing air from the lungs are said to be like plant roots drawing

[14] *Ti.* 70E; Hankinson (1991a: 199) notes that 'Galen's Platonising is neither slavish nor unthinking', as it comes with adaptations as well as the adoption of Peripatetic and Stoic elements when it is useful.

[15] *PHP* 6.3.2–4 de Lacy (5.520K). [16] *PHP* 6.3.5–6 de Lacy (5.520K).

[17] *PHP* 6.3.7 de Lacy (5.521K). For an extensive study of this claim as well as its Hippocratic pedigree, see Holmes (2017). Plato's *Ti.* 76E–77E is also relevant background here (see the later discussion for Galen's interpretation of the claim about plant sensory capacities). See also *Nat. Fac.* 1.6 (108–9, 24 Helmreich=2.11K), where Galen describes the genesis as starting with the casting of the seed either into the womb or into the earth, as there is no difference. His claim there is that the initial genesis is of the same kind in plants and animals.

[18] *PHP* 6.3.9 de Lacy (5.522K). [19] *PHP* 6.3.11–15 de Lacy (5.522–524K).

nourishment from the earth.[20] In both cases, offshoots spring from the governing parts, which is key to Galen's analogy.[21] He calls it a general principle, known to everyone with expertise in natural sciences: the greater is the source of the smaller,[22] and, even more so in animals than in plants.[23] It must therefore follow that the liver is the source (*rhizōsis*) of veins. This claim is also supported by a citation from Hippocratic *On Humours*,[24] stating that 'for as the earth is to the trees, so the stomach is to animals'.[25]

This analogy establishes that the liver is the anatomical source of veins. Then he moves on to the second step, that is, showing that the liver and veins are not just physically connected, but also that there is a physiological hierarchy between them. To establish this point, Galen uses as a foil the account that takes the liver to be the producer of blood but makes the heart the supplier of the power to veins. Such an account, he argues, is unreasonable, because the source of production ought to be the source of power too.[26] The liver, therefore, is not a servant to the heart but a 'leader and ruler' (ἡγεμόνος καὶ ἄρχοντος) in its own right.[27] This point is supported by the evidence from dissection that shows the liver, not the heart, to be connected to the veins in a way that points to their source. The vena cava, notably, is connected to the heart only by an offshoot branch. If the veins grew from the heart, they would be observed to branch off from the heart, just like the great artery growing from the left ventricle of the heart that splits into two branches, one going to the head and another one to the spinal column. This is not the case for veins, however.[28]

Thus, Galen establishes the liver as the *hēgemon* and moves on to the proof concerning the production of blood. Here, he aims to show that it must be attributed to the liver and not to the heart. The substance of the liver is, he argues, much closer to that of blood, and therefore, it is more proper for the production of the blood.[29] Subsequently, he also argues that

[20] *PHP* 6.3.16–18 de Lacy (5.524–5K), see also Anonymous Londinensis 6.13–33 Manetti (2011: 11–12) that attributes to Hippocrates the claim that we are rooted in air like plants in moisture.
[21] *PHP* 6.3.19 de Lacy (5.525); see also *Prop. Plac.* 10.1 (100 Lami Garofalo).
[22] *PHP* 6.3.20 de Lacy (5.525K).
[23] *PHP* 6.3.32 de Lacy (5.529K).
[24] Interestingly, Holmes (2017: esp. 383) has shown that the Hippocratic texts do not, in fact, ascribe the status of the soul to the vegetative functions, so citing Hippocrates in the context of this discussion is not entirely accurate.
[25] *PHP* 6.3.41 de Lacy (5.532K), tr. de Lacy (1978–84: 383); Hippocrates' quote is from *Hum.* 11 (170, 1 Overwien=5.491 Littré).
[26] *PHP* 6.4.1–2 de Lacy (5.532–3K); my discussion is brief, because there is already an excellent extensive analysis of this argument in Hankinson (1991a).
[27] *PHP* 6.4.9 de Lacy (5.535K), tr. de Lacy (1978–84: 385).
[28] *PHP* 6.5.2–5 de Lacy (5.538–9K).
[29] *PHP* 6.8.27–36 de Lacy (5.570–2K).

the heart is the source of pneuma-like and boiling blood, which indicates that the heart must be the seat of the spirited, not the vegetative soul.[30]

The argument from temperature not only supports his anatomical point but also leads to a significant physiological observation. Having noted that he has provided enough proof that the transmission of nutriment comes from the area of the stomach to the heart in *On the Natural Capacities*,[31] Galen argues that the seat for the spirited soul, but not the vegetative one, must necessarily be warm (which is true of the heart, not the liver area). Furthermore, the vegetative soul found in plants is much colder than the spirited soul in animals. In animals, these two souls are closer in warmth, and, overall, the vegetative soul found in plants is colder than the vegetative soul found in animals.[32] In animals, it has to be warm in order to make the nutritive fluid warm; at the same time, its heat must also be fairly gentle, since it is not the kind of boiling heat that is strong enough to make veins pulsate.[33] This claim marks the crucial distinction between the plant and the animal life: the heat. Animals are not merely extra warm plants, the warmth provided by the spirited soul is so great that it makes them possessed of an entirely different kind of vitality. The nature of the spirited soul and its domain (including the significance of heat) will be analysed in greater detail in Chapter 3. For current purposes, it is important to note that the domain of the liver is marked by a very low heat, distinguished by slow and barely perceptible pulsation.

With the arguments outlined in this section, Galen establishes that the ruling part of the vegetative domain in animals is the liver and outlines the anatomy of the domain of the vegetative soul. Using the scheme distinguishing the four types of parts discussed in Chapter 1, we can identify the governing part (the liver) and its offshoots (veins), connecting it with the rest of the body. There are also parts that are both self-managed and subject to the governance of the liver. The stomach, discussed in Chapter 1, is one such part. In order to understand how the double-ruling – the internal one and the 'external' one (in the sense of being governed by the principal organs) – takes place and how it results in

[30] *PHP* 6.8.39 de Lacy (5.573K).

[31] This seems to refer not to one specific argument but to a number of points that support such a view. *Nat. Fac.* 3.4 (211–15 Helmreich=2.152–7K); 3.7 (217–20 Helmreich=2.161–5K); 3.13 (236–249 Helmreich=2.187–204K) are some of the examples.

[32] This is one of the ways in which the liver does, in the end, differ from plants. Another is having a nerve inserted in it, just like all viscera of an animal, see *UP* 6.18 (1.365, 5–7 Helmreich=3.501K).

[33] *PHP* 6.8.53–55 de Lacy (5.576–7K), esp.: οὔτε γὰρ ἂν οὕτως θερμὸν εἰργάζετο χυμόν, εἰ μὴ καὶ αὐτὸ τοιοῦτον ὑπῆρχεν, οὔτ᾽ ἀσφύκτους ἂν εἶχε τὰς φλέβας, εἰ ζεούσης θερμασίας ἦν ἀρχή.

nutrition, the following section looks more closely at the process by which the body processes, distributes and absorbs nourishment.

2.2 The Vital Activities of the Liver

The liver is the governing part of the vegetative domain, and it is in charge of two related processes: nourishment and growth. The digestive system underpins both of them, and therefore it will be the starting point for investigating the scope and the nature of the activities of the vegetative soul. To the modern reader, the stomach might intuitively seem like the proper organ of digestion, but Galen actually describes the digestive system as a group of different organs working together. They all perform the same task – the breaking down of the nutriment – and the division of labour is surprisingly even. Possibly the clearest account of this process can be found in *On the Natural Capacities*. With an overarching aim to show that the process of nutrition is governed by natural capacities, Galen writes that several organs are necessary to carry out the process of digestion for the following reason:

> ἐπειδὴ γὰρ ἡ ἐνέργεια ταύτης τῆς δυνάμεως ἐξομοίωσίς ἐστιν, ὁμοιοῦσθαι δὲ καὶ μεταβάλλειν εἰς ἄλληλα πᾶσι τοῖς οὖσιν ἀδύνατον, εἰ μή τινα ἔχοι κοινωνίαν ἤδη καὶ συγγένειαν ἐν ταῖς ποιότησι, διὰ τοῦτο πρῶτον μὲν οὐκ ἐκ πάντων ἐδεσμάτων πᾶν ζῷον τρέφεσθαι πέφυκεν, ἔπειτα δ' οὐδ' ἐξ ὧν οἷόν τ' ἐστὶν οὐδ' ἐκ τούτων παραχρῆμα, καὶ διὰ ταύτην τὴν ἀνάγκην πλειόνων ὀργάνων ἀλλοιωτικῶν τῆς τροφῆς ἕκαστον τῶν ζῴων χρῄζει. ἵνα μὲν γὰρ τὸ ξανθὸν ἐρυθρὸν γένηται καὶ τὸ ἐρυθρὸν ξανθόν, ἁπλῆς καὶ μιᾶς δεῖται τῆς ἀλλοιώσεως· ἵνα δὲ τὸ λευκὸν μέλαν καὶ τὸ μέλαν λευκόν, ἁπασῶν τῶν μεταξύ. καὶ τοίνυν καὶ τὸ μαλακώτατον οὐκ ἂν ἀθρόως σκληρότατον καὶ τὸ σκληρότατον οὐκ ἂν ἀθρόως μαλακώτατον γένοιτο, ὥσπερ οὐδὲ τὸ δυσωδέστατον εὐωδέστατον οὐδ' ἔμπαλιν τὸ εὐωδέστατον δυσωδέστατον ἐξαίφνης γένοιτ' ἄν ... ὅτι δὲ καὶ τῷ ἄρτῳ καὶ πολὺ μᾶλλον θριδακίνῃ καὶ τεύτλῳ καὶ τοῖς ὁμοίοις παμπόλλης δεῖται τῆς ἀλλοιώσεως εἰς αἵματος γένεσιν, οὐδὲ τοῦτ' ἄδηλον. ἓν μὲν δὴ τοῦτ' αἴτιον τοῦ πολλὰ γενέσθαι τὰ περὶ τὴν τῆς τροφῆς ἀλλοίωσιν ὄργανα.
>
> For since the action of this capacity is assimilation, and it is impossible for anything to be assimilated by, and to change into anything else unless they already possess a certain community and affinity in their qualities, therefore, in the first place, any animal cannot naturally derive nourishment from any kind of food, and secondly, even in the case of those from which it can do so, it cannot do this at once. Therefore, by reason of this law, every animal needs several organs for altering the nutriment. For in order that the yellow may become red, and the red yellow, one simple process of alteration is

required, but in order that the white may become black, and the black white, all the intermediate stages are needed. So also, a thing which is very soft cannot all at once become very hard, nor vice versa; nor, similarly can anything which has a very bad smell suddenly become quite fragrant, nor again, can the converse happen ... Further, it is quite clear that bread, and more particularly lettuce, beet, and the like, require a great deal of alteration in order to become blood. This, then, is one reason why there are so many organs concerned with the alteration of food.[34]

In the long discussion that follows, Galen names the other two reasons, viz. the need to discharge superfluities (περίσσωμα) and the need to carry pabulum (κατατετμημέναι) in every direction. Digestion is effectively a very long and complex conversion process of foodstuffs into blood, and numerous parts are needed in order to perform various stages of this process. The egalitarian standing of all the parts involved in digestion is striking, and it naturally raises the question of the role of the liver. Why does this conveyor-like process need a *hēgemon*?

The answer is suggested by the arguments in *On the Doctrines of Hippocrates and Plato* and *On the Usefulness of Parts*, where Galen attacks Erasistratus' claim that the heart is the source of both arteries and veins. This claim, apparently made in the first book of *On Fevers*, must have been quite brief because Galen takes it upon himself to figure out possible motivations for making it and to reject them all in turn. Most pertinently, he complains that Erasistratus did not provide a clear account of the production of blood, despite the fact that it is more significant than the activity of the stomach. He supports this point by stating that, while it would be possible to survive if the stomach could not crush food, the same would not be the case if the activity of the liver – the production of blood – was damaged.[35] Given Galen's claim at the beginning of Book 6 of *On the Doctrines of Hippocrates and Plato*, stating that the motion of the liver is much harder to observe, it is clear that the liver is the distributor of the nutriment processed by the digestive system: it is in control of how much nutriment to send, as well as where and when to send it. This role alone would earn the liver the title of the *hēgemon*, but it has another important activity. In Book 4 of *On the Usefulness of Parts*, Galen describes the activities of the liver as follows:

[34] *Nat. Fac.* 1.10 (115, 12–116, 17 Helmreich=2.20–21K), tr. Brock (1916: 33–5).

[35] *PHP* 6.6.26 de Lacy (5.554K). In the case of damage to the stomach, one could survive on liquids. This claim is unpacked further against the background of Galen's understanding of parthood in Chapter 1.

Αὐτὸ δὲ τὸ ἧπαρ, ἐπειδὰν αὐτὴν παραλάβῃ πρὸς τῶν ὑπηρετῶν ἤδη παρεσκευασμένην καὶ οἷον ὑπογραφήν τινα καὶ ἀμυδρὸν εἶδος αἵματος ἔχουσαν, ἐπάγει τέλεον αὐτῇ τὸν κόσμον εἰς αἵματος ἀκριβοῦς γένεσιν. ἀλλ' ἐπεὶ τῶν κατὰ τὴν γαστέρα τὰ μὲν οὕτω μοχθηρὰ καθάπερ ἐν τῷ σίτῳ γῆ καὶ λίθοι καὶ τὰ τῶν ἀγρίων ὀσπρίων σπέρματα διεκέκριτο, τὰ δ' οἷον ἄχνη καὶ πίτυρον ἑτέρας καθάρσεως ἐδεῖτο, ταύτην αὖθις ἐπάγει τῇ τροφῇ τὴν κάθαρσιν τὸ ἧπαρ.

When the liver has received the nutriment already prepared by its servants and having the crude outline, as it were, and indistinct semblance of blood, it provides the final elaboration itself so that the nutriment becomes actual blood. The impurities corresponding to the earth, stones, and seeds of wild plants in the wheat were eliminated from the food in the stomach, but this stands in need of a second cleansing from the impurities corresponding to the chaff and bran in wheat, and it is the liver which accomplishes thus further purification of the nutriment.[36]

The liver, in short, performs the crucial final stage in the production of blood before sending it out for distribution throughout the rest of the body.[37] Evidently, Galen takes this step to be distinct from other digestive stages, because the loss of this stage compromises a body's ability to be nourished in the way that the loss of another part of the digestive system (e.g., the stomach) does not. To be precise, the liver, according to him, purifies the blood.[38] The vivid analogy to the processing of wheat grain spells this point out explicitly: the liver separates nutritious material from non-nutritious in the same way as farmers separate grains from bits of earth, stones and wild seeds. Galen, however, is unsatisfied with just one analogy and, noting that a comparison to liquid substance processing would be even clearer, describes young wine that is still fermenting, its dregs still sinking down while the fine parts rise to the surface. The upper portions are like the useful blood that the liver properly separates, before sending it out to the rest of the body. The residues from the final production of blood in the liver are divided into two types: the thin yellow one (received by the bladder) and the thick muddy one (received by the spleen).[39] After some further processing via such organs as kidneys,

36 *UP* 4.3 (1.197, 5–13 Helmreich=3.269K), tr. May (1968: 205).

37 It is evident that this is meant to be distinct from other digestive stages from the fact that, as mentioned earlier, the loss of this stage compromises a body's ability to be nourished in the way that the loss of another part of the digestive system (e.g., the stomach) does not.

38 The activity of the liver is parallel to the activities of the other two central organs, which elaborate the vital pneuma and the psychic pneuma. These processes will be discussed in Chapter 3.

39 *UP* 4.4 (1.198–9, 19–24 Helmreich=3.271–2K). These are the yellow and the black bile, respectively. The latter is an especially mysterious substance, and Galen does not theorise it in a consistent way; see Stewart (2018).

gallbladder, spleen and so on, the former is expelled from the body as urine and the latter as excrement.

Once the two non-useful residues are separated, and thus the blood is completely concocted by the innate heat, the bright red useful blood is sent out by the liver via the veins.[40] The supply of blood plays a crucial part in the healthy maintenance of the animal body because it is the key material component for the growth and regeneration of bodily tissues. In this way, nutrition and growth are effectively two aspects of the same function.[41] The liver, as the refiner and the distributor of blood via its offshoots (veins), stands at the centre of this process. Owing to the fact that it reaches the whole body by means of the veins, it is able to connect all the body parts via a single nutrition system and thus establish the means for an organism as a whole to grow and be nourished.

2.3 Natural or Innate Capacities

The anatomical account discussed up to this point is fairly straightforward. But understanding the processes of nutrition properly requires an account of how the liver is able to carry out its activities. In order to produce such an account, Galen has to dabble in a bit of *phusiologia*,[42] because the issue at stake is theoretical: it is a matter of the mechanism by means of which the liver distributes the blood. We know that it has its own motion that enables it to send the blood out, but what causes this motion?

In his time, Galen had a choice between two competing theories, each with very different implications for the understanding of human nature. The first is derived from the mechanistic model of physiology, advocated by the followers of Erasistratus and Asclepiades of Bithynia.[43] Second, the 'Hippocratic' model positing natural capacities could be called a vitalist alternative.[44] *On the Natural Capacities* presents an extensive rejection of the first option and support for the latter. All the arguments concerning

40 *UP* 4.4–5 (1.199, 9–22 Helmreich=3.272K).

41 The fact that natural growth also presupposes nutrition – so that expanding tissue does not merely distend but genuinely increase in size – is an important point in Galen's polemics against mechanistic theorists in *Nat. Fac.* 1.7. He uses the example of a children's game involving an animal's bladder to illustrate his point; see *Nat. Fac.* 1.7 (113, 9–19 Helmreich=2.17–18K). This passage is discussed further in Section 5.2.1.

42 For 'physiology' and *phusiologia*, see the discussion in the Introduction.

43 Although Galen generally focuses on the mechanistic aspect of the Erasistratean thought, the latter in fact combined both mechanistic and teleological explanations, as argued by von Staden (1997b).

44 In the sense that organic entities are governed by fundamentally different principles than the non-organic ones; in this case, those principles are natural capacities.

specific organs share the same key point in common: their activities are a result of their innate capacities.[45] These capacities are inherent in the homoeomerous tissues and are determined by the mixture of the four qualities: hot, cold, dry and wet.[46]

This point is crucial not only for the argument in this treatise but also for Galenic physiology in general: all the tissues in the animal body are endowed with innate capacities enabling them to perform certain actions without any external impetus. *On the Natural Capacities* outlines how the four natural capacities – attractive, alterative, retentive and expulsive – account for the processes in various organs, granting them a certain degree of functional sufficiency. As the four-fold division of parts discussed in Chapter 1 states, some parts are governing parts (ἀρχαί), others are capable of self-management (διοίκησις), while yet others are both self-managed and governed by the principles. Whatever degree of self-management a part might have, it must be owing to its innate capacities. These capacities allow the tissues to draw nutriment to themselves, assimilate it by altering its properties to those of their own while retaining it,[47] and to expel any matter that they can no longer process.

This account is a rival to mechanistic accounts. Much of *On the Natural Capacities* is dedicated to refuting Erasistratus' use of the *horror vacui* principle to explain all the processes pertaining to digestion and certain other physiological processes.[48] However, it is important to note that, at the end of the treatise, he clarifies that mechanistic explanations are not impossible, only inappropriate to certain cases. He explains at length the differences between mechanical attraction and capacity-based attraction, ascribing the former to cavities and the latter to tissues; he also notes various differences among them.[49] The point about the contrast is fairly apt: as far as he is concerned, the capacity-centred explanation is the proper one even when a phenomenon resembling *horror vacui* takes place, because such a phenomenon is also fundamentally explainable in terms of

45 *Nat. Fac.* 2.3 (159, 6–10 Helmreich =2.80K): εἰ μὴ γὰρ δύναμίς τις σύμφυτος ἑκάστῳ τῶν ὀργάνων ὑπὸ τῆς φύσεως εὐθὺς ἐξ ἀρχῆς δοθείη, διαρκεῖν οὐ δυνήσεται τὰ ζῷα, μὴ ὅτι τοσοῦτον ἀριθμὸν ἐτῶν ἀλλ' οὐδ' ἡμερῶν ὀλιγίστων. The use of the term τό ὄργανον indicates that the issue at stake is the complete activity of the parts (see Section 1.1.4.). See also *Nat. Fac.* 3.1 (204 Helmreich=2.143K); 3.9 (230 Helmreich=2.178K) and 3.12 (233 Helmreich=2.182K).

46 *Nat. Fac.* 1.3 (106, 4–6 Helmreich=2.7K).

47 As explained in the aforementioned passage *Nat. Fac.* 1.10 (115, 12–116, 17H=2.20–21K).

48 See, for example, *Nat. Fac.* 1.16 (145–150 Helmreich=1.60–67K). The attack against Erasistratus' explanatory model is developed through Book 2 and in parts of Book 3 as well. See also Vallance (1990: 63–78). For more on *horror vacui*, see Berryman (1997).

49 *Nat. Fac.* 3.15 (251–5 Helmreich=1.206–14K).

capacities. Although Galen's own understanding of physiology and human nature does not eschew the mechanistic explanation entirely, he takes them to be subordinate to the capacity-based explanations[50] that rely on the innate ability of tissues to manage themselves via four natural capacities.

It is the drawing of what is appropriate that initiates the process of nutrition. The following account in *On the Causes of Symptoms* provides a fairly detailed description of how it takes place:

> [ἡ φύσις] ἔδωκε δὲ καὶ τῆς ἐνδείας αἴσθησιν, ἵν' ἐξορμῶντα τὰ ζῷα πρός τε τὴν ἐδωδήν τε καὶ πόσιν ἐνὶ χρόνῳ πληρῶνται. καὶ καλεῖται μὲν ἡ τῆς τοιαύτης πληρώσεως ἔφεσις ὄρεξις, γίνεται δ' ἐπ' αἰσθήσει τῆς ἐνδείας, ὅταν αἱ μὲν φλέβες ἐξ αὐτῆς τι τῆς γαστρὸς ἕλκωσιν οἷον βδάλλουσαί τε καὶ μυζῶσαι, μὴ φέρουσα δὲ τὴν μύζησιν ἡ γαστὴρ, ἀλλ' οἷον διασπωμένη, τῆς ἀνίας ταύτης ἴαμα τὴν ἐδωδὴν πορίζηται. τρέπονται γὰρ αἱ φλέβες οὕτως ἐπὶ τὰ παρακείμενα σιτία, κἀξ αὐτῶν ἕλκουσι τὴν τροφὴν, οὐκ ἐκ τῆς γαστρὸς, καὶ συμβαίνει μετὰ τὴν προσφορὰν ἅμα τε τὰς φλέβας ἐπὶ τὰ σιτία τρέπεσθαι καὶ τὴν κοιλίαν εἰς ἑαυτὴν ἕλκειν ἐξ αὐτῶν ὅσον κεκένωται πρότερον ὑπὸ τῶν φλεβῶν. ἡ μὲν οὖν τῆς μυζήσεως αἴσθησίς ἐστιν ἡ πεῖνα· δύο δὲ ἄλλα, τὸ μὲν τοῦ βδάλλειν τὰς φλέβας ἡγεῖται, καὶ καλεῖται καὶ τοῦτο ὄρεξις ὁμωνύμως θατέρῳ, φυσικὸν ἔργον ὑπάρχον, οὐ ψυχικόν· αὐτῆς δὲ τῆς τοιαύτης ὀρέξεως ἡ κένωσις προηγεῖται καὶ γίγνεται πέντε συμπτώματα τὰ σύμπαντα κατὰ στίχον ἐφεξῆς ἀλλήλων τεταγμένα· κένωσις μὲν πρώτη, δευτέρα δὲ ὄρεξις ἡ φυσικὴ τῶν κενωθέντων μορίων, εἶτα ἡ μύζησις τῆς κοιλίας, εἶτα ἡ ταύτης αἴσθησις, εἶτα ἡ ὄρεξις αὐτῆς ἡ ψυχικὴ ἁπασῶν ὑστάτη.

> And it [nature] has given a perception of lack so that animals are stimulated to fill themselves with food and drink at one time. And the desire for such filling is called appetite, but it arises from the perception of lack whenever the veins draw from the stomach itself, as if to milk or suck, although the stomach does not bear the sucking, but is, as it were, 'distracted', providing itself with food as a remedy for this distress. In this way, the veins turn to the foods at hand and draw nourishment from them, not from the stomach. And after the taking of food what happens is that, at the same time, the veins turn themselves to the food and the stomach draws to itself from them as much as had previously been emptied by the veins. Hunger, then, is the perception of the sucking, whereas with regard to the other two, one leads in the milking of the veins, and this is also called appetite, having the same name as the other and is a physical action, not a psychical one. An emptying precedes such an appetite so there are altogether five symptoms arranged in order following one another. First there is the emptying; second is the physical appetite of the emptied parts; next is the sucking of the stomach; next is the sensation of this; last of all there is the psychical appetite of this.[51]

[50] See the discussion in Adamson (2014: 203–4).

[51] *Symp. Caus.* 1.7.3 (7.129–31K), tr. Johnston (2006: 227).

The main purpose of this passage is to provide an account of hunger, and it proves to be a fascinating insight into how the physical (produced by nature, φύσις) and psychic (produced by the soul, ψυχή) activities, governed by two distinct principal parts (the liver and the brain, respectively), are integrated. Their activities take place not contemporaneously: the psychic sensation follows physical appetite. For the sake of clarity, the current discussion is only preoccupied with the first part of the phenomenon, governed by the liver and consisting in the first three stages (as Galen lays them out in the final sentence of the passage). The psychic aspect of this phenomenon, that is, the question of how the αἴσθησις of the lack of nutriment is produced, will be discussed in Chapter 4, together with a broader discussion of the activities governed by the brain.

Hunger begins with a lack of nourishment, which produces what Galen calls a physical appetite (ὄρεξις ἡ φυσική). This appetite leads to the drawing from the veins, which in turn starts drawing from the stomach. At this point, the physical part of the hunger phenomenon ends. The language of 'milking' and 'drawing' suggests that the physical appetite is just a matter of tissues exercising the attractive capacity, and in fact, Galen typically describes vegetative capacities as the ability to attract what benefits and reject what harms.[52] One of the clearest formulations of the scope of such actions can be found in *On My Own Opinions*, and this passage also contains an enlightening elaboration of how he understands the distinction between the physical and the psychic.[53]

Animals, argues Galen, are capable of perceiving their environment owing to sense perception, while plants have perception only in a restricted sense. It seems impossible, he continues, that plants are able to attract what is appropriate and reject what is inappropriate without first recognising these two kinds. Therefore, this recognition (γνωρίζειν) must be some kind of a capacity. Then Galen explains that people misunderstand Plato's description of the nature of this capacity,[54] even though he makes it clear that plants have a different kind of perception (ἕτερον εἶναι γένος

[52] It is also important that these capacities are found throughout the body, in every part that is to be nourished, including, for example, the controversial spleen (*Nat. Fac.* 3.9 (229, 3–6 Helmreich=2.177–8K)).

[53] The distinction of capacities is certainly not invented by Galen; see Debru (2008: 266–7).

[54] There are two different ways of translating this part of the text. Boudon-Millot and Pietrobelli (2005: 212), and Nutton (1999: 123) read Galen as suggesting that Plato did not ascribe to plants γνωριστικὴν δύναμιν, while Wilberding (2014: n79) argues, on the basis of *Plat. Tim.* 11.15–16 Schröder, that Galen suggests that people misunderstand the kind of perceptive capacity plants have.

αἰσθήσεως ἐν τοῖς φυτοῖς).[55] The difference between cognitive capacities and vegetative perception is explained in the following sentence, where Galen notes that vegetative perception consists in the ability to perceive *only* these two impressions, accompanied by pleasure and pain. Plants are unable to perceive their environments in any other way, by contrast with the sensory-perceptual capacities of animals.[56]

Presumably, the key difference is that all the plants and animal parts that belong to the vegetative domain cannot *grasp* any object they come into contact with; their sensory capabilities are unlike sense perception, which is able to perceive various properties of the object. The vegetative soul, in other words, cannot sense what an object is *like* when it comes into contact with it. It can only register whether this object is beneficial or harmful and accept it or reject it accordingly. Although Galen does not say it explicitly, it seems reasonable to assume that the vegetative soul cannot perceive something as harmful and still accept it.[57] Therefore, its 'perception' is just a reaction; the kind of diagnostics the vegetative soul is able to perform consists in simply triggering one of the two possible reactions available to it: acceptance or rejection. This reading explains Galen's refusal to attribute sense perception to the vegetative soul. As far as Galen is concerned, it only 'perceives' a very small range of properties it comes into contact with. It does not have the capacity to distinguish between, for example, an apple and a piece of paper as such, although it could distinguish between (or, to put it otherwise, react differently to) 'nutriment' and 'non-nutriment'. When blood is delivered via veins to, for example, a muscle, it 'senses' beneficial material and accepts it.[58]

55 See Plato *Ti.* 77A. See also Das (2020: 57) and Wilberding (2014: 252–4).

56 *Prop. Plac.* 15.7 (142 Lami Garofalo). See also *MM* 7.6 (10.473K) where Galen describes the treatment by baths with an explanation that the nature extends to the pleasant and withdraws from what is not. See also the discussion in note 58.

57 Although such a scenario is conceivable if a body is in a diseased state. However, these are by definition abnormal conditions, in which capacities are not working the way they are supposed to. This reinforces the conclusion that, strictly speaking, natural capacities are not able to behave in such a way.

58 My reading of this passage is in agreement with Wilberding's (2014: 264) interpretation of these capacities as, effectively, a binary reaction. This interpretation has been criticised by Das (2020) on the grounds of making the attractive capacity in both animate and inanimate objects the same (this possibility is discussed in Wilberding (2014: 266), arguing that the difference lies in animate objects attracting and assimilating the material completely). Das proposes that sympathetic reaction, rather than the 'deterministic' model of alteration, underpins the 'choice' plants make, and this model is, broadly speaking, borrowed from the Stoic *oikeiōsis*. This criticism is not entirely compelling, as the four-quality theory is a much more fine-grained explanation than both the sympathetic reaction and

The fact that innate capacities exist in all the tissues of the body presents a conundrum when it comes to the liver, the *hēgemon* of the entire process of nutrition. The tissues of the liver either have the very same kind of natural capacities as all the other tissues or they have a special type. If it is the former, it does not have any capacities that would motivate its status as the *hēgemon*. In that case, the liver does not have the means to exercise any kind of power over the other parts. Alternatively, the liver, as the overseer of this whole process, might be endowed with some extra capacities, but nothing in its anatomy or activities suggests this. In fact, in *On My Own Opinions*, Galen explicitly describes the functioning of the vegetative soul in terms of natural capacities.[59] At the same time, the liver is also the seat of the vegetative soul. Galen uses the term 'soul' for what is present in the liver exclusively. This suggests that the difference between the activities of the liver and the natural capacities in other parts could be explained in a way that manoeuvres between the two options.

A further discussion of the special status of the liver can be found in a passage in *On My Own Opinions*, in the context of discussing the changes that take place either via one or two qualities or via entire substance acting. Having discussed the examples of these changes in drugs, Galen turns to natural processes, stating that they also occur either through just one or two qualities or through the whole substance acting. The examples of the latter are digestion and blood making in the liver, as well as nutrition and

the *oikeiōsis* style of perception in plants; therefore, in order to understand the details of these processes, we would have to return to the four-quality theory. At the same time, it is certainly true that Galen recognises a robust distinction between the animate and the inanimate. The disagreement between Wilberding's and Das readings hangs on both of them positing this threshold with the attractive capacity, so that what identifies something as animate or not is dependent on how its attractive capacity functions (to be precise, in Wilberding's reading it also depends on post-attraction assimilation). However, it would also be possible to argue on the grounds of *Nat. Fac.* 1.14 that the distinguishing feature of animate objects is the capacity of alteration, and the attractive capacity is subordinate to it. Having praised Epicurus for at least recognising the existence of attractive capacity in a lodestone (although getting the physics hopelessly wrong), Galen calls nature a craftsman and explains that the substance of things tends towards unity and alteration, because parts act and are acted upon by one another; then he adds that, with this assumption, 'it would not have been difficult to allow that this constructive nature has powers which attract appropriate and expel alien matter' (1.14 (134, 21–3 Helmreich=2.46K), tr. Brock (1916: 73)). I will argue later in this work that this Aristotle-derived view is crucial for Galen's understanding of vitality. For the current purposes, it is enough to note that even if the attractive capacity were the same in both animate and inanimate objects (and this section of *On the Natural Capacities* does not make it clear enough that it is, because Galen only explains how attraction takes place in living bodies, not in inanimate ones), this would not indicate that there is no distinction between plants and inanimate bodies, because, crucially, plants are capable of the innate change via alteration.

[59] *Prop. Plac.* 13.1 (120 Lami Garofalo).

growth. The latter take place in all the parts of the animal. Each part, Galen argues, functions in accordance with its natural capacities, and he reiterates that these are common to animals and plants, attracting what benefits and rejecting what harms. But to maintain a normal state, all the body parts are reliant on the liver for nutriment and recovery. He then contrasts these capacities with the capacities coming from the brain. The latter is constantly coming and going. Similarly, the capacity coming from the heart also does not remain in the other parts, but 'the capacities called natural remain innate in the substances of body parts'.[60]

The liver is unlike the other two governing parts of the body, because its activity is constant; it is constantly supplying the body with nutriment, unlike the heart and the brain whose capacities are not always activated. In this respect, the liver has much in common with ordinary tissues, but Galen nevertheless calls it the 'source' of the capacities. It must, therefore, have governing ability just like the brain and the heart, which distinguishes it from the ordinary parts, even if its activities are slower and steadier.[61] At the end of the passage, Galen goes on to reiterate that, according to him, the organisation of the body is maintained by the three principles, further showing that, for all their differences, the three seats of the souls have more in common with each other than with other parts. But what renders the capacities of the liver to be governing capacities, if, in many ways, they act like the capacities of any ordinary tissues?

The liver must be the overseer of all the vegetative capacities by virtue of constantly providing all the body with nutriment, which it does by sending out blood via veins. Such a reading solves the conundrum regarding the nature of the liver's governing power. All organs attract what is beneficial and reject what is harmful to them via their capacities, but only the liver reacts in this way to the body *as a whole*. The significance of this point becomes apparent if we consider the four-fold division of all the body parts discussed in Chapter 1, consisting of principles, their offshoots, self-managing parts (tissues), and the parts with their own capacities governed by principles via their offshoots, followed by the acknowledgement of the parts that have no governance, only genesis. The examples of the latter are hair and nails. The latter parts can be used as a foil for understanding the significance of the interconnectedness of the other parts. They must be in

60 *Prop. Plac.* 10.3 (102 Lami Garofalo):, τὰς δὲ φυσικὰς ὀνομαζομένας δυνάμεις ἐμφύτους μένειν ἐν ταῖς οὐσίαις τῶν μορίων.

61 These properties make them harder to be perceived as well; this point is very much in line with the opening of Book 6 of *PHP* discussed earlier.

possession of some natural capacities because they grow, but their growth is not connected to any other part and they do not participate in any of the processes together with the other parts. If all body parts were like that, there would hardly be a body, only an assembly of distinct entities. For a body to hold together, different parts need to be connected and 'governed' together by a central principal part. There is no unity among varied parts if there is no governance. Therefore, the governing parts play a key role in unifying the body, and the way that Galen divides the body into parts indicates how they are to be put together, so to speak.

It is important to note that nothing in Galen's texts suggests that the natural capacities of the liver are different in nature from the natural capacities of the other organs. The former operate on a larger scale than the latter, and, thus, they end up being more significant in scale, not by nature. Furthermore, this hierarchy can be seen in anatomy (the way that Galen understands human anatomy): the liver has a connection to the other organs via veins, which enables its managing role too. Since the vegetative soul does not have perception in the sense of cognition, it reacts via its own natural capacities to the natural capacities of the other organs. The liver can therefore be said to have second-order vegetative capacities, and it is by virtue of these that it can be called the seat of the soul and be categorised together with the seats of the spirited and the rational souls.

2.4 Two Theories of Embryonic Growth

The account of nutrition also serves as the introduction to the account of growth, as Galen takes these two activities to be closely connected: by attracting and assimilating nutriment, the body is not only nourished but also grows. As noted at the beginning of this chapter, Aristotle connects nourishment with reproduction: it is, after all, in the embryonic stages when animals grow most dramatically; in adults, growth occurs due to an increase of mass or owing to a healing injury. In some passages, Galen explains that the construction of an embryo, on the one hand, and the construction of tissues in wound healing, on the other, are to all intents and purposes the same process:

> Ὡς γάρ, εἰ καὶ κατ᾽ ἀρχὰς εὐθὺς οἷόν τ᾽ ἦν ἡμῖν γεννῆσαι ζῷον, οὐκ ἄλλῳ μὲν [οὖν] ἄν τινι λόγῳ τὴν γένεσιν αὐτοῦ τὴν πρώτην, ἄλλῳ δ᾽ ἂν ἐποιούμεθα τὴν ἐπανόρθωσιν, οὕτως, ἐπεὶ μηδέτερον τούτων αὐτοὶ πρώτως ποιοῦμεν, ἀλλ᾽ ἡ φύσις ἐστὶν ἡ καὶ δημιουργοῦσα πρώτη τὸ ζῷον καὶ νῦν ἰωμένη νοσοῦν, οὐκ ἄλλῳ μὲν τρόπῳ σάρκα πρότερον ἐδημιούργησεν, ἄλλῳ δὲ νῦν, οὐδ᾽ ἄλλῳ μὲν τρόπῳ τὴν τροφὴν ἐπὶ τῶν

> κυουμένων, ἄλλῳ δὲ νῦν ἐπισπᾶται, ἀλλὰ καὶ ταῦθ' ὁμοίως ἐργάζεται καὶ τρέφει καὶ διακρίνει καὶ ἀποκρίνει καὶ πάνθ' ἁπλῶς εἰπεῖν ὡσαύτως ἐργάζεται νῦν τε καὶ τότε.
>
> Thus, if we had the capacity to create an animal in the first place, the principles involved in that initial creation would be no different from those involved in its restoration. In reality, though, we are not primarily responsible for either of these tasks: it is Nature who first constructs the animal and subsequently heals it if it is sick. And so its method in that original construction of flesh is no different from its subsequent method; nor is its method for the absorption of nutrition in the foetus different from its subsequent method; this function, along with nutrition in general, the separation and excretion of substances – all the functions, in short – are performed in the same way now as in that initial creation.[62]

The tissues of an embryo grow in the same way as the tissues of an adult do: by attracting what is beneficial and rejecting what is not beneficial. However, the question of whether these capacities are fully sufficient for the conception of an embryo is a different matter. Explaining embryonic growth by means of the same process as the one that occurs in tissue restoration is economical, but it only works for accounting for the increase of the mass. The material for growth can be provided by the paternal seed, but what renders its arrangement?

Thus, for Galen, the attempts to conceptualise embryonic growth come with a set of distinct challenges. They are outlined in Book 1 of *On the Natural Capacities*, in the context of discussing the work of the alterative capacity in particular. Galen assigns a role to this capacity in the generation of the embryo, marking out a distinction between its manifestations in an embryo and a fully formed animal. In the former case, the capacity enables the coming-to-be of something new, whereas, in the latter case, the material is changed into something that already exists.[63] The process of embryonic formation is not entirely accounted for by means of the alterative capacity for the following reason:

> ἀλλ' ἡ μὲν γένεσις οὐχ ἁπλῆ τις ἐνέργεια τῆς φύσεως, ἀλλ' ἐξ ἀλλοιώσεώς τε καὶ διαπλάσεώς ἐστι σύνθετος. ἵνα μὲν γὰρ ὀστοῦν γένηται καὶ νεῦρον καὶ

[62] *Thras.* 26 (66, 18–67, 4 Helmreich=5.853K), tr. Singer (1997: 75–6).

[63] *Nat. Fac.* 1.8 (114, 8–15 Helmreich=2.19K), tr. Brock (1916: 31, slightly altered: 'For, when the matter which flows to each part of the body in the form of nutriment is being worked up into it, this activity is nutrition, and its cause is the nutritive capacity. Of course, the kind of activity here involved is also an alteration, but not an alteration like that occurring at the stage of genesis. For in the latter case something comes into existence which did not exist previously, while in nutrition the in-flowing material becomes assimilated to that which has already come into existence.'

φλὲψ καὶ τῶν ἄλλων ἕκαστον, ἀλλοιοῦσθαι χρὴ τὴν ὑποβεβλημένην οὐσίαν, ἐξ ἧς γίγνεται τὸ ζῷον· ἵνα δὲ καὶ σχῆμα τὸ δέον καὶ θέσιν καὶ κοιλότητάς τινας καὶ ἀποφύσεις καὶ συμφύσεις καὶ τἄλλα τὰ τοιαῦτα κτήσηται, διαπλάττεσθαι χρὴ τὴν ἀλλοιουμένην οὐσίαν.

Genesis, however, is not a simple activity of Nature, but is compounded of alteration and of shaping. That is to say, in order that bone, nerve, veins and all other [tissues] may come into existence, the underlying substance from which the animal springs must be altered; and in order that the substance so altered may acquire its appropriate shape and position, its cavities, outgrowths, attachments, and so forth, it has to undergo a *shaping* or *formative* process.[64]

Genesis involves not only alteration but also another capacity, namely the shaping one. This complicates the picture, since it becomes harder to determine whether the special alteration taking place in the embryo differs principally from nutritive alteration or whether it is different owing to the presence of the shaping capacity. The previous passage appears to suggest that two processes take place: alteration produces new tissues and the shaping capacity structures them. Galen comes back to the topic in the following book, in which he attacks Erasistratus for not recognising the importance of capacities in embryology, and explains the disparate activities of the alterative and shaping capacities as follows:

πῶς οὖν Ἐρασίστρατος αὐτὴν οὐκ οἶδεν, εἰ δὴ πρώτη μὲν αὕτη τοῦ σπέρματος ἐνέργεια τὸ σύμμετρον αἵματος ἐπισπᾶσθαι πρὸς ἑαυτό; σύμμετρον δ' ἂν εἴη τὸ λεπτὸν οὕτω καὶ ἀτμῶδες, ὥστ' εὐθὺς εἰς πᾶν μόριον ἑλκόμενον τοῦ σπέρματος δροσοειδῶς μηδαμοῦ τὴν ἑαυτοῦ παρεμφαίνειν ἰδέαν. οὕτω γὰρ αὐτοῦ καὶ κρατήσει ῥᾳδίως τὸ σπέρμα καὶ ταχέως ἐξομοιώσει καὶ τροφὴν ἑαυτῷ ποιήσεται κἄπειτ' οἶμαι δεύτερον ἐπισπάσεται καὶ τρίτον, ὡς ὄγκον ἑαυτῷ καὶ πλῆθος ἀξιόλογον ἐργάσασθαι τραφέντι. καὶ μὴν ἤδη καὶ ἡ ἀλλοιωτικὴ δύναμις ἐξεύρηται μηδ' αὐτὴ πρὸς Ἐρασιστράτου γεγραμμένη. τρίτη δ' ἂν ἡ διαπλαστικὴ φανείη, καθ' ἣν πρῶτον μὲν οἷον ἐπίπαγόν τινα λεπτὸν ὑμένα περιτίθησιν ἑαυτῷ τὸ σπέρμα.

How, then, was Erasistratus unaware of it, if the primary activity of the seed be to draw to itself a due proportion of blood? Now, this fluid would be in due proportion if it were so thin and vaporous, that, as soon as it was drawn like dew into every part of the seed, it would everywhere cease to display its own particular character; for so the seed will easily dominate and quickly assimilate

64 *Nat. Fac.* 1.5 (108, 7–15 Helmreich=2.10–11K), tr. Brock (1916: 19). The definition of genesis as involving both alteration and shaping (i.e., work done by the shaping capacity) is consistent in the treatise, for example, slightly later at *Nat. Fac.* 1.6 (108, 20–22 Helmreich=2.11K).

> it – in fact, will use it as food. It will then, I imagine, draw to itself a second and a third quantum, and thus by feeding it acquires for itself considerable bulk and quantity. In fact, the alterative capacity has now been discovered as well, although about this also Erasistratus has not written a word. And, thirdly the shaping capacity will become evident, by virtue of which the seed firstly surrounds itself with a thin membrane like a kind of superficial condensation.[65]

Notably, the alterative capacity essentially performs the same work here as in nutrition: it allows for the proliferation of matter. The shaping capacity, meanwhile, forms tissues. Although this act is only briefly described, it is worth unpacking Galen's claim here. The generation of the membrane around the seed is not a mere act of structuring pre-existing, already shaped organs. Separating a portion of matter to create layers in the embryonic tissue also allows its outermost structure to undergo a further, special alteration through which it becomes a membrane. This act, notably, amounts to design, neither explained nor *explicable* by means of qualitative alteration. In *On Seed*, Galen describes the same process:

> ἐν γὰρ τῇ πρὸς τὸ θῆλυ σπέρμα μίξει πολλαὶ τῶν πομφολύγων ἐῤῥάγησαν, ἐξ ὧν εἴσω τε καὶ πρὸς τὸ βάθος ἐχώρει τὸ πνεῦμα σώζειν ἑαυτὸ γλιχόμενον– οὐ γὰρ οἷόν περ ἀτμὸς ἦν, ἀλλ᾽ αὐτοκίνητος ἀρχὴ ζώου–, καθάπερ καὶ [αὐτὸ] τὸ περιέχον ὑγρὸν αὐτὸ κοιλίαν εἰργάσατο τῷ σπέρματι μεστὴν πνεύματος. ὅπως οὖν μηδ᾽ ἐντεῦθεν ἑτοίμως κενοῖτο, στεγανὸν ἑαυτῷ τὸν οἶκον ἐργάζεται τῆς περιειληφυίας αὐτὸ τοῦ σπέρματος ὑγρᾶς οὐσίας, ὅσον ἦν παχύτερόν τε καὶ σκληρότερον, ἀπωθούμενον εἰς τὴν ἐκτὸς περιγραφήν, ὅπερ ἔμελλεν ἐν τῷ χρόνῳ θερμαινόμενόν τε καὶ ξηραινόμενον ὀστοῦν ἔσεσθαι.
>
> For in the mixing with the female seed many of the bubbles burst, and the pneuma from them passed inside and deep down, in the desire to preserve itself – it was not a kind of vapor but was a self-moving source of the animal –; and likewise the surrounding fluid of its own accord formed within the seed a cavity filled with pneuma. Then to prevent its being readily emptied out, (the pneuma) makes for itself a tightly sealed chamber, pushing back to the outer circumference all that was thicker and harder in the seed's moist substance surrounding it; and this, when heated and dried, would in time be bone.[66]

The creation of the membrane leads to the creation of bone tissue by means of drying out and hardening. Through these processes, different organs are generated. While drying and hardening are qualitative alterations, the very act of pushing thicker material outwards is not. Galen

[65] *Nat. Fac.* 2.3 (163, 5–18 Helmreich=2.85–6K), tr. Brock (1916: 135, slightly altered).
[66] *Sem.* 1.8.5–7 de Lacy (4.540K), tr. de Lacy (1992: 91–3, slightly altered).

does not explain this process as arising from the interaction between qualities. Arguably, it would not be consistent with his elemental theory, since, on that account, only thin substances spread outwardly.[67] Furthermore, this passage contains certain teleological terminology: the membrane is generated so that the pneuma does not eviscerate. This implies rational thought, which indicates that, as Galen elsewhere claims, the seed contains the scheme of the Craftsman, although it is not clear in what manner.[68] The work of the alterative and shaping capacities, therefore, are consistently reported as being different. Furthermore, the presence of the shaping capacity at the time of embryonic formation is of critical importance. The alterative capacity simply cannot do the kind of work required there. More precisely, the alterative capacity is capable neither of rationalisation, nor, as a result, design.

In some passages, however, Galen describes the vegetative soul as a demiurge, a term that has strong connotations of creative capacity.[69] Does it mean that we ought to assign the fifth natural capacity to the vegetative soul, the shaping one, which is hardly ever mentioned together with the standard four? In order to settle this question, it is necessary to investigate more closely how Galen uses the term 'demiurge', including the scope and range of a demiurgic activity.

2.5 Galenic Demiurge(s)

There are a few references to the vegetative soul as a 'demiurge' in Galen. For instance, in *On Seed* he ascribes the same demiurge, the vegetative soul, to both an animal embryo and a growing plant.[70] In the late treatise *On the Formation of the Embryo*, he reaches *aporia* in regard to the question of who or what forms embryos.[71] Although seemingly inconsistent, these two claims could be using the term in different senses. Galen is well known for doing this when it comes to the term 'substance',[72] and he even alludes to the multiple meanings of a 'demiurge' in the treatise *On Seed*. Here, he discusses the question of why complete restoration of tissues is not

[67] *MM* 12.5 (10.843K).

[68] See, respectively, *Foet. Form.* 5, 11 Nickel (4.682K) and 6, 31 Nickel (4.700K) for both claims.

[69] For a major study of this notion and its use in a variety of texts, see O'Brien (2015); see also Vinkesteijn (2022) for an outline of some of the problems concerning the understanding of the creative capacities.

[70] *Sem.* 1.9.17 de Lacy (4.546K).

[71] In *Form. Foet.* 6, 31 Nickel (4.700K), he uses that exact term.

[72] For example, in *Sem.* 2.2.7 de Lacy (4.611K).

possible, even if all the materials necessary for such a restoration are, in theory, present. He explains this as follows:

> κατὰ δὲ τὴν πρώτην ἐκ τοῦ σπέρματος γένεσιν ἀθρόον μὲν ἔτι τὸ ὑγρόν, ἐξ οὗ τῶν ἀγγείων ἡ διάπλασις, ὁ δημιουργὸς δ᾽ αὐτοῦ διττός, ἥ τ᾽ ἐν αὐτῷ τῷ σπέρματι δύναμις ἥ τ᾽ ἐν τοῖς τῆς μήτρας ἀγγείοις, οἷς προσέπεσεν. ἐπὶ μὲν γὰρ τῶν ἑλκωμάτων ἀπορίᾳ δαψιλοῦς ὕλης ἀργὸς ἦν ἡμῖν ὁ τοσοῦτος δημιουργός· ἐπὶ δὲ τῆς ἐν τῇ μήτρᾳ τοῦ ζώου γενέσεως ἥ τε ὕλη δαψιλής, καὶ σύνεστιν αὐτῷ δημιουργὸς ἕτερος, οὐ ψαύων μόνον τῆς ὕλης, ἀλλὰ καὶ δι᾽ ὅλης αὐτῆς διαπεφοιτηκώς.
>
> But at the initial generation from semen the fluid out of which the vessels were fashioned was still in a mass, and its craftsman was two-fold: the power in the semen itself and the power in the vessels of the uterus on which (the semen) fell. In the wounded, for want of abundant material, the craftsman of this (latter) kind was useless to us; but in the generation of the animal in the uterus the material is abundant, and along with that craftsman there is another, not merely touching the material but permeating it through and through.[73]

Galen argues that some tissues cannot be completely regenerated due to the lack of material. For the current purposes, the more interesting aspect of this passage is the way in which demiurges involved in the formation of an embryo are presented. First, there is the seed and uterine blood vessels. In the final sentence, he also mentions the craftsman permeating 'through and through'. This description is a reference to a designing creation, to be contrasted with mechanistic generation and such processes as distension or external manipulation of matter without substantial alterations.[74] Galen himself appears to distinguish this as a different type of demiurgic activity altogether. It also appears to play a special role in the formation of embryos; in order to understand the scope of the capacities of the vegetative soul, it is necessary to determine the extent of its demiurgic role.

The designer that permeates through and through hails from the early Stoicism,[75] but Galen is surely more directly influenced by his contemporary Middle Platonist adoption of this concept. The Middle Platonists argued that the Hellenistic innovations were ideas already present in Plato's dialogues to a diligent reader.[76] Some support for such a stance

[73] *Sem.* 1.13.16–18 de Lacy (4.560–1K), tr. de Lacy (1992: 113).

[74] The contrast is made especially clearly in *Nat. Fac.* 2.3 (160, 10–14 Helmreich=2.82K), although it is arguably a common background assumption whenever alteration is discussed in opposition to mechanical production, as in, for example, *Hipp. Elem.* 3.18 de Lacy (1.430–1K). See also Hankinson (2017b: 259–63).

[75] Aëtius 1.7.24 Mansfeld and Runia=*SVF* 2.1027=LS 46A.

[76] Bonazzi (2016: 179–82).

can be gained from the dialogues that were, in one way or another, influential to the Hellenistic school, for example, Plato's *Timaeus* and Stoicism.[77] In this dialogue, the term 'demiurge' is applied to the divine designer who imposes order and thus generates the world of becoming. Notably, this demiurge is a rational, provident power designing the world teleologically, viz. for the sake of making it good.[78] Given how important Plato's authority in general and the *Timaeus* in particular are to Galen,[79] it is not surprising that he would use the term 'demiurge' to refer to such a designer. *On the Usefulness of Parts* is especially abundant with design references, although the notion of a nature-demiurge designing with intent is remarkably consistent throughout the corpus, as pointed out by Jacques Jouanna.[80] Here, the designer is referred to as a 'demiurge' (usually 'our demiurge' or 'the demiurge of animals') in singular nominative alone thirty-seven times.[81] It is quite clear that the Platonist-inspired cosmic designer generating in a perfectly rational and providential manner is the underlying concept.[82] The key refrain in this treatise is 'because it is better so', which mimics the *Timaen* description of the work of the divine designer, except that Galen uses it in reference not so much to *kosmos* as a whole but to all the parts of human anatomy, from brains to buttocks.

Interestingly, on some occasions, he also describes the parts themselves as demiurges. For example, the thorax and a certain bone are called 'demiurge' in *On the Usefulness of Parts*. The thorax is said to be the demiurge of voice and respiration,[83] but it is quite clear that this body part could not possibly have a designing capacity. The motions of the thorax, which will be discussed in greater detail in Chapters 3 and 4, are controlled by the nervous system; all they amount to is simple rising and falling of the ribcage. Similarly, the muscle is also described as the demiurge of motion.[84] It is worth noting that, in the same work, Galen explains that muscle is just flesh with nerves weaved through it, and it is the nerve that is really the cause of the muscular motion, so both of these cases are

77 There is also a general consensus in the scholarship that this dialogue was a significant influence in Stoicism, see for example, Powers (2013), Reydams-Schils (1997), Scade (2010) and Sedley (2007: 206–10).

78 *Ti.* 29A–30B.

79 See Das (2020, chapter 1) for an argument that Galen uses the *Timaeus* for lending theoretical support to and legitimizing his medical project. See also de Lacy (1972: esp. 36–9).

80 Jouanna (2013: 292–3).

81 The second highest number of occurrences of singular nominative of 'demiurge' is four (in references to *technē*), in *Thrasyboulos*.

82 Schiefsky (2007: 393).

83 *UP* 4.7 (1.203, 14–16 Helmreich=3.277K).

84 *UP* 17.1 (2.437, 21 Helmreich=4.347K).

based on the same anatomical facts.[85] In order to understand this sense of the term 'demiurge', it is necessary to turn to another major influence to Galen, Aristotle.

As pointed out by Jouanna, Aristotle's texts, whose influence on Galen is substantial,[86] play a rather significant role in shaping Galen's conception of a demiurge as well.[87] 'Demiurge' shows up often in Aristotle's biological works. Here, a demiurgic act is generally associated with generation,[88] elemental constitution and innate heat.[89] With the exception of the passages in which Aristotle is talking about artisans, the verb signifying the demiurgic activity is very often used in reference to the term 'nature' (φύσις).[90] The Aristotelian concept of nature as a demiurge is rather different from the Platonic demiurge. As James Lennox argues 'though the verbs of agency are often metaphoric extensions from the craft domain, the nature referred to as agent is simply an animal's formal nature.'[91] He shows that Aristotle consistently distinguishes formal and material nature in his biological works, such as *Parts of Animals*, and theoretical ones, such as *Physics*.[92] The formal nature, the soul, is identical to the animal's substantial being that includes the motive cause and the final cause.[93] The claims in Aristotle's biology that seem to refer 'demiurgic' acts in the Platonic sense of the term are better read as referring to formal nature, which explains both common essential features and structuring and maintaining particular parts.[94]

Arguably, in order to understand in more fine-grained detail how natural change takes place within this broad account of formal nature, it is important to look at the notion of agent and patient, which is adopted broadly in Aristotle's biological works but explained most clearly in his

85 *UP* 1.18 (1.44, 22–24 Helmreich=3.61K). *UP* 7.14 (1.413, 7–10 Helmreich=3.568K).

86 See the discussion of Galen's multi-faceted engagement with the Peripatetic tradition in van der Eijk (2009). For a larger study arguing for the importance of the Aristotelian background for Galen, see Kovačić (2001). See also Falcon (2021: 247–50), Gottschalk (1987: 1166–71), Lloyd (1991, chapter 17), Moraux (1984) and Singer (2014: 20–38).

87 Jouanna (2013: 308–9), in reference to Galen's portrayal of Hippocrates as the ultimate source of the knowledge of nature.

88 Esp. embryonic generation, see *GA* 1.18 (722b1); 2.4 (738b21).

89 *GA* 3.4 (755a19); *MA* 7 (702a7).

90 *GA* 2.22 (730b31); 2.6 (743b23); *IA* 12 (711a18); *PA* 1.5 (645a9). See Broadie (1987: 35–50) for the point that Aristotle does not psychologise his teleological explanations. Galen also often ascribes the demiurgic activity to 'nature', especially in *On the Usefulness of Parts*.

91 Lennox (2001: 184).

92 Lennox (2001: 185) refers to *Physics* 2.2, presumably especially to the discussion 193a30–194b–15).

93 *PA* 1.1 (641a25–7).

94 Lennox (2001: 187–200); on p. 200, Lennox notes that the latter is goal-oriented efficient cause, acting '*selectively* and *in accordance with instructions* inherited from its parents' (emphasis original).

theoretical treatise, *Physics*. At the beginning of Book 2 of his *Physics*, Aristotle famously provides a clear conceptual account of the acts performed by nature as follows:

> Τῶν ὄντων τὰ μέν ἐστι φύσει, τὰ δὲ δι᾽ ἄλλας αἰτίας, φύσει μὲν τά τε ζῷα καὶ τὰ μέρη αὐτῶν καὶ τὰ φυτὰ καὶ τὰ ἁπλᾶ τῶν σωμάτων, οἷον γῆ καὶ πῦρ καὶ ἀὴρ καὶ ὕδωρ (ταῦτα γὰρ εἶναι καὶ τὰ τοιαῦτα φύσει φαμέν), πάντα δὲ ταῦτα φαίνεται διαφέροντα πρὸς τὰ μὴ φύσει συνεστῶτα. Τούτων μὲν γὰρ ἕκαστον ἐν ἑαυτῷ ἀρχὴν ἔχει κινήσεως καὶ στάσεως, τὰ μὲν κατὰ τόπον, τὰ δὲ κατ᾽ αὔξησιν καὶ φθίσιν, τὰ δὲ κατ᾽ ἀλλοίωσιν· κλίνη δὲ καὶ ἱμάτιον, καὶ εἴ τι τοιοῦτον ἄλλο γένος ἐστίν, ᾗ μὲν τετύχηκε τῆς κατηγορίας ἑκάστης καὶ καθ᾽ ὅσον ἐστὶν ἀπὸ τέχνης, οὐδεμίαν ὁρμὴν ἔχει μεταβολῆς ἔμφυτον.

> Of things that exist, some exist by nature, some from other causes. By nature the animal and their parts exist, and the plants and the simple bodies (earth, fire, air, water) – for we say that these and the like exist by nature. All the things mentioned plainly differ from things which are not constituted by nature. For each of them has within itself a principle of motion and of stationariness (in respect of place, or of growth or decrease, or by way of alteration). On the other hand, a bed and a coat and anything else of that sort, qua receiving these designations – i.e. in so far as they are products of art – have no innate impulse to change.[95]

In this passage, he contrasts the entities existing by nature and the entities existing by craft, such as beds and coats. The key difference between these two is that the principle of change is internal to the natural entities, whereas in artefacts, it is external. The distinction is fairly straightforward, but it has some complex consequences when the Aristotelian definition of change is taken into consideration. Change necessarily involves two entities: the agent that initiates the change and the patient that changes.[96] In the case of artefacts, it is easy to apply this model: the artisan is the agent, and the artefact is the patient. In the case of organic entities, however, when only one entity is changing, it is not immediately obvious how to assign such roles. In Book 8 of *Physics*, Aristotle addresses this problem and offers the following solution:

> εἴ τι κινεῖ αὐτὸ αὑτό, πῶς κινεῖ καὶ τίνα τρόπον. ἀναγκαῖον δὴ τὸ κινούμενον ἅπαν εἶναι διαιρετὸν εἰς ἀεὶ διαιρετά· τοῦτο γὰρ δέδεικται πρότερον ἐν τοῖς καθόλου τοῖς περὶ φύσεως, ὅτι πᾶν τὸ καθ᾽ αὑτὸ κινούμενον συνεχές. ἀδύνατον δὴ τὸ αὐτὸ αὑτὸ κινοῦν πάντῃ κινεῖν

95 *Ph.* 2.1 (192b9–18), tr. Hardie and Gaye (1984: 329), from Barnes (1984).

96 See Waterlow (1982: 159–64). The discussion at the beginning of Book 3 of *Physics* (*Ph.* 3.1–3) outlines the central model.

αὐτὸ αὑτό· φέροιτο γὰρ ἂν ὅλον καὶ φέροι τὴν αὐτὴν φοράν, ἓν ὂν καὶ ἄτομον τῷ εἴδει, καὶ ἀλλοιοῖτο καὶ ἀλλοιοῖ, ὥστε διδάσκοι ἂν καὶ μανθάνοι ἅμα, καὶ ὑγιάζοι καὶ ὑγιάζοιτο τὴν αὐτὴν ὑγίειαν . . . τὸ μὲν ἄρα κινεῖ τὸ δὲ κινεῖται τοῦ αὐτὸ αὑτὸ κινοῦντος.

If a thing moves itself, in what sense and in what manner does it do so? Now everything that is in motion must be infinitely divisible; for it has been shown already in our general course on *Physics*, that everything that is in motion in its own right in continuous. Now it is impossible that that which moves itself should in its entirely move itself; for then, while being specifically one and indivisible, it would as a whole both undergo and cause the same locomotion or alteration; thus it would at the same time be both teaching and being taught, or both restoring to and being restored to the same health . . . Therefore when a thing moves itself it is one part of it that is the mover and another part that is moved.[97]

In the case of change within an organic entity, there is still the agent and the patient, but they are different *parts* or sections of that entity. In other words, the principle governing change is exactly the same in organic entities and artefacts; the difference lies in the number of discrete substances involved. In the case of artefacts, the agent and the patient are two numerically distinct substances. In the case of an organic entity, there is only one substance, and its parts act as the agent and the patient of change.[98] It might seem counterintuitive to use the language of demiurgic activity in the latter case as well as in the former, but, as Sarah Waterlow noted, the agent of change in a single substance conceptually resembles an artisan, for it does not change *qua* agent, for example, heating in fire is not a change of fire,[99] so this analogy is conceptually coherent. A demiurge in this sense is a part that acts as the agent of change within an organic entity, that is ultimately circumscribed by formal nature.[100]

Animal generation presents some of the more vivid examples of Aristotle's uses of these notions, and these uses were presumably especially important to Galen. The interaction between paternal and maternal contributions to an embryo are called the agent and the patient, respectively, in *Generation of Animals*, and the former is endowed with the ability to cause movement.[101] The motions of maternal and paternal

[97] *Ph.* 8.5 (257a31–b14), tr. Hardie and Gaye (1984: 430).
[98] Waterlow (1982: 210).
[99] Waterlow (1982: 242); see also Connell (2016: 123–7, 156–60) for the scope of craft analogy in embryology.
[100] See Gelber (2010, esp. p. 197); see also Kress (2023).
[101] *GA* 1.20 (729a28) and *GA* 4.1 (766b14–15).

contributions, as well as their effects on each other, play an important role in accounting for both the pattern of familial resemblance and the deviation from this pattern. While explaining the absence of family resemblance, Aristotle presents a conceptual analysis of agent/patient relationship that builds on *Physics* 2.1. In some cases, the movements causing familial resemblance relapse (λύεσθαι), and the agent is acted upon by its patient too. The example provided is of a knife that becomes blunted by that which it cuts, or heat that becomes cooled by that which it heats. With the exception of the prime mover, movers are moved in turn. Aristotle refers his readers to a non-extant treatise for further discussion, but this short analysis alone serves the purpose of explaining how paternal resemblance might not occur and how different parts can take on the resemblance of a different parent.[102] Ultimately, animal generation has to be explained in terms of formal nature, yet the agent/patient relationship plays an important role in explaining how various biological *motions* take place in this process.[103]

This sense of 'demiurgic' activity of the constituents of the human body fits Galen's description of various parts as 'demiurges' well. The expansion and contraction of muscles that cause the change in other organs (e.g., the expansion of the thorax moving the lungs, as discussed in Chapter 3) are demiurgic acts in this exact sense. The examples mentioned so far concerned structured organs, but this scheme applies to the homoeomerous parts as well. This point is important, given that the natural capacities are properties of tissues, that is, the homoemerous parts. One important passage comes from the treatise *On the Therapeutic Method.* Here, we find an illuminating conceptualisation of a demiurgic act in the context of therapeutics. The passage of interest can be found in the context of explaining how to treat shallow wounds and ulcers. In a brief theoretical interlude, Galen states the following:

> ἐπεὶ τοίνυν ἐν τοῖς κοίλοις ἕλκεσι πρόκειται γεννῆσαι τὴν ἀπολωλυῖαν σάρκα, δεῖ γινώσκειν τὶ περὶ σαρκὸς γενέσεως, ὡς ὕλη μὲν αὐτῆς αἷμα χρηστόν, ὁ δ' οἷον δημιουργός τε καὶ τεχνίτης ἡ φύσις. ἀλλ' οὐχ ἁπλῶς εἰπεῖν χρὴ φύσιν, ἀλλὰ προσθεῖναι τὴν τίνων καὶ ποῦ. δῆλον δὲ ὅτι τῶν ὑποκειμένων σωμάτων οἷς σὰρξ ἐπιτρέφεσθαι μέλλει, τούτων ἡ φύσις ἔσται

102 *GA* 4.3 (768b16–769a6); my discussion of the dynamics of hereditary resemblance in Aristotle is necessarily abbreviated, but see Connell (2016, especially chapter 9) for a more thorough discussion.

103 See Gelber (2010) for a more detailed study of the family resemblance problem in *Generation of Animals*, and the argument that Aristotle resolves it by positing not a subspecific form but agent/patient motions.

> δημιουργὸς τῆς γενηθησομένης σαρκός. ἀλλ' ἡ φύσις ἑκάστου τῶν σωμάτων ἐδείχθη κατά τινα θερμοῦ καὶ ψυχροῦ καὶ ξηροῦ καὶ ὑγροῦ κρᾶσιν ἀποτελεῖσθαι. δῆλον οὖν ὡς ἡ τούτων εὐκρασία κατὰ τὸ ὑποκείμενον μόριον ᾧ μέλλομεν ἐπιθρέψειν τὴν λείπουσαν σάρκα τὸν λόγον ἕξει τοῦ δημιουργοῦ.
>
> Accordingly, since in hollow wounds and ulcers our task is to recreate the flesh that has been destroyed, it is necessary to know about the generation of flesh, and that its material is useful blood, and that the 'demiurge' or 'craftsman', as it were, is Nature. But we must not simply say 'Nature' but add the nature of what things and how. It is clear that the flesh of the bodies underlying those wounds will be what causes growth, and the nature of these will be the 'demiurge' of the flesh that will be regenerated. But the nature of each of the bodies was shown to consist of a certain *krasis* of heat, cold, dryness and moisture. It is clear that the *eukrasia* of these [qualities] in the underlying part will have the ground of the 'demiurge' by which we will cause the growth of the flesh that is lacking.[104]

Galen's claim that the term 'nature' requires further explication echoes the previous passages and further supports the argument that the term 'demiurge' can be meant in different senses.[105] In this specific context, the subject is flesh, a homoeomerous part, and its nature lies in the *krasis* of the four qualities that is specific to flesh. The four qualities, when mixed, give rise to the natural capacities that are responsible for the activities of flesh. Strictly speaking, the warm and the cold are more active than the dry and the wet, but it is a special proportion of each of them that is responsible for the inherent natural capacities in the homoeomerous parts.[106] As noted earlier in this chapter, these capacities consist of rejecting what harms and attracting what benefits, ultimately resulting in the processes of nutrition and growth. Thus, in wounds and ulcers, the flesh, with the help of the nourishment from blood, will grow and eventually cover up the opening in the flesh. Galen notes that, under ideal conditions, this demiurgic process happens without medical intervention,[107] but in certain cases, drying medication needs to be used, adjusting the degree of drying capacity to the mixture of the patient.[108]

Equally illuminating are descriptions of the role that the demiurge plays – or fails to play – in pathological conditions. When explaining the difficulty in treating a dry febrile condition, Galen explains that 'there is no

[104] *MM* 3.3 (10.173–4K), tr. Johnston and Horsley (2011: 267–9).

[105] This is not the only place where he does so. See *PHP* 6.1.8 de Lacy (5.507K) where he notes that the phrase 'in accordance with nature' can be used in many ways.

[106] See *Nat. Fac.* 1.3 (105–7 Helmreich=2.7–9K). See also *MM* 8.1 (10.530K).

[107] *MM* 3.3 (10.174–5K). [108] *MM* 3.3 (10.178–9K).

difficulty in properly treating strong dryness of a body other than the fact that the nourishment it requires restoratively is not of a nature to assimilate itself, but needs the demiurge of what is actually nourishing it, which is weak'.[109] The dry condition is hard to treat for one reason only: its nourishment is not of such nature as to assimilate itself. Presumably, this is owing to the fact that wetness is a passive quality. The restoration of a healthy condition requires active work from the tissues (viz. the tissue must act as demiurges), but they are weak when in a dry condition. In other words, febrile conditions create a feedback loop: dried out tissues cannot assimilate the nourishment they need for rectifying excessive dryness and thus they keep on drying out.[110]

This passage is quite clear on the point that a demiurge is simply a catalyst triggering certain processes in an organic body. Before turning back to the question of the vegetative soul and its generative powers, it is worth remarking on the implications of this model. This model of organic (as opposed to artisan-like) change establishes grounds for organic unity in a way that is fundamentally different from the atomist accounts, like the ones Galen ascribes to Erasistratus and Asclepiades in his *On the Natural Capacities* and contrasts with the Hippocratic account grounded in the notion of natural capacities.[111] For Galen, it is crucial to recognise not only the external but also the internal type of demiurge. The physiological change takes place not because one discrete atom bumps into another discrete atom – in other words, when two distinct substances interact with each other, which is an interaction that can be modelled on mechanistic accounts.[112] Instead, physiological change takes place within a single substance (e.g., a person), when her parts act as agents (e.g., muscles) and patients (e.g., bones of the thorax), forming single, coherent unity. The key difference is that these are parts; not entities that primarily operate

109 *MM* 7.7 (10.497K), tr. Johnston and Horsley (2011: 297): οὐδὲ γὰρ οὐδὲ δι᾽ ἄλλο τι χαλεπὸν γίγνεται θεραπεῦσαι καλῶς ἰσχυρὰν ξηρότητα σώματος ἢ ὅτι χρῄζει μὲν ἀναθρέψεως, ἡ τροφὴ δ᾽ οὐ πέφυκεν ἑαυτὴν προσφύειν, ἀλλ᾽ αὐτοῦ δεῖται τοῦ τρεφομένου δημιουργοῦντος αὐτήν, ὅπερ ἐστὶν ἄτονον.

110 Natural aging and eventual death is also caused by the dryness of mixtures, see *San. Tu.* 1.2.6–7 Koch (6.4–5K).

111 Although he also mentions that Aristotle belongs to this tradition in *Nat. Fac.* 2.4 (165, 198 Helmreich=2.89K); see also *Hipp. Elem.* 5.1 de Lacy (1.448K).

112 The insensitivity of atoms and the impossibility that their interaction would produce sensation (which is a kind of alteration) are the key points Galen makes in his rejection of the 'Epicurean' account of pain at the beginning of *On the Elements According to Hippocrates*. The argument is discussed in greater detail in Chapter 4.

in accordance with the laws of physics in general, but the parts whose acts are primarily circumscribed within a specific, biological whole, viz. a living body. The parthood of the latter is fundamentally different from the former, and more importantly, lays the ground for the kind of unity that is necessary for organic life.

2.6 The Vegetative Soul as a Demiurge

The claim that the vegetative soul is a demiurge has to be read against the background of the Aristotelian tradition, especially its theorisation of vital motion and vital change. When Galen talks about the demiurgic regeneration of tissues, he is clearly referring to the inherent capacities in tissues to absorb nutriment and to grow. It is worth noting that this is already a kind of generative capacity, owing to the fact that it accounts for the expansion in mass when tissues grow. There is little reason to suppose that the generative activity of the vegetative soul in the embryo amounts to anything more. He does present the development of the embryo and the restoration of tissues as the same type of processes in principle,[113] but the most coherent and charitable way of reading this claim is with a reference to the growth of tissues. The tissues grow, in the sense of expanding in size, the same way in an embryo and an adult animal; after all, growth, together with nutrition, is the hallmark of the fundamental vitality, that is, the vegetative life. In so far as the vegetative capacities are capable of generation, they are ever-present in both the embryo and throughout the remainder of the animal's life, generating in the same way. However, they are also clearly not designing agents, because the vegetative process only increases (or restores) what is already in existence, rather than creating something entirely new. Galen explicitly states that there is more than one demiurge active in the womb. As well as the seed and blood, there is the designer that permeates through and through, generating a new substance, that is, the embryo. The generation of a new substance (in the Aristotelian sense of the word) requires the generation of the form, which is a domain of the shaping capacity whose substance (in the Stoic sense of the word)

[113] *Thras.* 26 (66, 18–24 Helmreich=5.853K), tr. Singer (1997: 75): 'Thus, if we had the capacity to create an animal in the first place, the principles involved in that initial creation would be no different from those involved in its restoration. In reality, though, we are not primarily responsible for either of these tasks: it is Nature who first constructs the animal and subsequently heals it if it is sick.'

Galen never identifies.[114] He is quite clear that the conception is a more complex process than tissue growth.[115]

Having noted the relatively primitive nature of the vegetative capacities, it is important to emphasise that the notion of the vegetative soul as a demiurge not only explains the body's ability to grow and heal itself (fundamental activities for maintaining life) but also provides a blueprint for the conceptualisation of organic unity. The ability of bodily tissues to perform certain activities is grounded in their elemental parts acting on each other, thus enabling the tissue to change by virtue of its inherent properties alone, viz. as an organic entity. As Galen explains, the vegetative soul is in charge of the growth of a child after birth,[116] up until the full formation of the internal organs, after which all three souls fully govern the animal.[117]

2.7 Concluding Remarks: On Vegetative Unity

In the four-fold division of parts presented in *Art of Medicine*, the key criterion for distinguishing different kinds of parthood is the ability to self-manage (διοικεῖν) and to govern (ἄρχειν) or be governed by the principal parts. In the case of the nutritive system, the governing part is the liver and its governing activities are enabled by its offshoots, the veins. The veins are spread throughout the body and are inserted into the parts made of homoeomerous tissues that possess natural capacities and, therefore, the capacity to self-manage. Some of the parts nourished this way, for example the stomach, belong to the nutritive system, while others, for example a leg muscle, do not. In the case of the latter, the connection to the nutritive system helps it to be nourished and grow (e.g., by restoring tissues). In the case of the former, however, there is more at stake, namely, the systematic unity.

Galen's nutritive system is like a conveyor belt: each part belonging to this system does a little bit of processing. The liver, as the *hēgemon*, stands at the end of the process, making the final conversion of foodstuffs into

114 *Nat. Fac.* 1.6 (111, 18–25 Helmreich=2.15K); 3.1 (205–6, 16–23 Helmreich=2.145K). This is also the third kind of demiurge mentioned in the passage from *Sem.* cited earlier, that which permeates through and through. See also the discussion of the plastic capacity in the chapter on the nervous system (Chapter 4).

115 See the discussion in Hankinson (2017b: 263–6); see also Hankinson (2006). The problem of the substance of the rational soul will be addressed again in Chapter 4; see the Introduction for the discussion of the scholarship on the problem of the substance of this soul.

116 *Prop. Plac.* 3.5 (68 Lami Garofalo).

117 *Prop. Plac.* 10.4 (102 Lami Garofalo).

useful blood and sending it out to the rest of the body via the veins. The nutritive parts (the stomach, the spleen, and so on) have a degree of independence *qua* their ability to self-manage. They can absorb and process the nutriment that is presented to them via their innate natural capacities. However, they are all connected in such a way as to produce that nutriment in the form of blood. At the risk of cliché, the whole is thus greater than the sum of its parts, because the parts work together to sustain themselves in a way they could not do individually: their tissues can absorb the nutriment that is presented to them, but only in combination with other parts, the whole nutritive system working as one, they can also produce that nutriment for themselves and the rest of the body. They are not only self-sufficient individually; when put together they constitute a self-sufficient whole: a body that is able to nourish itself. It is not merely the connection between parts (although that is also important) that renders them as parts of a single whole, but their activities that come together to form a single functionally unified entity.

At the beginning of this chapter, it was highlighted that Galen thinks of the vegetative aspects of life as plant-like, and an embryo in this sense is very much a plant-like entity. It is the development of the internal organs that turns this entity into an animal, and underscores the emergence of the more complex type of vitality. The development of these parts is not simultaneous but staggered. Just like many other philosophers and doctors, Galen maintained that the rationality does not properly manifest itself until teenage years.[118] The domain of the brain and the nervous system in general, thus, comes into play later in life. Before a person becomes a rational animal, one has to become an animal. And the animal nature is underpinned by the activities of the cardiac and pneumatic systems, which are explored in Chapter 3.

118 One of his bigger points of contention against Chrysippus the Stoic and his unified psychological model of the soul rests precisely on this point in *PHP* 5.1.10 de Lacy (5.431K). The mainstream Stoics ascribe affections to the rational part of the soul and, since it is not developed in children, they deny that children have affections. Galen criticises this view as sophist and praises Posidonius' adoption of tripartition. For a more detailed discussion of Posidonius' scheme and its Platonic influences, see Tieleman (2003a: 214–20).

CHAPTER 3

Respiration and Transpiration
The Cardiac System and Pneumatology

If the vegetative soul separates the organic plant life from the inorganic existence, then the spirited soul is the hallmark of the animal life, and just as the activities of the former are underpinned by the nutritive system, so the activities of the latter are by the cardiac system.[1] The workings of the cardiac system are centred around one key regulatory activity, breathing; it is the ability to breath that distinguishes animals from plants. The significance of breathing for animal vitality is evident from the fact that the deprivation of breath swiftly leads to the end of life. The explanation of this easily observable phenomenon posed a substantial challenge to ancient philosophers and scientists, and Galenic texts are excellent sources for debates and disagreements in this area. Galen opens *On the Usefulness of Respiration* with the observation that the usefulness of breathing is self-evident, as animals die quickly when deprived of breath.[2] He then sets out a variety of explanations of the phenomenon by his predecessors. The rest of the treatise consists of refutations of flawed accounts with arguments

[1] At the same time, it is quite important for Galen not to mistake it for the seat of the *hēgemonikon*. It is hardly an exaggeration to say that one of his most prominent lifelong projects was his rebuttal of various cardiocentrists. Aristotle was one of them (see *UP* 8.3 (1.451–3 Helmreich=3.623–5K), for a well-known, rhetorically charged criticism; see van der Eijk (2009: 274–6) for an accompanying discussion), although, on the whole, Galen spends more time engaging critically with the Stoics and Stoicising doctors, such as the Pneumatists. His grand treatise *On the Doctrines of Hippocrates and Plato* is focused on the attack on the Stoic philosopher Chrysippus, representing those who maintain that the *hēgemonikon* resides in the heart rather than the brain (see Tieleman (1996, 2003a) for Galen representations; see also Rocca (2003: 28–41) for the cardiocentrism in the Classical and Hellenistic philosophy and science). This debate shows up in other works too; in *MM* 13.21 (10.929K), Galen attacks the Pneumatists for locating *hēgemonikon* in the heart. He claims that their hypocrisy is evident when one sees that Athenaeus applies medicine to the head of a patient suffering from phrenitis rather than the chest.

[2] *Ut. Resp.* 1.1 (80 Furley and Wilkie=4.470K): Τίς ἡ τῆς ἀναπνοῆς χρεία; ὅτι γὰρ οὐχ ἡ τυχοῦσα, φανερὸν ἐκ τοῦ μηδὲ βραχύτατον ἡμᾶς χρόνον δύνασθαι διαρκεῖν ἀπολομένης αὐτῆς. Shorter reiterations of the simple observation that animals die when they cannot breathe can be found in other works too: *Prop. Plac.* 15.4 (138 Lami Garofalo); *Hipp. Elem.* 5.24 de Lacy (1.454K); *UP* 6.2 (1.302, 6–7 Helmreich=413K); *Foet. Form.* 5, 17 Nickel (4.685K). Galen is, of course, not the first to make this claim; see Debru (1996: 129–30).

supporting Galen's preferred view, namely that breathing is effectively a process of the heat regulation of the heart and, to some extent, resupply of the psychic pneuma. He associates this view primarily with Hippocrates.[3]

While to the contemporary mind, the heart is probably associated primarily with blood, in the Galenic framework, blood properly belongs to the nutritive systems and the liver that elaborates it.[4] The heart does participate in the circulation of the blood to the extent that the blood is located in arteries and the heart moves the arteries, but it has little to do with its proper activity, which is nutrition. The nutriment is sent out by the liver via veins.[5] Instead, it is the other material circulating in the arteries, the pneuma, that is subordinate to the activities of the heart specifically. Galen differentiates between three types of pneuma: vital, psychic and natural.[6] All three will be covered in this chapter, although special attention will be paid to the first two, not only because they are discussed most extensively, but also because there is more at stake with them.[7] As the name suggests, the vital pneuma is a key component to animal vitality that is maintained by breathing. The psychic pneuma, elaborated in the arteries and located in the brain and some nerves, plays an important role in accounting for psychic capacities, including the capacity for reasoning.[8] Some of the arguments against the cardio-centric

[3] As the following discussion shows, Galen only engages with medical names in this treatise and does not mention, for example, Aristotle and his view that respiration cools the cardiac system in *Juv.* 16 (475b15–20) and *Resp.* 21 (480a23–480b12). One possible explanation is that Aristotle's view closely resembles that of Diocles of Carystus, whose fragments on respiration, derived from Galen, are collected in van der Eijk (2001: 65–8). It has been suggested that Diocles was a pupil of Aristotle (especially advocated by W. W. Jaeger, see, for example, Jaeger (1938)), leading to an extensive scholarly debate covered in von Staden (1992), which found Jaeger's suggestion to be unlikely; for a current and more nuanced understanding of Diocles' connection to Peripatos (as well as other philosophers), see van der Eijk (2000–1: xxxiv–xxxviii).

[4] See the more detailed discussion in Chapter 2.

[5] See Chapter 2 for Galen's argument on this precise point.

[6] *PHP* 2.8.36–40 de Lacy (5.280–1K).

[7] When it comes to the role that pneuma plays in the brain/nervous system, Rocca (2003) presents a detailed and informative study. I make use of various points made there, especially regarding anatomy, although the focus of this chapter is the cardiac system and the vital pneuma, which plays the key role in conceptualizing animal vitality. For this reason, the discussion in this chapter will be centred around the notion of the innate heat as well as the Galenic division of the bodily parts in accordance with their viscosity, which is instrumental in accounting for the speed of animal vitality.

[8] *UP* 9.4 (2.13, 6–11 Helmreich=3.700K). Some of the arguments against the cardiocentric theory are specifically focused on the evidence of the location of the psychic pneuma. See, for example, *PHP* 2.4.40–42 de Lacy (5.237K), tr. de Lacy (1978–84: 125–7): 'For the present it is enough for me to only make this further statement, that if speech were produced when pneuma in the lungs is somehow shaped by the heart's pneuma and then imparts this shape to the pneuma in the

theory are specifically focused on the evidence of the location of the psychic pneuma. The study in this chapter explores the overlap of the domains of nervous and cardiac systems, thus building on the conclusions on Galen's understanding of vitality in Chapter 2 and laying the ground for the understanding of the overall unity of Galenic physiology.

This chapter consists of four large sections. Section 3.1 is dedicated to a study of the many ways in which Galen differentiates breathing, including respiration and transpiration, forced and unforced breathing. The aim of this section is to distinguish and clarify the ways in which, according to him, breathing takes place and which parts participate in which kinds of breathing. The other three sections are, broadly speaking, dedicated to the question of the physiological significance of breathing. They are organised around the three types of pneuma, although some subsections involve studies of other pertinent notions. Section 3.2 is, broadly speaking, dedicated to the study of the vital pneuma, and its leading preoccupation is the question of how, according to Galen, breathing maintains vitality or, alternatively, why animals die when deprived of breath. Apart from the study of Galen's position on this matter, this section also addresses the notion of the innate heat and discusses the significance of a rarely discussed division of parts into solids, fluids and pneumata. Section 3.3 focuses on the generation and activities of the psychic pneuma, including its role as an instrument of the soul. Section 3.4 briefly addresses the question of the so-called natural pneuma, of whose existence Galen was uncertain, before turning to the discussion of the significance of the cardiac system for the unity of the animal body.

3.1 Anatomy of the Breathing Process

In order to understand why breathing is the hallmark of animal vitality, we need to answer the question of what purpose it serves in the body, and Galen does provide an extensive discussion of this matter. However, before turning to this issue, it is worth spending a little time on the process of breathing itself. The anatomy of breathing can come across as a slightly tedious subject, but it hides a number of significant insights about Galen's attempts to theorise neatly a phenomenon that he recognises as complex and multifaceted.

windpipe, speech would not be immediately destroyed when certain nerves have been cut in the neck or the head.'

It is evident that breathing consists of different motions: animals can hold their breath, slow it down or speed it up, make it deeper or shallower and so on. These are just some types of conscious breathing, but most of the time, humans are not aware of their breathing at all. Such a range of motion was well observed by ancient theorists of the human body too. Doxographical sources offer a valuable glimpse into the popular explanations.[9] Galen's account of breathing survives in by far the most elaborate form, with multiple classifications.

The key distinction is between respiration (ἀναπνοή) and transpiration (διαπνοή). The former is defined as breathing via the larynx, the latter via the skin of the whole body.[10] Respiration is further divided into forced and unforced kinds, and this distinction, anatomical in nature, will be discussed later. The fundamental distinction in the theory of breathing, however, concerns voluntary and involuntary motion. According to him, breathing mostly falls under the dominion of the heart,[11] by and large, and therefore it is involuntary. He also argues that the intelligent design of the human body providently allowed for some control of breath via voluntary motion. This type of motion occurs in virtue of the soul, while the involuntary type occurs owing to nature, and they originate from the nervous and the cardiac systems, respectively.[12] The discussion of nutrition in Chapter 2 also produced a very similar kind of division, only in that case, the motions of nature were attributed to the vegetative soul. While in the case of nutrition, the distinction served to differentiate between the lack of nutriment in tissues and the perception of that lack, in this case, it differentiates between voluntary and involuntary breathing. The relevant background here is the *Timaeus'* tripartition of the souls that notably describes the two lower souls as a subdivision of the irrational soul.[13] In denoting both lower souls as 'nature', however, Galen applies the Stoic nomenclature to the Platonic concept.[14]

The contrast between the nature and the soul is a useful heuristic tool that helps to distinguish between the roles different organs play in any physiological process and therefore it is not entirely surprising that 'nature'

9 See, for example, Aëtius 4.22.2 Mansfeld and Runia, containing accounts of both voluntary and involuntary types of breathing put forth by Empedocles, Asclepiades and Herophilus.

10 *Comp. Med. Loc.* 9.10 (13.319K); *Hipp. Epid.* 5.5 (17b.252–3K); *Hipp. Vict.* 2 (15.180K); *Plat. Tim.* Fr. 17 (Larrain); *Symp. Diff.* 5.1 Gundert (7.75K).

11 *UP* 6.2 (1.301, 3–4 Helmreich=3.412K). See Debru (1996: 100–2) for the metaphorical language (and its historic background) Galen uses to describe the heart.

12 The voluntary motion is discussed in greater detail in Chapter 4.

13 *Ti.* 69C–D.

14 See Hankinson (1991a: n8); see also von Staden (2000: 102) for a suggestion that the Stoic terminology might have been inspired by the Alexandrian doctors.

applies to both the vegetative and the spirited domains. Furthermore, it is worth noting that Galen models these two domains in very similar ways too. One pertinent example is his account of respiration, outlined in *On the Causes of Respiration* as follows: when an animal breathes in through the nose, the air (ἀήρ) is drawn in, and a small part of it goes to the brain while the larger part of it is taken via the trachea to the lungs.[15] Nothing else is said of what happens to this portion of air in this treatise, but his other texts explain that it nourishes the psychic pneuma, and this point will be discussed later. The larger portion of air goes into the lungs via the trachea. The lungs are described as the great stomach of pneuma (ὁ δὲ πνεύμων οἷα βαθὺς γαστὴρ ὑπόκειται τῷ πνεύματι).[16] The language is evocative enough: the lungs process air just like the stomach crushes food. But the similarity does not end here. Galen continues by noting that the thorax steers (οἰακίζει) the lungs. Thus, both the stomach and the lungs are under dominion of other organs and recipients of external motion.

The position of the lungs, however, is more complex than the position of the stomach, which simply belongs to the system controlled by the liver. To the extent that the lungs are subordinate to the heart, they resemble the stomach.[17] But the fact that the lungs are steered by the thorax also indicates that they are subordinate to the nervous system too, since the thorax itself is moved by muscles and articulated by bones.[18] Strikingly, for Galen, the organ peculiar to respiration neither initiates nor controls respiratory motions.[19]

An indirect target of this Galenic point might be Herophilus' view. Although little survives of the Herophilean account, the extant evidence highlights that he maintained that the lungs have their own innate motion.[20] His account is an alternative to the Aristotelian account that

15 *Caus. Resp.* 2 (240 Furley and Wilkie=4.466K). For the distinction of the surrounding air and the air that is breathed in, see also *Thras.* 18 (55, 12–15 Helmreich=5.837K).

16 This language most likely predates Galen, because Ps. Aristotle's *De Spiritu* 481a28–30 reports Aristogenes as claiming that pneuma is nourished by respiration, when air is *digested* in the lungs (Ἀριστογένης . . . τροφὴν γὰρ οἴεται καὶ τὸ πνεῦμα πεττομένου τοῦ ἀέρος ἐν τῷ πνεύμονι). For the authorship and medical significance of this treatise, see Lewis and Gregoric (2015).

17 Even to the extent that it is not an absolutely vital organ. It is worth remembering that some of the breathing takes place as transpiration (discussed later in greater detail), which forgoes the lungs completely. Galen also describes an experiment of covering the mouth of a boy, thus preventing him from lung respiration, and the boy staying alive, owing to respiration through skin; *Ut. Resp.* 5.2 (124 Furley and Wilkie=4.504–5K).

18 *Caus. Resp.* 2 (240 Furley and Wilkie=4.466K).

19 In *Ut. Resp.* 5.4 (126 Furley and Wilkie=4.506K), Galen states that the lungs are the first organ of respiration, but in so far as it is moved by the thorax, it is, properly speaking, second.

20 Aëtius 4.22.3 Mansfeld and Runia; Ps. Galen *Hist. Phil.* 103=T143c von Staden, see also von Staden (1989: 259–62).

posits the rise and fall of the innate heat as the source of respiratory motion.[21] In a sense, Galen goes back to the Aristotelian model in making the lungs subject to the external mover, although this mover now is the nerves and the muscles, rather than the heart. This naturally renders respiration voluntary. The strength of Galen's account is that it can explain very easily how animals are able to modify the breath, including holding it, deepening it, slowing it down and so on. When accounting for such a range of motions, he uses both philosophical and anatomical knowledge. The overall conceptualisation of the phenomenon is built on a famous philosophical motif.

Galen outlines the causes of respiration in the treatise *On the Causes of Respiration* as follows: the capacity of choice, the instruments (organs) that aid this capacity and the purpose (*chreia*) for which the former two are necessary.[22] He comes back to this tripartite formula at the very end of the treatise, reiterating it with a rather poetic simile: 'Choice is like a charioteer who moves the reins and the horses; the nerves are like the reins, and the muscles are like the horses; similarly the use is the desired end of respiration, as victory is of chariot racing.'[23] This imagery appears to be built on the famous chariot simile in Plato's *Phaedrus*.[24] This dialogue is of great importance to Galen,[25] so it is no wonder he uses this motif here too.

Yet there are clear differences between the Platonic and the Galenic chariots. The key aspect of Plato's simile is the conflict between the horses, leading to the disorderly and painful motion of the chariot.[26] A Galenic charioteer, by contrast, would be enjoying a leisurely ride most of the time as there is no conflict between muscles.[27] The parts do not have different

[21] I am following von Staden (1989: 259–61), on the basis of Aristotle's *Resp.* 20–1 (479b17–480b30).

[22] *Caus. Resp.* 1 (240 Furley and Wilkie=4.465–6K). This appears to be a formulaic claim, cf., for example, *Diff. Puls.* 4.2 (8.714K), for the same type of formulation but in reference to the causes of the pulse. See also the discussion of the significance of this formulation in Chapter 4. For a discussion of the notion of *chreia* and how it differs from activities, see Furley and Wilkie (1984: 58–69).

[23] *Caus. Resp.* 7 (244 Furley and Wilkie=4.469K), tr. Furley and Wilkie (1984: 245): ἡ μὲν γὰρ προαίρεσις ἔοικε τῷ κινοῦντι τὰς ἡνίας καὶ τοὺς ἵππους ἀναβάτῃ· ταῖς δ' ἡνίαις τὰ νεῦρα ἐοίκασι, καθάπερ καὶ ἵπποις οἱ μύες· οὕτω δὲ καὶ ἡ χρεία τὸ ἔσχατον ὀρεκτὸν καθέστηκε τῆς ἀναπνοῆς, ὥσπερ ἡ νίκη τῆς ἡνιοχικῆς.

[24] See esp. *Phdr.* 253D–257A. On the importance of the *Phaedrus* to Galen, see Rocca (2006: esp. 50–1) and Tieleman (2020).

[25] For a more thorough discussion, see Rocca (2006), and more recently, Tieleman (2020).

[26] *Phdr.* 246A–B.

[27] In principle, there is room for such a conflict, because respiration involves organs from different systems, which, in the Platonic model in the *Phaedrus*, have conflicting desires. Galen makes no note of such a conflict here, and it is quite clear why: it is hard to see how respiration could be explained by a presence of a conflict. Furthermore, Galen generally seems to think of human nature,

desires that might pull them in different directions. Only a disease or an injury to one of the parts would disrupt the physiological process carried out in this manner.[28]

The emphasis on the muscles is undoubtedly intentional, because in another treatise, *On Problematical Movements*, Galen explains the significance of the intercostal muscles for respiration, which he describes as the discovery made by his recent predecessors to which he himself added.[29] According to him, until the time of his teachers, the diaphragm was considered to be the most important organ of respiration.[30] Galen, however, claims he discovered the importance of the intercostal muscles by means of dissection. He explains how he showed that the upper part of the thorax is moved by muscles stretching down from the neck, and the middle parts by the intercostals. These paired muscles expand and contract the thorax, while other muscles only make it expand. He experimented with ligating the nerves moving these muscles, thus depriving the thorax of motion without opening it.[31] He notes that this demonstration, which he taught to his friends too,[32] is the best proof for respiration being voluntary: 'For the thorax immediately becomes immobile and the animal soon dies with its head thrown back, since, although it wishes to breathe, it cannot move its thorax.'[33]

3.1.1 Forced and Unforced Respiration

These muscles, then, play the role of the horses in the chariot simile. As already mentioned, Galenic horses are not in conflict with one another. The reason for this is the fact that each muscle is assigned a different

at least on the physiological level, as consisting of parts cooperating in harmony. This problem is addressed more extensively in Chapters 4 and 5.

28 See van der Eijk (2017: esp. 239) for the Galenic concept of disease as merely a possible – but not unavoidable – interruption of the overall well-designed human physiology.

29 *Mot. Dub.* 2.7–13 (128, 21–30, 12 Nutton). This treatise survives only in Latin and Arabic translations. For an in-depth discussion of the textual tradition and translations, see Nutton and Bos (2011: 18–89). I will be citing the Latin translation.

30 *Mot. Dub.* 2.8 (128, 25–6 Nutton).

31 The procedure, including advice on the choice of surgical instruments, is covered in detail in *AA* 8.4 (732–44 Garofalo=2.667–75K).

32 On the public nature of Galen's demonstrations of these dissections, see Salas (2020: 27–34).

33 *Mot. Dub.* 2.12–13 (130, 8 Nutton) tr. Nutton and Bos (2011: 131): *inmobilis enim fit thorax confestim et animal mox moritur curvatum quidem quia desiderans inspirare, non potens autem movere thoracem*. The claim is followed by a remark stating that these things were discovered by Galen's predecessors, although he was able to add to them. Among these predecessors are certainly the Alexandrian doctors, especially Herophilus (see also Chapter 4). For a biographic discussion of Galen's engagement with the topic, see Debru (1996: 18–23).

movement and thus is responsible for a different kind of respiration. This becomes especially clear in Galen's account of forced (βίαιος) and unforced (ἀβίαστος) respiration in *On Causes of Respiration*. In *On the Doctrines of Hippocrates and Plato*, he describes the former as occurring in sickness or during intense physical exercise and the latter as occurring in a healthy and calm state of the body.[34] The two types of respiration have two parts each, so there are four parts altogether as well as four groups of muscles performing these motions.[35] They are as follows: in the case of unforced respiration, the diaphragm is responsible for breathing in and the abdomen muscles for breathing out.[36] In the case of forced respiration, the muscles around the hollows of the shoulder blades and the inner intercostal muscles are responsible for breathing in. The outer intercostal muscles, meanwhile, are the proper organs for forced breathing out.[37]

As already noted, Galen's choice to adopt the *Phaedrian* chariot motif might seem not entirely fitting. The key point of the original is to exemplify the conflict, but the conflict in the case of respiration is hardly possible, as muscle motions cannot be at odds with each other *per se*. A closer look at the way in which Galen describes the forced and unforced motions shows that his use of the simile is more likely motivated by the need for a unified explanatory device. He is using the simile not as an illustration of a conflict but as an illustration of a control mechanism. The question of control is, after all, key to the account of respiration.

However, the scope of the controlled motion is not always clear. The unforced respiration especially does not seem to sit easily in the category of voluntary action. Much breathing via the lungs is done, after all, without intention or any thought at all. Galen himself notes that some people think that breathing during sleep shows respiration to be involuntary.[38] He does not agree with this view, as the description of the dissection at the end of Section 3.1 shows: nerve ligature in muscles stretching from the neck down evidently stops respiration, making it a voluntary act. However, he does not entirely dismiss the ancient knowledge of assigning the key role to the diaphragmatic breathing either. The key passage here comes from

[34] *PHP* 2.4.32–5 de Lacy (5.234–5 K); this brief discussion also makes a reference to *Causes of Respiration* at 2.4.38 de Lacy (5.236K).

[35] *Caus. Resp.* 5 (242 Furley and Wilkie=4.468K).

[36] The diaphragm is full of nervous tissue, so it moves like a muscle; *Caus. Resp.* 2 (242 Furley and Wilkie=4.467K). See *Us. Puls.* 7.1 (218 Furley and Wilkie=5.172K), where breathing out is described as a passive relaxation of the expanded thorax. See also *UP* 5.14 (1.289 Helmreich=3.595K).

[37] *Caus. Resp.* 5 (242 Furley and Wilkie=4.468K).

[38] *Mot. Dub.* 10.3 (164, 10–13 Nutton).

Anatomical Procedures, which states that the movement of breathing is initiated from below by the diaphragm, which expands and contracts in accordance to its own tension and relaxation, thus initiating respiration. The respiration in the lower thorax, therefore, is said to be a physical, not a psychic act.[39]

Although this claim appears to contradict the demonstration cited at the end of Section 3.1 (showing that once certain nerves are ligated, the dissected animal dies of suffocation, which demonstrates that nerves control respiration), it is not entirely the case. The key point here is the relationship between the motions of the diaphragm and the organs controlling respiration. While Galen highlights the significance of the diaphragm for breathing (also praising anatomists for discovering it), this organ is not fully responsible for respiration according to him: it causes movement only in the lower part of the thorax, while the upper part and the intermediate parts are moved by the intercostal and the neck muscles.[40]

This leads to two possibilities: the unforced respiration via the diaphragm is, in fact, involuntary. If this is the case, then the question arises as to why the vivisected animal dies: why does the involuntary respiration via the diaphragm not continue when the nerves of the upper muscles are ligated, keeping the animal alive? Evidently, the movement of the lower thorax cannot be sufficient for a full breath. But if that is the case, then how can animals breathe while asleep?

A solution can be found by employing the differentiation of parts. The diaphragm has its own motion, which is called physical rather than psychic. It is, therefore, a self-managing part, whose activities are enabled by its own innate natural capacities. It also has muscles and nerves connecting it to the governing part of the nervous system, the brain.[41] The diaphragm, therefore, belongs to the category of parts that are both self-managing and governed by the principal parts.

The tension and relaxation of the diaphragm originate in its natural capacities (just like 'drawing' in the veins and the stomach; the account of

[39] *AA* 8.2 (718 Garofalo=2.657K): Τῆς δ' ὅλης αὐτοῦ κινήσεως ἐναργῶς ἐξηγοῦνται κάτω μὲν αἱ φρένες αὐταὶ [τε] κατὰ τὴν ἑαυτῶν ἔντασίν τε καὶ χάλασιν ἐναλλὰξ γιγνομένην εὐρύνουσαί τε καὶ συστέλλουσαι τὸ ταύτῃ πέρας, ἐπισπώμεναί τε κάτω μὲν διὰ τοῦ ξιφοειδοῦς χόνδρου τὸ στέρνον, ἄνω δέ πως ἀτρέμα καὶ πρόσω τὰς νόθας. καὶ τήν γε δόξασαν εἶναι φυσικὸν ἔργον, οὐ ψυχικὸν, ἀναπνοήν.

[40] *Mot. Dub.* 2.9 (128, 29–31 Nutton).

[41] The tissues of the diaphragm are described in *AA* 5.5 (496 Garofalo=2.503–4K) and 5.8 (520–8 Garofalo=2.520–6K).

hunger, which also consists of both physical and psychic motions, serves as a useful analogy here). The nerves 'sense' it, producing a psychic reaction in the brain, which in turn triggers the motion of the motor nerves in the neck and intercostal muscles. This reaction is voluntary, but it need not be a product of intent, just like, for example, raising one's arm to shield the eye from bright light or pulling away from a barking dog. The motions of the diaphragm, thus, trigger the motion in the nerves that move the upper thorax. In this way, the entire thorax can move even during sleep. Once the nerves in the muscles controlling the upper thorax are ligated, these muscles cannot move, and the vivisected animal suffocates, indicating that the diaphragmatic motion cannot compensate for the loss of motion in the upper thorax. Thus, even unforced respiration belongs to the genus of voluntary motion. Furthermore, the presence of the nerves, the reigns of muscles,[42] means that unforced breathing can be altered and changed by will. This activity does require intent, and it is an important part of the overall human design that certain activities can be controlled intentionally. Presumably, both forced and unforced respiration is voluntary not because it requires an act of will to initiate it but because it can be subjected to the will. This activity fundamentally differentiates any subtype of respiration from the fully involuntary breathing that takes place in the arteries. Transpiration, the involuntary arterial breathing, will be discussed in Section 3.1.2.

3.1.2 *Transpiration*

Transpiration, breathing through the whole body, is an important example of the body's innate ability to intake the air without deliberate action, via pulsating arteries. Transpiration is somewhat less prominently discussed than respiration, and there are few side-by-side comparisons between them, but the existing ones show that they share many key features.[43] In *On the Usefulness of the Pulse*, Galen argues that 'what respiration does for the heart alone is done by the pulse for the warmth that

[42] This discussion, as well as the whole treatise, ends with a brief examination of the nerves involved in respiration, all of which grow from the spinal medulla; *Caus. Resp.* 6 (244 Furley and Wilkie=4.468–9K). The nervous system will be discussed in greater detail in Chapter 4.

[43] *On the Usefulness of the Pulse* begins with the question of whether the purpose of the pulse is the same as that of respiration or something else. Many doctors maintain it, yet, Galen warns, it is important not to accept such claims uncritically; after all, the ceasing of pulse will not result in death, unlike the ceasing of respiration; *Us. Puls.* 1.2 (194 Furley and Wilkie=5.149K).

is all over the body'.[44] The purpose of transpiration and the attendant notion of the innate heat will be discussed in Section 3.2, together with the purpose of respiration. Before turning to this discussion, it is important to briefly cover the physiological process of transpiration.

Whereas respiration, as discussed earlier, is governed by the nervous system,[45] the expansion and contraction of arteries is prompted by the heart.[46] Both processes follow the same pattern: just like in respiration, so too in the pulsation of arteries, expansion draws in pneuma, while contraction expels the residues of burning humours. The significant difference is the involuntary nature of the cardiac motion and the voluntary nature of the nervous motion. Galen presents the discussion of the origin of the former in a polemical context.

Just as in the case of respiration, Galen presents his account as an alternative to the flawed Erasistratean view that mechanistic processes account for the activities of the arteries, emphatically maintaining that arteries 'do not expand because they are filled; they are filled because they expand'.[47] The innate capacities of tissues, rather than mechanistic processes, govern transpiration. Delving into the precise nature of the motion of arteries, Galen further seeks to determine whether expansion or contraction, or both expansion and contraction, ought to be considered the activities of the arteries. He concludes that both respiratory and transpiratory organs have innate contrary capacities.[48] They are used when the residues from the burning of the humours build up, causing a desire in the animal to blow out the breath forcefully. In a healthy state of the body, breathing out is sufficient.[49] These motions are just like those of respiration, the only difference being the source: pulse is moved by the physical (or vital) capacity, respiration by the psychic.[50]

A more extensive critique of the mechanistic account of transpiration can be found in Book 8 of *On the Doctrines of Hippocrates and Plato*, and this attack is especially notable because it concerns one of Galen's two intellectual inspirations, Plato. In a fairly rare instance of criticism, Galen

44 *Us. Puls.* 3.3 (206 Furley and Wilkie=5.161K), tr. Furley and Wilkie (1984: 209), slightly altered replacing 'breathing' with 'respiration'. See also the reiteration of this point at 4.1 (208 Furley and Wilkie=5.163K).

45 *Us. Puls.* 6.2 (216 Furley and Wilkie=5.169K).

46 *Us. Puls.* 4.2 (210 Furley and Wilkie=5.164K).

47 *Us. Puls.* 5.4 (214 Furley and Wilkie=5.168K), tr. Furley and Wilkie (1984: 214). For a discussion of Erasistratus' views, see von Staden (2000: 92–4)

48 *Us. Puls.* 7.1 (220 Furley and Wilkie=5.172–3K).

49 *Us. Puls.* 7.2 (220 Furley and Wilkie=5.173K).

50 *Us. Puls.* 8.1 (226 Furley and Wilkie=5.179K).

points out that Plato made a mistake in conflating the causes of transpiration for respiration and not following Hippocrates in this respect.[51] According to him, Plato also did not recognise the role that the capacity of attraction (which can also be observed while sucking water via a reed) plays in the process of transpiration. Galen cites a long passage from the *Timaeus* with the following faulty account: all breathing occurs via a circular pattern of motion that takes place when one substance (a certain amount of pneuma) pushes out another substance (another amount of pneuma). As there is no void, the third substance is necessarily drawn in, and so the cycle continues.[52] This explanation is mechanistic, as Galen notes, it does away with the capacity of attraction as an explanatory device.[53]

The example of sucking water via the reed hints that the critique of Plato is, indirectly, also a critique of the atomist doctors. This example is not mentioned in the *Timaeus*.[54] Sucking through a reed is the standard example found at the beginning of the treatises on pneumatics by Hero of Alexandria and Philo of Byzantium.[55] It demonstrates the working principle of a siphon, a foundational mechanism of pneumatic devices. The account of respiration in the *Timaeus* uses the principle of *horror vacui*, just like the operation of a siphon, as the central explanatory tool for respiration.

Galen himself, meanwhile, makes the attractive capacity the key explanatory tool. Respiration, Galen explains, is due to the sucking and pushing motion exercised by the thorax and muscles. Whereas the motion of the thorax is voluntary, the motion of the heart and arteries – pulsation – is not,[56] and 'by their dilation the arteries draw into the body the outside air through the openings that extend to the skin, for three purposes: to cool, to fan, and to generate psychic pneuma'.[57] When they contract, the arteries squeeze out smoky and sooty humours.

51 *PHP* 8.8.1–2 de Lacy (5.708K) and 8.8.12 de Lacy (5.710K). The target passage here is presumably *Ti.* 79B–80C; see Furley and Wilkie (1984: 7–9). See also de Lacy (1972: 33–5) for an overview of Platonic errors and the grounds for his inferiority to Hippocrates, according to Galen.

52 *PHP* 8.8.15–17 de Lacy (5.710–11K)=*Ti.* 79A–C.

53 The difference between the two will be discussed in the process of examining the pneumatic system. See Section 3.5 for the conclusion regarding this.

54 There is, however, a mention of cupping in the *Timaeus* (*Ti.* 79E–80A). Both practices are often used as examples when arguing for the existence of *horror vacui* (see, for example, Ps. Alexander of Aphrodisias *Pr.* 2.59; for further discussion of this passage, see Meeusen (2020: 94)). Perhaps Galen misremembered which one was mentioned in the *Timaeus*.

55 Hero *Spir. proem.* 86–91 Schmidt. Philo of Byzantium's *Pneumatica* survives in fragments and translations; Arabic translation of 4.a describes wine tasting via a tube; see Prager (1974: 130).

56 *UP* 7.9 (1.399, 13–14 Helmreich=3.549K), see also Chapter 4.

57 *PHP* 8.8.7 de Lacy (5.709K), tr. de Lacy (1978–84: 529).

Thus, the body is supplied with air not only via two different sets of organs but also via two different motions: one psychic and one physical, voluntary and involuntary, respectively. The reason why two types of breathing are necessary for the body is laid out clearly at the end of *On the Usefulness of Respiration*. Whereas all of the body is able to breathe sufficiently through the arteries, there are two special organs of breathing, the lungs and the nostrils, serving two central organs – the heart and the brain, respectively.[58] Galen proceeds to explain the importance of the system that moderates the innate heat for the sake of the maintenance of life as follows:

> τῶν μὲν οὖν ἄλλων ὀργάνων αἱ βλάβαι τῶν ἐνεργειῶν μικραί, τῶν δ᾽ εἰς αὐτὴν τὴν ζωὴν διαφερόντων μεγάλαι, τῶν δ᾽ οὐ μόνον εἰς αὐτὴν τὴν ζωὴν διαφερόντων, ἀλλὰ καὶ πρὸς τὰ ἄλλα λόγον ἀρχῆς ἐχόντων μέγισται. τοιαῦτα δ᾽ ἐστὶν ἐγκέφαλός τε καὶ καρδία. ὥσθ᾽ ἡ τούτων τῆς κατασκευῆς βλάβη παραχρῆμα βλάψει τὴν ζωήν. ἀλλ᾽ οὐδὲν ὑπαλλάττειν αὐτὴν οἷον τέ ἐστιν ἑτοιμότερον ἀμέτρου θερμασίας. ὥστε ἄμφω δέδεικται διὰ τοῦ λόγου τοῦδε, τό χρήσιμον τῆς συμμέτρου θερμασίας <καὶ> τὸ ἐν τῇ ἀναπνοῇ εἰς αὐτήν.
>
> Injuries to the activities of other organs are minor; injuries to those essential to life are great; but injuries to those that not only are essential to life but also have the status of principles with respect to the others are the greatest: and such are the brain and the heart. So injury to the composition of these will immediately injure life. But nothing is able to change it more readily than immoderate heat. So both the value of heat in moderation and of breathing in regard to this have been shown by the argument.[59]

Thus, Galen makes it quite clear that both types of breathing are required to maintain the vitality. Respiration helps to ensure the proper heat regulation in the key governing organs, while transpiration serves the rest of the body. This conclusion naturally raises the further question of how breathing contributes to the functioning of the body. In other words, what purpose does breathing accomplish to make it so crucial to vitality that even a relatively brief cessation poses the risk

[58] *Ut. Resp.* 5.4 (126 Furley and Wilkie=4.506K).

[59] *Ut. Resp.* 5.6 (128 Furley and Wilkie=4.508K), tr. Furley and Wilkie (1984: 129). Galen also wrote a separate treatise specifically dedicated to the topic of the innate heat, but it is not extant; see Durling (1988) for a reconstruction of the lost treatise. The very notion of the innate heat, of course, precedes Galen. An extensive study dedicated to this notion in antiquity is Mendelsohn (1964).

of death? Galen's attempts to answer this question are discussed in Section 3.2.

3.2 The Vital Pneuma and the Purpose of Breathing

When it comes to breathing, Galen outlines succinctly the most important puzzle at the very beginning of *On the Usefulness of Respiration*: the great usefulness of respiration is evident from the fact that animals are unable to survive once their respiration is in some way obstructed. But what makes respiration so fundamental to animal vitality? Galen starts his enquiry by presenting an overview of the prominent theories of his predecessors.[60] Asclepiades maintained that breathing is the source of the soul. According to Praxagoras, it is a kind of nourishment for the soul. Philiston and Diocles claimed that breathing is useful for the cooling of the innate heat. Hippocrates' view is a kind of combination of the latter two views: the use of breathing is both nourishment and cooling. Finally, Erasistratus stated that its purpose is to replenish arteries. Galen notes that some of these views, although they appear different, have the same outcome. For example, claiming that breathing strengthens the innate heat and claiming that it fans the innate heat amounts to the same view: breathing maintains the innate heat.[61] Thus, all the listed theories pertain either to the substance of the inspired air or to its quality.[62] If pneuma is called either nourishment or the substance of the soul or the filling of arteries, then animals breathe in order to supply substance to their bodies. Fanning, strengthening or cooling, meanwhile, concerns quality, and in that case, animals breathe for the sake of some qualitative alteration by means of pneuma. Thus, Galen narrows down the focus of the treatise to the question of whether pneuma is useful because of its substance or because of its quality.[63]

60 That Galen's selection and report is quite odd in general was noted in van der Eijk (2001: 63–4), with a suggestion that Galen might have been engaging with a doxographic tradition.

61 *Ut. Resp.* 1.2 (80 Furley and Wilkie=4.471K).

62 Although this appears to be a Galenic classification, see Lewis and Gregoric (2015: 144–5) for an argument that *De Spiritu* is a predecessor for this division. Strictly speaking, in Galenic text, the Asclepiadean theory could be put into the third category, because it has more far-reaching consequences than any of the other substance theories. Yet Galen puts Asclepiades' theory aside (ultimately grouping him with the substance theorists) as impossible to investigate due to the fact that the substance of the soul is unknown. He acknowledges that there appears to be a connection between the soul and breathing, because breathing maintains life, but it is not something that one can understand fully without knowing the substance of the soul.

63 'Both' is also an option and, to an extent, Galen's account ends up being a combination of these answers, although he clearly thinks that the primary purpose is the latter.

From early on in the treatise, it is quite clear that Galen favours the latter. His advocacy of his preferred option consists of giving explanations of certain scenarios in a polemical manner. For example, the investigation begins with the argument that humans suffocate when they breathe in and hold the breath. This shows that the use of breathing is not just the substance of air but also some of its qualities.[64] But presenting an explanation is not enough; Galen also sets out to refute the rival accounts.

His main rival in this case, and mostly throughout the rest of the treatise, is the Alexandrian doctor Erasistratus. His explanation is steeped in a distinctively Erasistratean understanding of human physiology, and thus, Galen is killing two birds with one stone: advocating both his account of respiration and his understanding of the principles governing human physiology. According to Erasistratus, a person suffocates while holding breath with lungs full of air because the heart cannot draw air from the lungs when breathing stops. The heart cannot draw the air owing to the principle of *horror vacui*.[65] If the heart draws in some air, the place previously occupied by that air would become empty, which is impossible.[66]

Galen pivots his rejection of the Erasistratean account on the attack of *horror vacui*. The rebuttal consists of three arguments. Only the last is presented as his own, the first two criticisms come from unnamed critics of Erasistratus. First, they point out that he only proves that the void does not exist *en masse* while the possibility that it might be dispersed throughout the solid bodies remains.[67] Second, these critics point out that the substance could stretch out in all directions, thus filling up greater space. This criticism is less obvious and deserves to be unpacked. Erasistratus' *horror vacui*-driven physiology relies of the constant replacement of matter as an operating principle. The impossibility of void motivates the replacement of one amount of matter by another amount of matter, and this change constitutes various physiological processes.[68] The critics, however, point

[64] *Ut. Resp.* 2.1 (82 Furley and Wilkie=4.473K).

[65] I am describing this as a principle because, as Berryman (1997) shows, there is no good evidence to suppose it was a theory; see also Berryman (2009: 166–70) for some problems with the conjecture about the unity of this theory, originally proposed by Diels (1893). See also Debru (1996: 53–60) and Vallance (1990: 62–78).

[66] *Ut. Resp.* 2.1 (84 Furley and Wilkie=4.473K).

[67] *Ut. Resp.* 2.2 (84 Furley and Wilkie=4.474K), see also *Nat. Fac.* 2.6 (173, 10–19 Helmreich=2.99K) and Adamson (2014: 204–5) for the reconstruction of Erasistratus' argument.

[68] Constant change is, of course, a premise in Galenic medicine as well, except that it is the qualitative change of mixture, triggered by various external and internal factors; see, for example, *San. Tu.* 1.5.5–6 Koch (6.14K).

out that, in principle, there is no reason to suppose that one amount of matter is being replaced with another rather than, for instance, that very same amount of matter stretches over a larger space, thus becoming thinner. The air could move from the lungs to the heart by extending.[69] Although he presents this argument, Galen is not necessarily an advocate of the stretching-matter explanation. A little later in the treatise, he puts this option aside, saying that this debate is too inconclusive on both sides.[70] But these arguments of the critics are enough to show that Erasistratus' views have a history of refutations, and then Galen adds one of his own to this collection.

His argument is more anatomical than philosophical. Galen points out that Erasistratus' scenario would entail the heart not moving the entire time when the breath is held, but this is not the case.[71] He also eliminates the possible objections and alternative accounts, namely, the counter-argument of the followers of Erasistratus stating that the heart only draws from the great artery rather than from the lungs,[72] and the argument that the heart does not contract or dilate but only oscillates, associated with Asclepiades and his followers.[73] The Erasistrateans are refuted by drawing attention to the fact that the valves of the heart prevent it from drawing the blood from the great artery, and this point was shown by Erasistratus himself.[74] In addition to this, Galen points out that, according to Erasistratus' own anatomy, nothing ought to prevent the heart from drawing air from the lungs, because he agrees that the thorax is moved voluntarily, which means that it ought to be possible to constrict the thorax on all sides and move the air from the lungs to the heart while keeping the upper part of the thorax closed.[75] In order to refute the Asclepiadeans, Galen presents an overview of the movements of arteries during the suspension of breathing, showing that it is impossible for arteries to either stop working (as would be the case

69 Especially given that it is a λεπτομερὲς body. This term, especially prominent in Galenic pharmacology (see Debru 1997), is also applicable to pneuma; see *MM* 12.5 (10.843K).
70 *Ut. Resp.* 2.5 (86 Furley and Wilkie=4.476K).
71 *Ut. Resp.* 2.5 (86–8 Furley and Wilkie=4.476–7K).
72 *Ut. Resp.* 2.3 (86 Furley and Wilkie=4.475K).
73 *Ibid.* Galen calls this view foolish and already refuted by Athenaeus, while providing his own refutation nonetheless.
74 *Ut. Resp.* 2.4 (86 Furley and Wilkie=4.475–6K). See also Adamson (2014: 199–200).
75 *Ut. Resp.* 2.6 (88 Furley and Wilkie=4.477–8K). To reinforce the conclusion that it is, in fact, possible for the air to move from the lungs to the heart while holding one's breath, Galen offers an experiment. One only needs to breathe in, hold the breath and notice that the heart beats during that time.

if the heart merely oscillated) or that the movement in the arteries doubles in such cases.[76]

These refutations support the main argument of the treatise, namely, the heart requires not the substance but the quality of pneuma. The argument is further reinforced by counterfactuals: if the opposite were true, the large quantity of air breathed in (i.e., overabundance) would not cause greater distress.[77] The desire to breathe out while holding one's breath shows that one requires more than just the substance of pneuma.[78] The expansion of heart and arteries while a person is holding breath shows that there is no lack of pneuma in the body, and therefore suffocation takes place not by the lack of its substance but its quality.

Not all of the scenarios Galen presents are preoccupied with anatomy. One of the more vivid case studies is the phenomenon when people suffocate in the Charonian pits, newly whitewashed houses and so on.[79] The Erasistratus-style explanation is that the air is so thin in these places that it cannot be contained in the arteries, and consequently death due to the lack of pneuma ensues. Galen rejects this explanation by arguing that it provides no reason why the air becomes thin in these conditions to begin with, or how arteries cannot contain air, or that there is not a different cause that is harder to discover. Furthermore, the motion in the arteries in these conditions is not observed to be changing.[80] His own explanation – that the quality of pneuma in these locations is altered, making respiration impossible – fits the bill much better. Thus we again arrive at the conclusion that the respiration maintains vitality primarily owing to the elemental qualities of pneuma rather than its substance.[81]

[76] *Ut. Resp.* 2.9 (92 Furley and Wilkie=4.480–1K). He also attacks the Erasistrateans who – against Erasistratus' own views – appear to be unable to determine that the arteries are emptied out during the suspension of breathing (*Ut. Resp.* 2.10 (94 Furley and Wilkie=4.482K)).

[77] *Ut. Resp.* 2.7 (90 Furley and Wilkie=4.479K).

[78] *Ut. Resp.* 2.8 (92 Furley and Wilkie=4.480K).

[79] *Ut. Resp.* 4.3 (112 Furley and Wilkie=4.496K). See also *UP* 7.8 (1.392, 25–393, 6 Helmreich=540–1K), tr. May (1968: 346–7):

> Now when it becomes necessary to account for suitable and unsuitable qualities in air, Erasistratus for some reason or other says that they are caused by its thinness or thickness and supposes that this is the reason why people die in Charonian caverns or in houses freshly coated with lime, and why some die of [inhaling] the odor of burning charcoal or other such vapors, viz. they die because the air, being too thin, cannot be retained in the body.

[80] *Ut. Resp.* 4.3 (114 Furley and Wilkie=4.497K).

[81] As ever with Galen, there is a caveat to this. Galen hastens to add that he only rules out that the replenishment of the substance of pneuma is the sole use of respiration. He intends to show that humans suffocate when deprived of breath because the substance of the psychic pneuma is not replenished, and therefore his argument so far does not rule out the possibility that the psychic pneuma is nourished by respiration; see *Ut. Resp.* 2.11 (96 Furley and Wilkie=4.484K).

3.2.1 *The Innate Heat: The Flame Model*

Having determined that pneuma must act qualitatively, Galen sets out to elucidate the details: what are the qualities that pneuma supplies? One might suppose that pneuma acts by cooling,[82] because of the desire to breathe in deeply during febrile illnesses. However, the desire to breathe in occurs during chilling diseases as well.[83] After an interlude,[84] Galen considers what is common in all of the views that maintain that the primary use of respiration is qualitative change.[85] He states that, although these theories are not all clear or articulate, they all refer to the preservation of the innate heat, modelled on the phenomenon of the flames in the following way:

> ταύτας γὰρ ἐναργῶς ὁρῶμεν οὕτως ταχέως ἀπολλυμένας, ὅταν ἀποστερηθῶσιν ἀέρος, ὥσπερ τὰ ζῷα, καθάπερ δηλοῦσιν αἱ τῶν ἰατρῶν σικύαι καὶ πάνθ' ὅσα στεγανὰ καὶ κοῖλα περιτεθέντα τῆς <τε> διαπνοῆς αὐτὰς εἴρξαντα ῥᾳδίως κατασβέννυσιν. ἂν τοίνυν εὑρεθῇ, τί ποτε φλόγες ἐν ταῖς τοιαύταις διαθέσεσι πάσχουσαι σβέννυνται, τάχα ἂν εὑρεθείη, τί ποτέ ἐστιν ὃ παρὰ τῆς ἀναπνοῆς ἀπολαύει χρηστὸν ἡ ἐν τοῖς ζῴοις θερμασία.
>
> For these we clearly see perishing when they are deprived of air, just as quickly as animals; as is shown by the cupping instruments of medical men, and by all closed and hollow vessels, which readily extinguish the flames when, placed about them, they cut them off from the draught. If it could be discovered what happens to flames in these circumstances to quench them, it would perhaps be discovered/what that useful something is in breathing, from which the natural heat in animals profits.[86]

This is a striking passage, primarily because Galen puts a finger on the exact issue at stake. The reason why a covered flame goes out and the reason why animals die when deprived of breath is the same from a

82 This is the view of Diocles and Philiston, described at the beginning of the treatise.

83 *Ut. Resp.* 3.2 (98 Furley and Wilkie=4.484–5K).

84 He launches an attack on unnamed doctors who maintain that the body always requires chilling from breathing but to a different extent. This stance, however, is dismissed on the grounds of methodological inconsistencies rendering the position hard to evaluate. The contradiction is as follows: commenting on the Hippocratic saying from *Prognostics* that the cold breathed out of the nose and mouth is fatal, these doctors end up concluding that, in certain chilled conditions, breathing is not necessary at all (*Ut. Resp.* 3.3 (100 Furley and Wilkie=4.486K)). Instead, breathing kindles by fanning, which, Galen points out, is a different kind of action altogether (*Ut. Resp.* 3.4 (100 Furley and Wilkie=4.486–7K)).

85 To be more elaborate, it is the thermal balance in the *krasis* brought about by the regulating qualitative change, as the discussion in this section shows.

86 *Ut. Resp.* 3.5 (102 Furley and Wilkie=4.487–8K), tr. Furley and Wilkie (1984: 103).

biochemical point of view. Although Galen could not possibly have known the precise details, the process of combustion in a candle and respiration in an organism's cell starts when fuel (let us say, a piece of wood and glucose, respectively) reacts with oxygen, releasing by-products (thermal heat, light and water in combustion, and water, carbon dioxide and energy in the case of respiration). The deprivation of oxygen naturally stops both chemical reactions.

As Galen does not explain explicitly how he conceives the similarities of the two processes, one might be justified in concluding that this analogy is just a lucky accident. And indeed, any doctor in antiquity would have lacked the means to explain the biochemical reaction. It is nonetheless hard to deny the easy observability of the fact that healthy animal bodies are warm, while ill or dead bodies are cold, and the loss of breath (and nutriment) leads to the latter state. Thus, a conjecture that there is a process in animal bodies analogous to the burning of a flame is likely based on observation.

Galen, moreover, theorises the nature of the 'burning' process in the human body on the basis of various empirical observations. Using this method, he argues that respiration must both kindle and extinguish the warmth in the body, the innate heat. He starts by listing the ways in which flames can be extinguished,[87] including baths, excessive fanning, too much stuff heaped onto them or the lack of sustenance. In order to continue, the innate heat must not be increased to an extreme degree, nor must it be cooled by fanning, nor deprived of sustenance. These conditions are ensured by the two-fold motions, just like the motion of flame that moves not only upwards but also downwards, for sustenance.[88] It is destroyed when it is deprived of matter or one of its motions. For this reason, he concludes, every flame requires its surroundings to be cold in due proportion,[89] because excessive heat or cold quenches it.[90]

[87] See Debru (1996: 140–2) for the relevant Aristotelian background and the argument that Galen's model is more fleshed out.

[88] *Ut. Resp.* 3.6 (102–4 Furley and Wilkie=4.488–9K).

[89] The 'due proportion' is generally an important concept in ancient physiology, even if it might strike the modern eye as vague. See *San. Tu.* 1.5.1–12 Koch (6.13–15K), where Galen claims that all medical sects agree that health is *summetria* of some kind, even though they disagree of what exactly. The influx and the outflux of food and air are the central processes that any medical theory had to explain. See Debru (1996: 163–6) for a discussion of how the term is used in the preceding medical tradition.

[90] Although he meant to discuss the phenomenon of flames only at this point, Galen gets ahead of himself and also adds that the cupping instrument is one of the ways of making the inward motion of the flame excessive by preventing the air – overheated by the innate flame – from going outside. This remark foreshadows the explanation of the cycles of the innate heat.

The heat and its environment form a kind of small ecological system, maintained for as long as there is a *summetria*, as certain proportionality, in their qualities. In addition to the qualitative maintenance, there is also nourishment. In the living beings, the innate heat is kindled from blood (the standard nutriment).[91] This point is also illustrated with a lamp analogy as follows: the heart is like the wick, the blood is like the oil and the lungs are like the lamp cover.[92] Respiration both fans and cools the innate heat to an appropriate degree, while the motion helps to empty out the 'smokiness' from the 'combustion of the blood'.[93] At this point, Galen adds that this is not a science or demonstration but a persuasive account.[94] The main reason to choose this explanation is that its rivals are weaker and suffer from some fatal flaws.[95]

3.2.2 Bipartite Motions

Although the existence of the innate heat is rarely debated among the ancient theorists, its origins are. *On Tremor, Rigor, Palpitation and Spasm* presents a polemical defence of the Galenic account. While discussing rigor, an affection of the innate heat, he contrasts two theories accounting for the phenomenon of heat in the body. The first type of account is

[91] The whole process of nutrition, including the crucial role of blood, is described in *Nat. Fac.* 1.10–11 (115–119 Helmreich=2.20–6K); see also the discussion in Chapter 2.

[92] He adds that breathing out serves to empty out the smoky vapour, just like in the account of transpiration and respiration in *On the Doctrines of Hippocrates and Plato.*

[93] This motion is technically transpiration, as it happens in the arteries; see the later discussion about the differences between respiration and transpiration.

[94] Towards the end of the treatise, he concedes that he found no conclusions that follow necessarily; instead, his theory is based on persuasive conclusions and the fact that it has no counterexamples (*Ut. Resp.* 4.5 (116 Furley and Wilkie=4.498K)). Then Galen provides a couple of cases that his theory is able to explain, for example, breathing more deeply during exercise is due to the increase of heat in those who move more vigorously (*Ut. Resp.* 4.5 (116 Furley and Wilkie=4.498K)). The same reasons motivate the desire to breathe deeply when suffering from burning fevers (*Ut. Resp.* 4.5 (118 Furley and Wilkie=4.499K)). In addition to these, Galen's theory accounts for why children breathe more deeply and rapidly. Interestingly, he notes that the theory that breathing is the nourishment of the psychic pneuma helps to explain this phenomenon, because growing children need more nourishment (*Ut. Resp.* 4.6 (118 Furley and Wilkie=4.500K); see also *PHP* 8.7.8–13 de Lacy (5.703–5K)). He adds that this is a more general principle and one can find people living in hotter climates breathing more deeply and rapidly. Similarly, those who have just eaten or drunk breathe more deeply due to the constrained diaphragm as do pregnant women and those who suffer from water or phlegm in the stomach, liver or spleen (*Ut. Resp.* 4.7 (120 Furley and Wilkie=4.501K)). On Galen's notion of the persuasive, see Chiaradonna (2014), who argues that this notion derives from Empiricism, and Tieleman (forthcoming), who shows how the academic inheritance in this use of the term underpins the concept of fallibilistic science methodology.

[95] *Ut. Resp.* 3.10 (108 Furley and Wilkie=4.492K).

atomistic, and Galen introduced it polemically, by stating that he does not posit corpuscles and pores as the elements of the body (οὐκ ὄγκους καὶ πόρους ἡμῶν στοιχεῖα τιθεμένων τοῦ σώματος). This statement is a clear reference to Asclepiades, his followers and other comparable atomist doctors,[96] whose account of fevers was discussed earlier in the treatise. The theories of this kind maintain that the innate heat comes from friction or motion.[97] Without delving into details, Galen introduces the second – his own – account as follows: 'we suppose the whole body breathing and flowing together, the heat not acquired nor subsequent to the generation of the animal, but itself first and original and innate. This is nothing other than the nature and soul of life, so that you would not be wrong thinking heat to be self-moving and constantly moving substance.'[98]

Galen paints a clear contrast between the mechanistic and the vitalist understanding of the human body. The innate heat is not a product of a mechanistic process but a fundamental, primal part of animal physiology. His point is the same as in the arguments advocating for the existence of the innate natural capacities,[99] although in this case the issue at stake is not so much capacity as the elemental quality itself. The most striking aspect is calling the activity of this elemental quality 'the soul' and 'the nature'. The term 'soul' presumably ought to be understood as the spirited soul, the crux of animal vitality. The distinguishing feature of animal life, then, is the heat in the body. It is not, however, the only property that separates animals from plants. The more extensive description in another passage of the same treatise shows another way to understand the centrality of heat to animality, that is, motion.

[96] See *Trem. Palp.* 6 (7.615K), where Galen not only names Asclepiades as someone who denies the existence of the innate capacities and instead posits corpuscles and pores for explaining the origins of fever, but also notes that Asclepiades ought not to be singled out, for there are more doctors claiming the innate heat to be a product of a clearly identifiable mechanistic process.

[97] Seemingly the same view is rejected in *PHP* 7.7.4 de Lacy (5.702K). Here, more details are supplied, indicating that it is the friction of the particles of pneuma in the arteries that is supposed to produce the heat in an animal's body.

[98] *Trem. Palp.* 6 (7.616K), tr. Sider and McVaugh (1979: 199): ἀλλὰ τὸ μὲν ὅλον σῶμα σύμπνουν τε καὶ σύῤῥουν ἡγουμένων, τὸ θερμὸν δ' οὐκ ἐπίκτητον οὐδ' ὕστερον τοῦ ἡγουμένων, τὸ θερμὸν δ' οὐκ ἐπίκτητον οὐδ' ὕστερον τοῦ ζώου τῆς γενέσεως, ἀλλ' αὐτὸ πρῶτόν τε καὶ ἀρχέγονον καὶ ἔμφυτον. καὶ ἥ γε φύσις καὶ ἡ ψυχὴ οὐδὲν ἄλλο ἢ τοῦτ' ἔστιν, ὥστ' οὐσίαν αὐτοκίνητόν τε καὶ ἀεικίνητον αὐτὸ νοῶν οὐκ ἂν ἁμάρτοις.

[99] The capacities (*dunameis*) of the air, he explains, are just like the capacity of the numbing fish to numb anyone who touches it. This is not an uncontroversial theory, as Galen notes that some doctors deny that such qualities and capacities exist. *Ut. Resp.* 4.4 (116 Furley and Wilkie=4.497–8K). See also the references to Galen's attack on Erasistratus in *On the Natural Capacities* cited earlier.

A key aspect of the innate heat is its motion, and this motion is sustained by the two-fold directions. If it moved only inwards or only outwards, it would soon extinguish itself. The motion downwards allows the heat to gain sustenance, and thus it is kindled. Moving upwards, it disperses in all directions, thus quenching itself.[100] By being at one moment kindled, at another quenched, it persists. The underlying causes of both motions are elemental properties. The motion upwards is due to the inherent hot quality in the innate heat; its ability to move downwards, meanwhile, is due to a portion of cold in its mixture. The result is a self-sufficient cycle as follows:

> κατὰ μὲν τὸν πρῶτον λόγον τοῦ θερμοῦ, τοῦτ᾽ ἔστι αὐτοκίνητον αὐτοῦ, καὶ τούτου μάλιστα δεῖται πρὸς τὰς ἐνεργείας· μεγάλην δ᾽ ὅμως αὐτῷ χρείαν καὶ τὸ ψυχρὸν παρέχει. πέφυκε γὰρ τὸ μὲν θερμὸν εἰς ὕψος αἴρεσθαι καὶ συμπροσάγειν αὐτῷ τὴν τροφήν· εἰ δὲ μὴ τὸ ψυχρὸν ἐμποδὼν ἐγένετο, καὶ ἐπὶ μήκιστον προῆκε. γίνεται δ᾽ ἐμποδὼν τὸ ψυχρὸν τῇ τοιαύτῃ τοῦ θερμοῦ κινήσει, ὡς μὴ ἀπόλοιτο ἐκτεινόμενον. κίνδυνος γὰρ ὑπὸ κουφότητος καὶ τῆς πρὸς τὸ ἄνω ὁρμῆς ἀποστῆναι τῶν σωμάτων αὐτό. ἀλλὰ τὸ ψυχρὸν ἐπέχει τε καὶ κωλύει, καὶ τῆς ἄγαν ταύτης κινήσεως ἀφαιρεῖ τὸ σφοδρόν.

> Owing to the primal principle of heat, it is self-moved, and this is very necessary for its activities; but the cold is equally of great usefulness to it as well. For the heat is disposed by nature to rise upwards and bring together with it nourishment, and if the cold did not come in its way, it would escape to the greatest heights. But the cold does stand in the way of this motion of the heat, so that it would not be destroyed by dispersing. For there is danger of it leaving bodies due to its lightness and inclination to move upwards. But the cold holds, hinders and reduces the strength of this excessive motion.[101]

This passage gives an outstandingly clear account of how elemental properties govern the self-sustaining cycle of the innate heat. The property of coldness allows motion downwards towards the sustenance, and the property of hotness allows motion upwards, which, dispersing the heat, sustains the equal temperature. At the same time, the passage confusingly does not identify the substance (in the Stoic sense of the term) of the innate heat. What material or tissue exactly contains the elemental

[100] *Trem. Palp.* 6 (7.616–7K).

[101] *Trem. Palp.* 6 (7.617–18K), tr. after Sider and McVaugh (1979: 200). It is worth noting that the phrase '*kata proton logon*' is standard in Galen, and it refers to the original design and purpose of a part set by the designing demiurge; see van der Eijk (2020: 83–4). See also discussion of the notion of a demiurge in Chapter 2.

composition that allows for this motion? Pneuma must be a part of the answer. In *On the Doctrines of Hippocrates and Plato*, Galen writes that most heat in a body is to be found in blood and pneuma.[102] Yet this must be only a partial answer. When, immediately following this passage, he turns to discuss the illness of the innate heat, he gives the list of afflictions caused by the predominance of the heat as follows: inflammations, erysipelas, herpes, carbuncles, burning fevers and all the feverish affections.[103] The list contains localised afflictions of various tissues (most unrelated to respiration). Thus, the substance of the innate heat cannot be only pneumatic in nature. All the tissues have to constitute the substance of the innate heat for these diagnoses to be possible. Yet most tissues do not have a circular motion described in the preceding passage. This potential contradiction can be resolved with the help of another, not yet discussed, division of the body into parts. It helps to explain that the innate heat, although residing in all the tissues, does not manifest itself in the same way in all of them.

3.2.3 *Fevers and the Viscosity of Parts*

The division of parts in question separates the body into solids, fluids and pneumata.[104] It is not a common distinction, primarily only found in the context of describing afflictions of the innate heat, especially fevers. At the same time, the study of fevers is no niche subject; it forms an important part of ancient medical lore. Unlike the contemporary understanding of a fever, the ancient notion encompassed a variety of conditions that involved elevated body heat. Galen defines it as an increase of heat that harms the healthy activity or functioning and causes distress, noting that an increase of heat in the body without these symptoms does not constitute a febrile state.[105] Such a diagnosis was common and, in the world where means for effective temperature regulation were not available, signified a potentially life-threatening condition. He dedicates a significant part of his *On the*

[102] *PHP* 7.7.7 de Lacy (5.703K).

[103] *Trem. Palp.* 6 (7.618K): φλεγμοναὶ μὲν οὖν καὶ ἐρυσιπέλατα καὶ ἕρπητες καὶ ἄνθρακες καὶ τὰ καυσώδη καὶ φλογώδη καὶ πάντα τὰ πυρετώδη πάθη.

[104] Although Galen consistently maintains that the division of the body into solids, fluids and pneumata is Hippocratic (see note 49 in the Introduction; see also Gundert (1992, 2000: 15)), the specific view that the pneuma is a substance affected first and thus it plays the key role in health and illness is also the central doctrine of the Pneumatists; see Ps. Galen *Int.* 9.6 (22, 12–17 Petit=14.699K).

[105] *MM* 8.1 (10.532K).

Therapeutic Method to distinguish and classify different types of fevers,[106] and his discussion makes it clear that the treatment of these illnesses can be very difficult, owing to the fact that some of them profoundly affect the constitution of the body.[107] Consequently, the treatment must take into account multiple factors, making sure that it does not result in accidental injury to another vital system.[108] One of the clearest discussions of the way in which fever can injure vitality can be found in the small treatise *On the Differences of Fever.*

At the beginning of this treatise, Galen divides fevers, which he defines as heating against nature, in reference to their substance: (1) in accordance to more or less; (2) the matter in which the heat against nature is located; and (3) the direction of the movement of the heat.[109] Noting that the first type is a very familiar way of identifying fevers (and other illnesses), he focuses on explaining the difference between the last two. The second type refers to the cases when the body of the heart itself is taken over by the heat against nature or when humours are clinging to the ventricles of the heart.[110] The third type refers to the cases when the pneumata in the body are overheated, but the solids and fluids are not.

Thus, he implicitly differentiates between the fevers according to what type of tissue they settle in. This reading can be corroborated with a claim in *On the Therapeutic Method* where he states this explicitly, also adding an important piece of information: it is possible for one type of fever to change into another type.[111] The changes of heat in different tissues explain not only how one type of fever changes into another but also how all the different types originate, and both of these explanations refer to the same division of bodily matter into solids, fluids and pneumata. Galen introduces it as follows:

106 A useful summary and overview can be found in Brain (1986: 10–13); as in most other areas, Galen presents himself as a follower of Hippocratic fever lore. See Yeo (2002) for a discussion of how Galen reads and reinterprets Hippocratic *Epidemics 6*. A common (although not uncontroversial) fever treatment in ancient medicine was bloodletting; Brain (1986: 158–72) also contains an illuminating discussion of the possible benefits of this treatment.

107 *MM* 8.1 (10.533K). Fevers can also be very light and in *San. Tu.* 1.5.27–9 Koch (6.19–20K), he employs this example for criticising doctors for the claim that seeds of diseases (τὰ σπέρματα τῶν νόσων) are present in people. Using the case of the light fever, Galen argues that health and disease have to be defined in reference to pain and harm to the vital functioning (κατὰ τὸν βίον ἐνεργείαις).

108 *MM* 9.10 (10.637–8K). This passage makes some important claims regarding the unity of central physiological systems, for which see Section 5.3.1.

109 *Diff. Feb.* 1 (7.275K).

110 In *Cur. Rat. Ven. Sect.* 5 (11.264–5K), this condition is identified as fever arising from the putrefaction of humours.

111 *MM* 9.1 (10.600K).

ῥᾴστη μὲν οὖν ἡ ἐκ τῶν ὑγρῶν εἰς τὸ πνεῦμα μετάληψις τῆς θερμότητος, ἧττον δ' ἑτοίμως τῷ πνεύματι συνεκπυροῦται τὰ ὑγρά. καὶ μέν γε καὶ τὸ στερεὸν σῶμα τοῖς ὑγροῖς τε καὶ ἀερώδεσιν ἑτοιμότερον μεταδίδωσι τῆς θερμασίας ἢ αὐτὸ παρ' ἐκείνων λαμβάνει· πᾶσα μὲν γὰρ ἡ λεπτομερὴς οὐσία ῥᾷον ἀλλοιοῦται τῆς παχυμεροῦς· ἔστι δὲ λεπτομερεστάτη μὲν ἡ τοῦ ἀέρος, παχυμερεστάτη δὲ ἡ τῶν στερεῶν σωμάτων, ἐν τῷ μεταξὺ δὲ ἀμφοῖν ἡ τῶν ὑγρῶν.

And while the change of heat from fluids into pneuma is most easy, the fluids heat up less readily than the pneumata. And indeed, the solid body gives a share of heat to the fluids and airy [substances] more readily than it takes from the others; for all the fine substance undergoes qualitative change more easily than the thick; and the finest substance is that of air, while the thickest is that of the solid bodies, and in between these two is the substance of the fluids.[112]

The passage describes the speed with which differently textured tissues undergo thermal change: pneuma changes quickly, solid parts slowly, and fluids somewhere in between. The behaviour of tissues is determined by their textural properties. The finer the tissues are, the more readily they undergo changes. As a result, they transmit heat to each other asymmetrically, namely a solid part can heat up pneuma easily but not the other way around. The alterations in pneuma cause the bipartite motions of the innate heat. In healthy states, the solid parts undergo the heating and cooling cycle, with the very minute motion, if any. The liquid parts are presumably more prone to motion, but not significantly so. When pneumata comes into contact with the solid and the liquid parts in which the heat is, let us say, kindled, it is heated too. However, owing to the very fine texture, pneuma is also more volatile, and this heat also results in more motion, prompting it to move outwards, which ultimately manifests itself as an exhalation. Pneuma, thus, enables the bipartite 'motion' of the innate heat in the parts that do not move themselves, by moving kinetically on behalf of them, prompted by the qualitative alteration in these parts. The interactions between tissues generate a single phenomenon: the temperature of the body or the innate heat. It is the combined warmth of all the body parts that is manifest to tactile sensation.[113] The bipartite motions of the pneuma correspond with qualitative changes in solid and liquid parts, producing a single unified thermal state in the body.

[112] *Diff. Feb.* 2 (7.277–8K), tr. mine. See also *CC* 4.2–4 Lyons and *Us. Puls.* 7.7–8 (224–6 Furley and Wilkie=5.178K).
[113] *Temp.* 1.6 (21, 5–9 Helmreich=1.541–2K).

It is important that it is pneuma that moves and not any of the other parts. The excessive heat and 'motion' resulting from it is pathological, especially in solid parts. A passage from *Advice for an Epileptic Boy* illustrates this point clearly. In this passage, Galen prescribes an exercise regime to an epileptic boy, noting that the master ought to keep it moderate or, to be more precise, prescribe it proportionately (συμμέτρως). This term clearly refers not only to numerically expressible proportion but also functionality. The exercise has to be moderated with two purposes in mind: warming up the body and not overheating it. The former is necessary to rid the body of superfluity (τὸ περιττόν), that is, the by-products of nutrition. This process is carried out by the capacities in the tissues of numerous internal organs.[114] Galen's advice indicates the body needs to be warmed up so that this process, primarily dependent on the alterative capacity, can take place. The other pathological extreme is overheating. Once a body is exercised to this state, the solid parts of the body are affected, and their shapes melt together (τῶν στερεῶν σωμάτων καὶ συντήκει τὴν ἕξιν), with the molten humoral matter (τὰ συντήγματα) gathering in joints and muscles and causing pain as well as fatigue.[115]

The solid parts require some innate heat in order to carry out qualitative alteration, but they also undergo change and even, in some sense, motion under the circumstances of excessive heat. Owing to the thickness of these parts, their 'motion' is fairly minute, primarily consisting in the dislocation of 'melting' tissues and the deformation of the functional shapes of organs, but it has a dangerous effect. This particular pathology is caused by motion, but excessive heat in the body can be brought about by numerous external and internal circumstances, including emotions.[116] Presumably, the reason why the division of parts in accordance to viscosity primarily appears in discussions of fevers is as follows: they are the illnesses of heat regulation and the stakes of healthy heat regulation are most clear in pathological cases.

The flow of pneuma into and out of the body is, therefore, crucial for its healthy functioning, and some portion of pneuma must reach every part of the body very regularly. While some of this flux takes place by means of respiration, pneuma also enters the body by means of involuntary motion of the arteries. The following section explores further the

[114] *Nat. Fac.* 1.10–11 (115–119 Helmreich=2.20–6K). [115] *Puer. Epil.* 3 (11.362–3K).
[116] For example, grief and sleeplessness in *MM* 10.5 (10.687K).

differences between transpiration and respiration as well as summarises the significance of the vital pneuma that is active in both processes.

3.2.4 The Innate Heat in Transpiration

As noted earlier in this chapter, pneuma is supplied via two ways: by means of respiration and transpiration. In his expositions of transpiration, Galen makes it clear that it serves the same purpose, that is, heat regulation. Unlike respiration, which is primarily focused on the heart, transpiration supplies the entire body. Galen's primary point of contention is the mechanistic accounts of this type of breathing, and he especially criticises Plato for offering such an account in the *Timaeus* already mentioned earlier in this chapter. According to Galen, transpiration is enabled by the innate capacities of the tissues, not *horror vacui*. In the process of the same critique, he describes the circular pattern of motion that transpiration consists of:

> τὴν τοῦ τροχοῦ περιαγωγὴν οὐχ ἁπλῆν δεῖ νοεῖν, ἀλλ᾿ ἐξ ἐναντίων κινήσεων συγκειμένην, ὅταν μὲν ἐπὶ τὸ δέρμα τὸ ἔμφυτον ὁρμήσῃ θερμόν, ὠθουμένου τε καὶ περιελαυνομένου τοῦ ἐκτὸς ἀέρος εἰς τὸ σῶμα διὰ τοῦ στόματος, ὅταν δ᾿ αὖ πάλιν ὁρμήσῃ διὰ τοῦ στόματος ἔξω φέρεσθαι, περιωθουμένου τοῦ περιέχοντος ἡμᾶς ἀέρος εἰς τὸ σῶμα διὰ τοῦ δέρματος, ὡς ἐνέργειαν μὲν εἶναι [διὰ] τῆς φύσεως ἡμῶν τὴν ἐκπνοὴν καὶ διαπνοήν, πάθος δὲ τὴν εἰσπνοήν, οὐ μόνον τὴν διὰ τοῦ στόματος, ἀλλὰ καὶ τὴν διὰ τοῦ δέρματος.
>
> The turning of the wheel must not be thought of as simple but as a combination of opposite motions: when the innate heat initiates a motion toward the skin, the outside air is 'pushed' and 'moves in a circle' into the body through the mouth; but when the innate heat initiates a contrary motion of air outward through the mouth, the air enveloping us is 'pushed around' into the body through the skin. As a result, exhaling and transpiring are activities of our nature, whereas inhaling, not only through the mouth but also through the skin, is an affection.[117]

Reading this passage alone makes it hard to appreciate Galen's contrast between the *Timaen* circular and his own dual motion, owing to the fact that this description is so terse. The excerpts from other aforementioned treatises help to fill in crucial details here. The emerging picture is remarkably similar to the account of respiration discussed earlier, which is not unexpected, given that both transpiration and respiration follow a very similar pattern. The passage describes how two types of breathing take

[117] *PHP* 8.8.18–19 de Lacy (5.711–12K), tr. de Lacy (1978–84: 533).

place in a body at the same time, in accordance with the cycle of the innate heat.

First, the heart, being the source of the heat,[118] sends it out through the arteries, and it radiates towards the skin. At this point, the body is heated and requires cooling. The thorax moves, pulling air into the lungs through the mouth. The intake of cold air cools the body. The action of the thorax is enabled by muscles and nerves, so it is voluntary, governed by the nervous system. Having cooled down, the body starts the second part of the cycle, which is kindling. First, the air is breathed out from the lungs. At the same time, the capacity to attract what is beneficial is activated in the heart. The heart makes the arteries expand, pulling the air in. There is no mention of the contraction of the arteries in this passage, but it must occur after this expansion, expelling the by-products of 'burning'.

In the last sentence, Galen employs the distinction between activity and affection. The activity is a motion originating from the object itself, whereas affection is a motion originating elsewhere.[119] Inhaling through the mouth is said to be affection, because the expansion of the lungs, the organ of the cardiac system, is controlled by the organ of the nervous system, viz. the thorax. Exhaling is natural because it allows the lungs to come back to their default position and shape. Transpiration, or breathing through the skin, works similarly. The main difference is that it is the heart, the direct governor of the cardiac system, that makes the arteries expand,[120] and in contracting they return to their original state, as do the lungs.[121] However, just as the injury to the parts moving the thorax results in suffocation, so the stoppage of pores results in a fever.[122]

[118] *Ut. Resp.* 5.4 (126 Furley and Wilkie=4.506K).

[119] This definition can also be found in *PHP* 6.1.5 de Lacy (5.506–7K); *Loc. Aff.* 1.3.4 Gärtner (8.32K).

[120] The arterial tissue is capable of some pulsation too. *Art. Sang.* 7.4–8.2 (176–8 Furley and Wilkie=4.731–2K); *Us. Puls.* 5.5 (214 Furley and Wilkie=5.168–9K); *Cur. Rat. Ven. Sect.* 6 (11.269K) for the heart and pulsation, see also *AA* 7.8 (654 Garofalo=2.614K).

[121] See the argument in *Us. Puls.* 7.1–2 (220 Furley and Wilkie=5.173K) that an expansion is the activity; it is also worth noting, however, that the contraction of arteries can be forced and unforced, just like breathing out via the lungs; *Us. Puls.* 7.2 (220 Furley and Wilkie=5.173K). This ties in with the previous point about Galenic polemics in *On the Natural Capacities*. The contraction of arteries moves pneuma in a mechanical motion, and Galen criticises Erasistratus for using it in physiological explanations while himself adopting it in certain cases. Yet here the key difference emerges. The mechanistic motion of the arteries is only a secondary effect of the expansion originating from the innate capacities of the tissues of the arteries/heart. This motion is owed to the natural capacities arising from the mixture of that particular tissue (for the mixture of the heart and its pathologies, see *Ars Med.* 10–11 (301, 14–309, 7 Boudon=1.331–7K)). The natural capacities are, then, at the very core of animal physiology and therefore they must take the most prominent role in any explanation of it.

[122] *MM* 8.2 (10.535K) and *MM* 8.4 (10.564K) that specifically mentions transpiration.

Ultimately, transpiration and respiration are similar in their fundamentals, despite being carried out by different organs, and they both serve the same purpose: the maintenance of the innate heat. The two types of breath, as noted, are necessary for ensuring that the thermal conditions are kept at optimal levels, since any deviation can quickly result in illness and death. These points explain why breathing is the hallmark of animal vitality.

Despite his hesitations earlier in *On the Usefulness of Respiration*, Galen ultimately states that this conclusion – that the use of breath is the preservation of the innate heat – is not only plausible but the truth itself.[123] The innate heat, as well as the pneumatic system that regulates it, ensures the conditions in which not only the nervous system but also the nutritive system can function. The regulation of the innate heat is, ultimately, the regulation of the elemental alteration that constitutes animal vitality. The process of breathing distinguishes the latter from the vegetative vitality. At the same time, there is much in common between the two domains: the language describing the respiratory anatomy maps onto the nutritive anatomy, while the innate capacities govern both involuntary breathing and nutrition.[124] Yet animal bodies are capable of motion, not only in terms of kinetic movement but also internal changes, all of which are enabled by a larger degree of heat and the internal bodily structure that enables the optimal distribution of that heat.

Vitality can be understood either as a certain kind of motion or, more fundamentally, as a certain series of qualitative changes or alterations. The predominance of any of the elemental qualities would bring about change, but the change into coldness, wetness and dryness leads to stagnation. Only heat is the ever-propelling property, ever 'rekindling' and restarting the change.[125] Yet even heat needs to be moderated by the other properties in order not to disperse itself in its activity. Breathing and the quick elemental alteration that comes with it, introduces the kind of speed of motion in animal bodies that are not possible in plants. While employing the Platonic pattern of tripartition, Galen distinguishes the spirited and the vegetative souls not just by their desires, but by the ways in which their

[123] *Ut. Resp.* 5.7 (128–30 Furley and Wilkie=4.508K).

[124] In the very last sentence of *On the Natural Capacities*, the treatise that discusses nutrition most extensively, he specifically refers to transpiration (not respiration), that is, the diastole of the arteries as absorbing pneuma and fine blood (but not liquids in the stomach and intestines). Natural capacities explain both the absorption of nutriment and the absorption of pneuma for heat regulation. *Nat. Fac.* 3.15 (256 Helmreich=1.214K).

[125] The connection between heat and motion is well embedded in ancient Greek philosophical and scientific thought; see Betegh (2019) for a more detailed discussion.

domains move. Borrowing the general scheme from the Platonists, Galen gives an exceptionally detailed account of the functioning of the soul domains. His association with the medical tradition undoubtedly helps to accomplish this task, but it is also worth noting that Galen uses the medical inheritance philosophically.

Crucial to the differentiation between animal and plant motion is what he calls the Hippocratic division of the parts into solids, fluids and pneumata. While it is true that the division is mentioned in the Hippocratic sources, Galen turns it into his own conceptual tool that helps to model the speeds of the qualitative changes in the body with reference to the viscosity of the affected tissues. These models have a practical purpose: they are crucial for his differentiation and treatment of fevers, but they also undoubtedly show that Galen thought of the body, especially the animal body, in terms of the movements of the tissues and the ways in which alterations were enabled by these motions. The speed of vital pneuma enables qualitative maintenance of heat at a suitable pace, but there is an even more subtle type of pneuma, the psychic pneuma, whose even more complex motions enable the psychic capacities.

3.3 The Psychic Pneuma and Its Purpose before Galen

Galen divides pneuma into three types: vital, psychic and natural. The pneuma discussed so far is of the first type. It is present in the arteries and it plays an instrumental role in heat regulation and, thus, in animal vitality. The psychic pneuma is also present in arteries but it has a distinct activity and a set of properties enabling that activity.

When theorising the psychic pneuma, Galen is engaging in a long-standing tradition that makes a connection between breathing and intelligence, starting with the Hippocratic works.[126] In *On Sacred Disease*, the brain is described as having the greatest power in humans. In a healthy state, it is the interpreter of things caused by air, since air supplies it with intelligence.[127] The air, according to this passage, is necessary for the

[126] See the discussion in Lloyd (2007: 136–40), which covers not only Hippocratic texts and some Presocratics, but also shows the provenance of the terminology and the theories concerning air, winds and pneuma in the Archaic poetry. See also von Staden (2000).

[127] *Morb. Sacr.* 16 (16.1–2 Grensemann=Littré 6.390), tr. von Staden (1989: 249): 'I think the brain has the greatest power in humans, for when it is healthy it is our interpreter of things caused by air (air, you see, provides intelligence)'. Κατὰ ταῦτα νομίζω τὸν ἐγκέφαλον δύναμιν ἔχειν πλείστην ἐν τῷ ἀνθρώπῳ· οὗτος γὰρ ἡμῖν ἐστι τῶν ἀπὸ τοῦ ἠέρος γινομένων ἑρμηνεύς, ἢν ὑγιαίνων τυγχάνῃ τὴν δὲ φρόνησιν ὁ ἀὴρ παρέχεται.

functioning of the brain. This claim, however, can be read in two ways: either there is something special inherent in the air that enables the brain to act or the air simply acts as a channel, and the brain stops functioning when deprived of air because it is cut off from the supply of the necessary material. In other words, the air could be an agent of cognition or it could be an instrument. Given the way in which air is described as a vehicle/supplier for all sense perceptions, the second option seems to be a more apt interpretation. As will be argued later, Galen's views are developed along these lines too, but this understanding of the connection between the air and intelligence is by no means uncontested.

Earlier in this chapter, Galen's report of Asclepiades' identification of pneuma with the soul in *On the Usefulness of Breathing* was mentioned. The Asclepiadean view, at least the way in which Galen describes it, appears to explain the soul and intelligence in terms of pneumatic activities.[128] Galen often identifies Asclepiades with the Epicureans and atomists, so this claim was motivated by a mechanistic understanding of human physiology. At the same time, the view identifying intelligence and pneumatic activities can be found in the texts and theories to which Galen is much more sympathetic. A fragment of Aristotle's early work *Peri Philosophias*, states that the *nous* is ethereal.[129] Arguably, this Aristotelian description can be associated with the Greek tradition traceable back to such figures as Diogenes of Apollonia who posited the existence of the intelligent, designing air.[130] By the time Galen was active, the association of pneuma and intelligence was ubiquitous, but there was a fairly wide range of options for interpreting this association, each of which brought distinct philosophical consequences and commitments. The following section contains an argument that Galen's view ends up being in line with the claims made in the Hippocratic passage, but the way in which he arrives at such a conclusion is distinctly Galenic.

3.3.1 The Generation and Nourishment of the Psychic Pneuma

The origin of the psychic pneuma as well as its distinctive characteristics are covered in both *On the Doctrines of Hippocrates and Plato* and *On the*

[128] This appears to be a Stoic-influenced position (Hankinson 2008a: 235–6, for example), but Asclepiades is typically described by Galen as an Epicurean, an interpretation supported by scholarship; see Leith (2012).

[129] Fr. 27 Ross. See also Clark (1975: 202).

[130] See Tarrant (2017: 65).

Usefulness of Parts. In Book 9 of the latter, Galen adds that he was right to point out that the vital pneuma in the arteries is used for the generation of the psychic pneuma in the brain,[131] after noting that the retiform plexus is more elaborate than the varicose plexus because of the necessity of greater elaboration of the psychic pneuma in the brain than in the reproductive organs.[132] A more elaborate description of how the vital type of pneuma turns into the psychic type can be found in Book 3 of *On the Doctrines of Hippocrates and Plato*, where he states:

> ὥσπερ γὰρ αὐτὸ τὸ σῶμα τῆς καρδίας ἐξ ἑαυτοῦ διαστελλόμενόν τε καὶ συστελλόμενον ἐν μέρει τάς ὕλας τε ἕλκει καὶ αὖθις ἐκπέμπει, κατὰ τὸν αὐτὸν τρόπον ὁ ἐγκέφαλος ἐπειδὰν προέληται τοῦ περιεχομένου κατὰ τὰς ἑαυτοῦ κοιλίας πνεύματος, ὃ δὴ καὶ ψυχικὸν ὀνομάζομεν, ἐπιπέμψαι τινὶ μορίῳ, τὴν εἰς τοῦτ᾽ ἐπιτήδειον κίνησιν κινηθεὶς οὕτως ἐπιπέμπει. γένεσις δὲ τῷ πνεύματι τῷδε τῷ κατὰ τὰς κοιλίας αὐτοῦ τάχα μέν τις ὀλίγη καὶ ἐκ τῶν εἰς αὐτὰς περαιουμένων γίγνεται φλεβῶν, τὴν πλείστην δὲ καὶ κυριωτάτην αἱ κατὰ τὸ δικτυοειδὲς πλέγμα τὸ κατὰ τὴν τοῦ ἐγκεφάλου βάσιν ἀρτηρίαι χορηγοῦσιν, αἵτινες ἀπὸ τῆς καρδίας ἀναφέρονται. ὥστ᾽ εἴ τις βούλοιτο τοῖς ἀληθέσι συνάπτειν τὸν μῦθον, ἐν τοῖς κάτω μέρεσι κυηθεῖσαν τὴν φρόνησιν, τουτέστι τὸ πνεῦμα τὸ ψυχικόν, ἐν τῇ κεφαλῇ φήσει τελειοῦσθαι καὶ μάλιστά γε κατὰ τὴν κορυφήν, ὅτι κατὰ ταύτην ἐστὶν ἡ μέση καὶ κυριωτάτη τῶν ἐγκεφάλου κοιλιῶν.

> Just as the body of the heart, as it alternatively dilates and contracts of itself, draws matter in and sends it out again, in the same way the brain, when it chooses to send to some member a portion of the pneuma contained in its own ventricles, which we call psychic (pneuma), executes the motion suitable to this end and this sends pneuma. Perhaps in some small part this pneuma in its ventricles is generated from the veins that end in the ventricles; but the major and principal production (of pneuma) is supplied by the arteries in the *rete mirabile* at the base of the brain, and these (arteries) come up from the heart. Therefore, if a person wishes to fit the myth to the facts, he will say that wisdom, that is, psychic pneuma, after being conceived in the lower parts, reaches full development in the head, especially the top of the head, because that is the location of the brain's middle and most important ventricle.[133]

131 *UP* 9.4 (2.12, 20–13, 2 Helmreich=3.700K).

132 *Rete mirabile*, the retiform plexus is a dense structure of blood vessels below the brain (*AA* 13.9 (Duckworth 1962: 174–5), but it is not actually found in humans. The existence of such a structure in humans is conjectured on the basis of the observations of bovine anatomy (see Rocca 2003: 249–53) and predates Galen, possibly originating with Herophilus' followers; see Rocca (2003: 203–5). On animal dissection for the study of human anatomy, see Rocca (2003: 67–78); Salas (2020: 158–68). The varicose plexus consists of the testicular blood vessels.

133 *PHP* 3.8.29–32 de Lacy (5.355–6), tr. de Lacy (1978–84: 231).

This passage presents a clear picture of how the psychic pneuma is generated: it is the vital pneuma that has been elaborated in the arteries, especially those in the *rete mirabile*. The generation of the psychic pneuma is gradual: it is conceived in the lower parts of the body and, as it raises through the body, it reaches its full development at the top of the head. Having started developing in the lower parts, it becomes increasingly finer and, as a result, more changeable as it travels up. The key points of this account are reiterated in *On the Usefulness of Parts*, where Galen notes that it is possible that the psychic pneuma 'is a sort of exhalation of useful blood'.[134] He also indicates that it differs from the rest of the pneumata as it is significantly more elaborated and finer.[135]

The psychic pneuma undergoes not only generation but also nourishment. In fact, its nourishment, alongside the thermal regulation, is said to be the reason for why humans breathe (respire, to be precise) at the beginning of *On the Causes of Respiration*.[136] The same claim is also made in *On the Usefulness of Respiration*, as mentioned earlier. The question of how exactly the psychic pneuma received its nourishment (τροφή), however, is a matter of debate. Having noted that the psychic pneuma must be nourished and there seems to be no other source for it than respiration, Galen also acknowledges the theory – not improbable and furthermore advocated by many doctors and philosophers – that its nourishment could come from the vapours rising from the blood. He compares the schools of Erasistratus and Hippocrates on this point. The latter maintains that the psychic pneuma is nourished by breathing in the air, whereas the former maintains that pneuma comes to the brain from the heart via the arteries.[137] Galen rejects Erasistratus' theory with the following experiment. When the arteries of the neck are ligated, an animal's breathing or motion are not affected, which shows that the brain does not need pneuma to be brought from the heart. The nourishment for the psychic pneuma, it

[134] *UP* 6.17 (1.361, 17–18 Helmreich=3.496K); tr. May (1968: 324). He also adds that a more elaborate description of this process is given in the other writings.

[135] *UP* 16.10 (2.420, 17–19 Helmreich=4.323K). Presumably, the generative process leads to the psychic pneuma being highly susceptible to alteration, making it more appropriate material for the activities it carries out from the brain; the connection between the psychic pneuma and the brain tissue are discussed in Chapter 4.

[136] This claim can be cross-referenced to other Galenic works as well, see, for instance, *UP* 7.9 (1. 396, 8–10 Helmreich=3.545K).

[137] *Ut. Resp.* 5.1 (122 Furley and Wilkie=4.502K).

follows, primarily comes from the air breathed in through the nostrils, just like Hippocrates says.[138]

The process of nourishment raises some questions. Most importantly, one might reasonably wonder what happens to the two types of pneuma (the elaborated psychic and the freshly breathed-in vital) once they arrive at the brain. Is 'nourishment' just a matter of the two pneumata mixing? If that is the case, then the dilution of the elaborated pneuma with the freshly breathed-in air seems to be a potential problem. Two pieces of information suggest that this is not the case. First, the fact that Galen puts an emphasis on the middle ventricle is important.[139] If pneuma is elaborated *especially* in the middle ventricle, then the air breathed in through nostrils also undergoes this process. The psychic pneuma is always a kind of altered, elaborated pneuma regardless of whether it comes from outside via the nostrils or from within the body via the arteries.

Second, there is no reason to suppose that the term nourishment is meant in a different sense from the conventional one. In that case, Galen's theorisation of nutrition supplies all the necessary information for understanding what is at stake in the nourishment of the psychic pneuma. Galen carefully distinguishes this generation and nourishment in *On the Natural Capacities*. In this context, he primarily talks about the workings of the nutritive system, but the concept can be applied in this context too.[140] He defines generation as a process during which underlying material substance is altered and shaped into an organ, giving it a form; thus, a new entity is generated. Nutrition, meanwhile, is effectively an addition of matter to the parts without anything new coming into existence.[141]

138 *Ut. Resp.* 5.2 (122 Furley and Wilkie=4.503K). See also *MM* 12.5 (10.839K), where the psychic pneuma is said to draw nourishment both via nostrils and from the *rete mirabile*. While rejecting the Erasistratean claim that the brain requires the supply of pneuma from the heart, Galen does not seem to completely rule out the possibility that arteries might contribute to the nourishment of the psychic pneuma in some way. Towards the end of the treatise, he hypothesizes that if it turned out that the psychic pneuma needed the vapour arising from blood as nourishment (which is plausible), his account of breathing as a process primarily dedicated to regulating the innate heat would still apply. The vapours, in that case, arise from the blood being heated in due proportion, being neither too cold nor too hot and, consequently, not smoky (*Ut. Resp.* 5.5 (126 Furley and Wilkie=4.506K)). The main way of feeding the psychic pneuma, however, is respiration via the mouth and nostrils.

139 He does not do this consistently, however. See, for example, *UP* 9.4 (2.14–5 Helmreich=3.702K), where it is implied that the long elaboration in the arteries produces pneuma by itself, as no additional step or organ is mentioned. It is more likely that this is not a contradictory account but only a shorter way of describing the process, because elsewhere in the very same treatise Galen states that the anterior ventricles prepare pneuma too (*UP* 8.10 (1.481, 8–10 Helmreich=3.663K)).

140 See the explicit comparison of the two in *San. Tu.* 1.2.14 Koch (6.6–7K).

141 *Nat. Fac.* 1.8 (114 Helmreich=2.19K).

As shown in Chapter 2, nutrition is a gradual process during which various tissues attract what benefits them and alter it into the same type of matter they are composed of, thus absorbing the nutrients into themselves. The nourishment of the psychic pneuma is also not a simple mixing of the two pneumata, but the alteration and absorption of the fresh pneumatic matter into the psychic pneuma.

The psychic pneuma is generated in the arteries, but, as it rises, it absorbs some of the air breathed in through the nose and mouth, thus replenishing its substance. Presumably, respiration also supplies the necessary qualitative change. After all, if the elaboration of pneuma makes it finer, it effectively means that it becomes more heated too, thus raising the risk of it dispersing. The respiration through the nose, therefore, resupplies some of the dispersed matter and, at the same time, this fresh air introduces some coolness, thus tampering and stabilising the psychic pneuma.

Once the psychic pneuma is fully elaborated in the brain, the latter sends it out by dilating, as the passage from *On the Doctrines of Hippocrates and Plato* indicates. This claim is elaborated with a more detailed anatomical description in *On the Usefulness of Parts*. The two anterior ventricles are responsible for the 'physical' motion, such as inspiration, expiration and the sending of the psychic pneuma out from the brain as well as its elaboration.[142] While the pneuma reaches them via the arteries, these ventricles send out the psychic pneuma via some of the nerves.[143] Although Galen does not emphasise it, there is a notable systematic circularity in the processes he describes: the heart receives pneuma by means of respiration, which is an activity controlled by the nervous system; in turn, it sends out the vital pneuma via the arteries, and the portion of pneuma that ends up elaborated in the *rete mirabile* becomes the psychic pneuma that the brain will use to send commands for the motion of the muscles controlling respiration.

The latter stage is especially interesting from a more philosophical point of view. It raises the question of the role that pneuma plays in perception and intelligence more generally,[144] especially whether pneuma could, in

[142] *UP* 8.10 (1.481, 6–10 Helmreich=3.663K).

[143] *UP* 8.11 (1.482, 14–18 Helmreich=3.665K). See also *PHP* 7.4.1–3 de Lacy (5.611–2K) where Galen explains that he is uncertain whether all the nerves have passages through which the psychic pneuma flows.

[144] I use 'intelligence' as a general term for the activities of the governing part located in the head, as listed in *PHP* 7.3.2 de Lacy (5.600K), including imagination, memory, thought, sensation, voluntary motion and so on (ἥ τε φαντασία καὶ ἡ μνήμη καὶ <ἡ ἀνάμνησις, ἐπιστήμη τε καὶ> νόησις καὶ διανόησις, ἐν δὲ τῷ πρός τι τῆς τ' αἰσθήσεως ἡγεῖσθαι τοῖς [τ'] αἰσθανομένοις τοῦ ζῴου μέρεσι καὶ τῆς κινήσεως τοῖς κινουμένοις καθ' ὁρμήν).

some sense, constitute them. Galen does entertain such a possibility, and his arguments, although covered quite extensively in the scholarship already,[145] are worth addressing for the sake of having a complete account of pneumatic physiology.

3.3.2 *The Psychic Pneuma as an Instrument: Two Arguments*

This section covers two arguments containing the most pertinent claims about the nature of the psychic pneuma for current purposes. The first one is a well-known argument showing that this type of pneuma is only an instrument of the soul, and the second one is an argument about the properties that enable the psychic pneuma in particular to perform its role as an instrument.

The clearest argument that the psychic pneuma is an instrument of the soul can be found in *On the Doctrines of Hippocrates and Plato.*[146] It follows a description of a vivisection of the animal brain. Galen notes that removing the bone and pulling aside dura mater does not impact the animal's sensation and voluntary motion. Even cutting the brain itself does not result in such a loss unless one reaches the ventricles. Cutting the posterior ventricle results in the gravest injury, while the cuts to the middle ventricle are somewhat less harmful, and the cuts to the anterior ventricles increasingly less so. The effects of pressure on the ventricles follow the same pattern.[147] On the basis of this observation, Galen builds the following disjunction. The psychic pneuma in the ventricles of the brain

[145] See, for example, Hankinson (2006: 234–7); Rocca (2021); Singer (2020: 267–72); see also Debru (1996: 145–54), containing an analysis built primarily on the works on breathing.

[146] *PHP* 7.3.30 de Lacy (5.609K), see also *Ut. Resp.* 5.1 (120 Furley and Wilkie=4.501–2K). This passage is also referred to later in *On the Usefulness of Respiration*, when Galen uses the disjunction, stating that pneuma in the cavities of the brain is either the substance of the soul or its primary organ in order to establish that the purpose of respiration is the maintenance of the innate heat. For if it is the case that the second part of the disjunction is true, then the brain contains within itself the substance of the soul, which must be either the innate heat or pneuma or the form of the composition (κατασκευή) as a whole or something incorporeal. One of these four options must be by necessity the primary organ of motion, and must keep the soul unaffected yet dissolve when one of the primary organs suffers (*Ut. Resp.* 5.7 (130 Furley and Wilkie=4.509K)). He states that an animal dies either because the composition of the brain is injured or pneuma in the brain is injured or only the heat is damaged. Yet the rapid damage to the composition can only occur through excessive heat. The same is true of the natural heat. Pneuma, meanwhile, can also only be destroyed either by means of emptying of substance or by means of excessive heat. However, the cessation of breathing does not empty the whole substance of the pneuma, unlike the brain injury (*Ut. Resp.* 5.7 (130 Furley and Wilkie=4.509–510K)). The only remaining option is the regulation of the heat. This is the primary use (*chreia*) of breathing, while the nourishment of the psychic pneuma is the second (*Ut. Resp.* 5.8 (132 Furley and Wilkie=4.510K)).

[147] *PHP* 7.3.15–18 de Lacy (5.605K).

must be either the first home of the incorporeal soul – *if* it is incorporeal – or the soul itself, *if* it is corporeal. Interestingly, the disjunction fails to produce results *qua* disjunction. As the argument progresses, both of these propositions are ruled out by the fact that the animal regains the capacities of voluntary motion and sensation once the ventricles are closed up. Galen concludes that the soul dwells in the body of the brain, whatever its substance might be,[148] while the psychic pneuma acts as the instrument of the soul.[149]

Subsequently, Galen provides the following motivation for his conclusion. When the psychic pneuma escapes from the ventricles, it does not deprive an animal of life, but only makes it lose – temporarily – the capacity for voluntary motion and sensation. If pneuma itself were the soul, the animal would die once it escaped, because the loss of substance would result in the complete and irreversible loss of life. However, the observation that the loss of the psychic pneuma results in only a temporary loss of capacities indicates that its significance is only instrumental. On the basis of this reasoning, it follows that the soul dwells in the body of the brain (its exact substance remaining undetermined) with the psychic pneuma as its instrument.[150]

Ultimately, the role of the psychic pneuma is comparable to the role of other organs, defined by Galen as parts with a complete activity, such as muscle, the instrument of voluntary motion.[151] The injury to the muscle in a limb will necessarily result in the loss of the ability to move that limb voluntarily, despite the fact that the muscle itself is not the cause of the motion (this argument will be covered in detail in Chapter 4). As the discussion in Chapter 1 showed, Galen approaches parthood as primarily functional. What makes some body parts irreplaceable is having the kind of activity (or a set of properties) that cannot be partially covered by other body parts. It is owing to its irreplaceable firmness that a bone, for example, is a necessary instrument of walking, whereas the stomach is not a necessary instrument of nutrition.

[148] Galen disavows any knowledge of the substance of the soul, especially that of the rational soul *in Form. Foet.* 6, 32–34 Nickel (4.701–2K) and, repeatedly, in *Prop. Plac.* 3.1 (64 Lami Garofalo); 7.1 (86 Lami Garofalo); 15.1–2 (136–8 Lami Garofalo). See the discussion in the Introduction.

[149] See also *Hipp. Epid.* 5.5 (17b.247–8K).

[150] *PHP* 7.3.19–22 de Lacy (5.606K); see also *PHP* 7.3.27 de Lacy (5.608K), where Galen writes that it is evident that the pneuma is not the soul from the fact that it collects back once it has been emptied from the brain after an injury. See also Rocca (2003: 177–8) who uses the term 'physiological agent' to denote the instrumental role of pneuma.

[151] *UP* 16.2 (2.380, 12–14 Helmreich=4.270K). See also discussion in Chapter 1.

At the same time, the psychic pneuma is also not entirely comparable to the parts called 'instruments' discussed in Chapter 1. Whereas there is only one type of bone tissue in the body, and this tissue is irreplaceable owing to its status as a self-managing part, there is another substance very similar to the psychic pneuma, that is, the vital pneuma. Could the latter cover some of the activities of the latter? Galen must think that it could not, given his definition of an 'instrument'. In order to answer this question, it is necessary to look more closely at the second argument that shows how he postulates the special properties and the activities of this pneuma.

The starting point of this investigation is the claim that the psychic pneuma is instrumental in voluntary motion and sensation, and the motion of the brain sends it out for these purposes.[152] Thus the psychic pneuma appears to act as a means of communication between the brain and the rest of the body as well as the outside world.[153] Not all nerves contain pneuma, but the optic nerve has clear channels for it,[154] and therefore the eyesight is the best case study of the psychic pneuma.[155] According to Galen, the outside air and the psychic pneuma, although presumably different in some aspects of their composition, share corresponding capacities that allow them to form a smooth 'line' for sensory signal transmission.[156] The crucial question is how this transmission takes place. One of the more informative descriptions of this process can be found in the discussion of the anatomy of the eye in *On the Usefulness of Parts*, where he states:

> ἀλλ' ἐπὶ μὲν τῶν ὀφθαλμῶν, κἂν ὅτι μάλιστα στεγανοὶ πανταχόθεν ὦσι, ῥᾳδίως ἐπὶ τὴν ἐν αὐτοῖς ἐγκεφάλου μοῖραν ἡ παρὰ τῶν ἔξωθεν χρωμάτων ἀλλοίωσις ἀφικνεῖται. λεπτὸς μὲν γὰρ καὶ λευκὸς καὶ καθαρὸς ὁ κερατοειδής, ὥστ' οὔτ' ἂν αὐτὴν οὔτε τὴν δι' αὐτῆς ὁδοιποροῦσαν ἀλλοίωσιν ἀποστέγοι. μετ' αὐτὸν δ' εὐθέως τὸ κρυσταλλοειδὲς ὑγρὸν

[152] See *PHP* 3.8.29–32 de Lacy (5.355–6K).

[153] Although the precise details are not so clear and, in Book 7 of *On the Doctrines of Hippocrates and Plato*, Galen explicitly states that he does not have an exhaustive answer. He writes that it is not clear whether pneuma is native to each nerve and is struck by the pneuma arriving from the brain or whether pneuma flows to them directly from the brain. He then proclaims he has no answer and mentions the third possibility, the qualitative change of continuous parts. This view is hinted at by those who posit the capacity without substance, calling it a 'flow of capacity'. The example provided is that of the sun sending out light through the air while remaining in the same place itself. Galen then adds that it is not clear whether this account implies that the capacity flows all the way from the brain to the limbs via the nerves or the substance of pneuma or if it falls on the nerves, alters them so violently that this change is further transmitted to the lower limbs (*PHP* 7.4.1–3 de Lacy (5.611–2K)).

[154] *UP* 8.6 (1.463, 9–10 Helmreich=3.639K).

[155] See also the discussion in Chapter 2.

[156] *Hipp. Prog.* 1.23(18b.72K).

> κατ᾽ αὐτὴν τὴν κόρην, ᾧ συμφυής ἐστιν ἡ ἐν ὀφθαλμοῖς ἐγκεφάλου μοῖρα. καὶ δῆλον ἤδη, διὰ τί μὲν ἀποβλαστάνει εἰς ὀφθαλμοὺς ἐγκεφάλου τις εἰλικρινὴς οὐσία, διὰ τί δ᾽ ἐν τῷ διεκπίπτειν ἐπυκνώθη, διὰ τί δ᾽ αὖθις ἐν ταῖς χώραις τῶν ὀφθαλμῶν ἐλύθη πλατυνθεῖσα, καὶ διὰ τί μόνη πασῶν αἰσθητὸν κέκτηται τὸν πόρον.
>
> As regards the eyes, even though they are covered as closely as possible on all sides, alteration from external colours easily reaches the part of the encephalon [the retina] contained in them. For the hornlike [membrane – the cornea] is so thin, clear, and pure, that it closes off neither this part nor the alteration that passes through it, and after the cornea, directly at the pupil, comes the crystalline humour [the lens], to which the part of the encephalon contained in the eye adnate. It is now clear why some of the unaltered substance of the encephalon forms offshoots to the eyes, why these become denser as they issue [from the cranium], why they are again resolved and flattened out in the orbits, and why they are the only ones of all [such offshoots – the cranial nerves] to have a perceptible channel.[157]

The eyesight is effectively just a transmission of an alteration in the air and pneuma. The anatomy of the eye is designed for this purpose. In order for a person to see, the external alteration of the air needs to reach the brain. Galen considers the retina to be an offshoot of the brain, and once an impression reaches this part, perception can take place. Before reaching the retina, an impression passes through the cornea and the lens, both of which are extremely clear and thus do not obstruct the transmission of the alteration. All parts of the eye anatomy, from the optic nerves to the lens, are described as extremely fine, pliable and enabling the transmission of the sensory impressions. Why is the psychic pneuma necessary in this process as well?

The answer must lie in the exceptional pliability of the pneumatic body. The superfine texture of the psychic pneuma makes it a unique tissue. In this respect, it exceeds not only the most subtle sensory nervous tissues but also the vital pneuma that primarily transmits thermal alterations. Since the psychic pneuma is elaborated to a great degree in the *rete mirabile* and the ventricles, it is hotter and drier than other tissues, which consequently renders it also extremely pliable. In fact, it must be the finest and most alterable tissue in the body. The significance of the pneumatic body is made especially clear in the division of the body into solids, fluids and pneumata and the discussion of the speed of their alteration.

Arguably, the model of body heating via three tissues is an illuminating parallel to how the psychic pneuma interacts with the nerve tissue too.

[157] *UP* 8.6 (1.466, 20–467, 9 Helmreich=3.643–644K), tr. May (1968: 403). See also Ierodiakonou (1999) for Galen's account of colour vision, positioned against Aristotle.

Tissues of different viscosity are affected at different rates, with pneumata showing extraordinary plasticity. Therefore, no matter how subtle a nerve is, it would have a lot of difficulty registering an alteration of the external impression to the same extent that the psychic pneuma does. Thus, the this pneuma acts as a material mediator of external impressions to the nervous system. Just as vital pneuma conducts heat, so the psychic pneuma serves as a conductor of alterations that constitute perception. The psychic pneuma, therefore, is the perfect tool of transmission: it is so subtle as to pick up and transmit the finest details of the external world, while its special heat allows it to affect the much denser nervous tissues.

This reading of the role of the psychic pneuma is corroborated by the observation that the quantity of pneuma affects the quality of perception. If one closes one's eye, one is able to see better because, Galen explains, more pneuma comes to the open eye.[158] The sight is equally hindered if there is less pneuma coming from above, in a proportional manner.[159] This claim indicates that pneuma acts via its quantity in the process of perception, although it does not rule out that it acts in some other manner as well.[160] Thus, the psychic pneuma has various distinct properties that render it irreplaceable by other parts, even other types of pneuma that, by virtue of being hot and less fine, could not play the same role in sense perception. Traditionally, the psychic pneuma has some connection not merely with sense perception but also with intelligence, as noted at the beginning of this chapter. Galen engages with these ideas as well.

3.3.3 Intelligence

When it comes to understanding Galen's notion of intelligence, one of the most useful passages is the description of the parencephalis in *On the Usefulness of Parts*. Having referred to his previous work in which he showed that pneuma is contained throughout the brains and not just in

158 *UP* 10.14 (2.109, 14–18 Helmreich=3.836K); also in *Symp. Caus.* 1.2.2 (7.89K) and *PHP* 7.4.11–12 de Lacy (5.614K). See also Boudon-Millot (2012: 563) for the broader discussion of Galen's proof that pneuma fills the cavity of the pupil.

159 See *UP* 10.5 (2.73, 1–5 Helmreich=3.784K), where the shrivelling of the cornea due to old age causes this phenomenon.

160 It is worth noting that this is partly why the constant nourishment of the psychic pneuma is necessary. A certain amount of pneuma is necessary for carrying out the activities well, and therefore constant resupply ensures that there is no lack of it.

its ventricles, Galen moves on to discuss the Erasistratean account of intelligence. According to him, although Erasistratus was right to claim that the parencephalis was more intricate in its structure than the brain itself, he was wrong to attribute the cause of the intelligence to this structure for the following reasons:

> πολύπλοκον δ' εἶναι φάσκων ἐπ' ἀνθρώπων μᾶλλον ἢ τῶν ἄλλων ζῴων αὐτήν τε ταύτην καὶ σὺν αὐτῇ τὸν ἐγκέφαλον, ὅτι περίεστιν αὐτῶν ἄνθρωπος τῷ νοεῖν, οὐκέθ' ὁμοίως ὀρθῶς μοι δοκεῖ γιγνώσκειν, ἐχόντων γε δὴ καὶ τῶν ὄνων πολύπλοκον ἱκανῶς τὸν ἐγκέφαλον, οὓς ἐχρῆν ὅσον ἐπὶ τῇ σκαιότητι τοῦ τρόπου παντάπασιν ἁπλοῦν τε καὶ ἀποίκιλτον ἔχειν αὐτόν. ἄμεινον δ' ἦν ἄρα τῇ τῆς οὐσίας εὐκρασίᾳ τοῦ νοοῦντος σώματος, ὅ τι ποτ' ἂν ᾖ τοῦτο, τὴν σύνεσιν ἕπεσθαι νομίζειν, οὐ τῇ ποικιλίᾳ τῆς συνθέσεως. οὐδὲ γὰρ τῷ πλήθει τοῦ πνεύματος τοῦ ψυχικοῦ χρῆναι δοκεῖ μοι μᾶλλόν περ ἢ τῇ ποιότητι τὴν ἀκρίβειαν τῆς νοήσεως ἀναφέρειν.
>
> On the other hand, when he says that the *epencranis* itself and along with it the brain are more complex in humans than in other animals because human intelligence is greater than theirs, it seems to me that his understanding is no longer so correct; for even donkeys have an exceedingly complex brain, whereas, judging by their stupidity it ought to be perfectly simple and uncomplicated. Hence it would be better to think that intelligence depends on the good temperament of the substance of the thinking body, whatever this body may be, and not an intricacy of structure. Indeed, it seems to me that accuracy of intellect should be ascribed not to the quantity of the psychic pneuma but rather to its purity.[161]

Erasistratus, according to this account, maintained that intelligence increases proportionally with the complexity of the brain and the parencephalis (which he called *epencranis*).[162] Galen refutes this position with a counterexample. Donkeys, allegedly the most stupid of animals,[163] also have highly complex brains and parencephalises. Instead, Galen suggests, intelligence ought to be linked proportionally to the *krasis* of the substance of the *thinking body*. The use of the 'τοῦ νοοῦντος σώματος' rather than a specific organ helps to avoid committing Galen to any specific claim about the substance of the soul.[164]

[161] *UP* 8.13 (1.488, 17–489, 2 Helmreich=3.673–4K), tr. May (1968: 418), slightly altered.

[162] This organ is cerebellum; the term 'parencephalis' originates from Aristotle's texts. See also Leith (2020) for a discussion of Erasistratus on the brain. Erasistratus also had an account of the psychic pneuma, see von Staden (2000: 93–6), who argues that Galen's account of the psychic and the vital pneuma, although more detailed, might be indebted to Erasistatus (112). See Rocca (2020: 279–80).

[163] See *San. Tu.* 1.10.21 Koch (6.52K), where donkeys are used as an example of an irrational animal.

[164] Consistent with his disavowal of such knowledge, as discussed in the Introduction.

He nevertheless mentions the qualitative constitution of one bodily tissue, the psychic pneuma. There is, presumably, no contradiction here: Galen is not attributing a greater role to the psychic pneuma than that of the necessary instrument. A body part is a necessary instrument if its loss incapacitates the process of which it is a part. The damage to the necessary instrument, especially if it is great, has the same effect to the process as the damage to the thinking body itself, whatever it may be.

Galen's strategy here is parallel to his refutation of Erasistratus' account of the usefulness of respiration. He attacks Erasistratus for stating that the usefulness of respiration lies in supplying the substance of pneuma, that is, animals need a certain amount of pneuma to function. According to Galen, it is the quality of the pneuma that matters, because the vital pneuma helps to maintain vitality by fanning and kindling the innate heat. Erasistratus clearly envisions pneuma as a substance whose presence animates the bodily processes in a corporeal way,[165] and so it acts via its mass, making its amount critical for healthy functioning of the body.

In this case, Erasistratus posits not so much the mass as the intricacy of construction as the explanation. Given his commitment to *horror vacui*, presumably his view is motivated as follows: as psychic processes are very complex, the motion of the material underpinning them must be complex too, and thus an exceedingly complex brain structure is needed to account for them. Galen's rejection begins with a simple observation that human brain anatomy is not, in fact, more complex than what is found in the stupidest of animals. Then he proposes an alternative, the same one he used for the account of respiration. Intelligence is better explained as dependant on the qualitative characteristics of the thinking body rather than its structure. Likewise, the precision of the intellectual activity depends on the qualitative characteristics of the psychic pneuma, rather than its quantity.

Better quality of the instrument of the soul naturally allows for better functioning.[166] It is not difficult to conjecture what Galen might have in mind here. When balanced, the psychic pneuma might, for instance, allow for a more precise grasp of the matters at hand. A mixture that is too wet or too cold is prone to stagnation and might manifest itself as the inability to

165 A view that is in line with his commitment to the *horror vacui* as playing an important role in accounting for human physiology, see von Staden (2000: 92–3).

166 The quality of the instrument depends on the mixture of its tissues; arguably, *That the Capacities of the Soul Follow the Mixtures of the Body* is making a related, if not the same, point. It is somewhat difficult, however, to situate the treatise in its precise polemical context, which makes it challenging to interpret it; see the extensive discussion in Singer (2013a: 33, 2013b 340–69).

notice details or grasp matters clearly. A mixture that is too hot, meanwhile, is prone to dissipation, it could manifest itself as the lack of focus or inattentiveness.

The effects of heating of the body by means of emotions and their pathological effects are discussed fairly extensively by Galen,[167] but they generally concern not so much the qualitative constitution of the psychic pneuma as the heating of the body overall.[168] It has been pointed out in scholarship that Galen generally accounts for strong emotions, such as anger, as heating.[169] These emotions cause motion that heats the pneuma, thus making it finer.[170] Finer pneuma is harder to contain and more liable to dispersing. If pneuma disperses, the body is deprived of the activities that it enabled.[171] The dispersion of pneuma pathologically has the same effect as emptying the pneuma from the ventricles of the brain in the experiment discussed in Book 7 of the *On the Doctrines of Hippocrates and Plato*. Although the main point of that passage is to show that the psychic pneuma is the instrument of the soul, it also shows that the loss of an instrument results in the loss of the capacity, even if temporarily.[172]

By including the category of the psychic pneuma in his pneumatology, Galen firmly plants himself within the tradition that often made a connection between psychic capacities and respiration, especially pneuma. His theorisation of the role that the psychic pneuma plays is, however, quite original. He is certainly indebted to the Aristotelian tradition, but whereas Aristotle makes pneuma a special kind of substance whose particular properties makes it specifically suited for perception,[173] Galen adopts a different approach. It is true that it is an especially refined version of

[167] The emotion, as the domain of the spirited soul, is understood as a physical phenomenon in Galen, see (Havrda 2017); the problem of the substance of the soul only concerns the rational soul; for a more extensive discussion of the emotions and the bodily states, see Singer (2017).

[168] Emotion is a kind of heating in the body that can lead to pathological heating and illness, see *San. Tu.* 1.8.16 Koch (6.40K), where Galen argues that strong emotion (anger, grief, etc.) risks fevers; while the weakness of spirit can produce a variety of ill bodily effects through the lack of the innate heat. See the discussion in Hankinson (2014) of the ways in which the irrational domain can affect the rational by means of heating.

[169] See Trompeter (2018: 195–7).

[170] *MM* 12.5 (10.841–3K).

[171] *Trem. Palp.* 5 (7.600K) tr. Sider and McVaugh: 'For warm things rarefy the pneuma and render bodies fine and soft. But cool things thicken, bring together, and force the pores of bodies to close; they thicken and solidify the pneuma and make it turbid. It is, therefore, easily retained, unable to dissipate both because of its own thickness and because of the denseness of the bodies surrounding it.'

[172] *PHP* 7.3.14–22 de Lacy (6.604–6K). See also Hankinson (2006: 235–6).

[173] To be precise, the ability to expand and contract (*MA* 10 (703a19–27)), which distinguishes them from automata (*MA* 7 (701a2–20)); see also Berryman (2002) and Corcilius and Gregoric (2013). For Aristotelian model of respiration and pneuma, see Debru (1996: 44–7).

pneuma, but its significance lies not so much in its fineness as the role it plays in the process, the role of a necessary instrument with distinct activities irreplaceable by other parts. In other words, the point is not so much that the psychic pneuma has properties uniquely suited for sense perception, but that it has the properties suited for perception in the particular anatomical arrangement. Its placement is just as important, if not more important, as the capacities it derives from its mixture. Therefore, its significance depends not only on the kind of substance it is but also on where in the body it is placed, in other words, on the kind of *part* it is. In parallel to the problem discussed in Chapter 1, the psychic pneuma is significant because it is more like a bone than a stomach. It is the structure of the vital processes of the body that makes it a uniquely crucial component of perception.

3.4 The Natural Pneuma

The vital and the psychic pneuma are the most important types for the healthy maintenance of human physiological processes. On some occasions, however, Galen also mentions the third type, the natural pneuma. This kind of pneuma is a bit of a mystery, as Galen talks about both its existence and properties with a high degree of uncertainty. As a result, there is little scholarship on the natural pneuma. Julius Rocca's study of this pneuma is the only more extensive work published recently, and it shows that Galen manages to avoid committing to anything definite about it.[174] Why was he mentioning something so uncertain to begin with? The answer seems to lie in the preceding medical tradition that distinguished between natural and psychic types of pneuma,[175] prompting Galen to consider the existence of the former type too. He did not engage with the tradition unreflectively, however. Here, I argue that his claims about the natural pneuma show that he was thinking about its possible existence systematically, in parallel to his theorisations of the other types of pneuma. Ultimately, while Galen's conjecturing on the possible existence of the natural pneuma comes up with few firm conclusions, it reveals much about his approach and especially his tendency to systematise the human body.

[174] Rocca (2012: 638–41); Temkin (1973: 107) shows that later Galenists embraced it and claimed the existence of three types.

[175] Attributed to 'the ancients' in Ps. Galenic *Int.* 9.2 (20, 20–1 Petit=14.697K); see von Staden (1989: n52, 253–4; 2000: n61, 65); see also Singer (2020) for the argument that Galen was more influenced by medical rather than philosophical traditions of theorising pneuma.

In the context of discussing fainting in *On the Therapeutic Method*, Galen briefly summarises his arguments on the three types of pneuma and their sources. First, he claims to have shown clearly that the brain is the source of the psychic pneuma that is nourished by respiration and the *rete mirabile*. He calls his demonstration (ἡ ἀπόδειξις) of the vital pneuma not equally clear, while also noting that it is not unpersuasive (οὐ ἀπίθανόν) that it is located in the heart and arteries, nourished by respiration and blood. Both of these points are in line with what he says about these two types of pneuma, including some degree of uncertainty about the vital pneuma in other works, and his arguments have already been discussed in this chapter. He then adds that 'if there is also such a thing as the natural pneuma, it would be contained in the liver and veins',[176] adding that the substances of capacities were discussed fully in *On the Doctrines of Hippocrates and Plato*.

This description gives the impression that the lower the source of pneuma is, the harder it is to ascertain its properties and its existence. This tendency is, of course, incidental: the difficulty of learning about the natural pneuma has little to do with how high it is located in the body; instead, its obscurity comes from the methodological difficulties that arise when studying the entire nutritive system to which this type of pneuma belongs. After all, Galen wrote that it is harder to show that the liver is the centre of the nutritive system than to demonstrate that the heart and the brain control their respective systems.[177] Nutrition controlled by the liver takes place gradually, and the results of its deprivation appear slowly too. Ligating veins, therefore, does not achieve the same kind of obvious results as ligating nerves or arteries. As much as this problem pertains to the study of the liver itself, it becomes an even more insurmountable obstacle when it comes to the finest substances in the liver-governed complex, the natural pneuma.

This passage also makes it clear that Galen models the possible existence and source of the third type of pneuma in accordance with the properties and activities of the three central organs. Just like the brain and the heart have a type of pneuma in their domains, so the liver too might have one. If this were the case, this type of pneuma would be sent out via the veins. If Galen is applying the tripartite model thoroughly, then he must think that the natural pneuma must be connected with nourishment in some

176 *MM* 12.5 (10.839–40K): εἰ δέ ἐστί τι καὶ φυσικὸν πνεῦμα, περιέχοιτ᾽ ἂν καὶ τοῦτο κατά τε τὸ ἧπερ καὶ τὰς φλέβας.

177 *PHP* 6.3.1–6 de Lacy (5.519–21K); see also the discussion in Chapter 2.

way. Just as the pneuma in the brain is instrumental to psychic activities and the vital pneuma to vital heat-regulating activities, so the natural pneuma in the liver, the ruling organ of nutrition,[178] must be tied to nutritive activities. And, indeed, if we follow Galen's reference to *On the Doctrines of Hippocrates and Plato*, we can find evidence corroborating this line of reasoning.

Galen alludes to the third type of pneuma very briefly in *On the Doctrines of Hippocrates and Plato*. In a polemical context against cardiocentrists,[179] notably the Stoics, he focuses on their argument that the ruling part is the source of pneuma and then adds the premise that this source is the heart. He takes this argument apart, pointing out that the Stoics assume what is under investigation regarding the psychic pneuma. If their claim concerns the vital pneuma, it does not follow that both pneumas have the same source. He then praises Erasistratus for distinguishing between the sources of the two pneumas, and he goes on to say that 'if they say that neither of these pneumas is meant in the argument, but rather the so-called material pneuma, which is analogous to dry and moist nutriment, they will learn about this too from Hippocrates: "The source of the nourishment of pneuma is mouth, nostrils, windpipe, lungs, and breathing generally."'[180]

The identification of this third type of pneuma with nutriment is presumably a Galenic addition, given the fact that the subdivision of pneuma into types is not Stoic to begin with. Galen is saying that if the cardiocentrists suppose that the heart is the source of the nutritious pneuma, they are wrong, because, as Hippocrates says, pneuma is nourished by the respiratory system. The way he describes the natural pneuma indicates that it does have some bearing on nourishment in providing dry and moist nutriment, although this is not the kind of nourishment that pertains to the heart. Just like the vital pneuma maintains the innate heat by both kindling and quenching it, so the natural pneuma, if it existed, would maintain the proper level of nutriment by supplying both moist and dry properties.

178 *PHP* 6.3.5–6 de Lacy (5.520–1K); *Cur. Rat. Ven. Sect.* 6 (11.269K). See also Harris (1973: 352) and the discussion in Chapter 2.

179 For more on this, see Tieleman (2009: 288–93).

180 *PHP* 2.8.39 de Lacy (5.281K), tr. de Lacy (1978–84: 165): εἰ δ' οὐδέτερον μὲν τούτων τῶν πνευμάτων ἠρωτῆσθαι κατὰ τὸν λόγον ἐροῦσι, τὸ δὲ ἀνάλογον τῇ ξηρᾷ καὶ ὑγρᾷ τροφῇ, τὸ προσαγορευόμενον ὑλικόν, ἀκούσονται καὶ περὶ τοῦδε παρ' Ἱπποκράτους· 'ἀρχὴ τροφῆς πνεύματος στόμα, ῥῖνες, βρόγχος, πνεύμων, καὶ ἡ ἄλλη διαπνοή'. See also Hippocratic *Alim.* 30 (82, 10–11 Heiberg=9.109 Littré).

Generally, the property of moistness is associated with nutriment.[181] According to the general principles of the four-element theory that Galen espouses, heat always consumes moisture, which results in dryness. The cold, although consuming nothing, produces moistness.[182] When discussing replenishing bodies for health in *Thrasybulus*, Galen notes that when there is a loss of dryness, nourishment must be given,[183] while the 'cooking' of the moistness produces dryness. It is also worth noting that excessive dryness prevents the homoeomerous tissues from absorbing nutriment.[184] It follows that the balance of the two properties would result in the regulation of nourishment in the body. The natural pneuma, thus, could be conceived as the regulator of these properties, in the same way as vital pneuma is involved in the regulation of the balance between the hot and the cold.

The principles of the four-element theory would also allow a conjecture that the natural pneuma would be denser than the other two types. Nourishment and the properties connected to it are generally associated with density.[185] The same conjecture can be made on the ground of this pneuma originating from the lower part of the body. Bearing in mind that the psychic pneuma is generated by going upwards in the body and gradually becoming finer, the natural pneuma, with its source located below the heart and the lungs, might be much less (or not at all) elaborated and, therefore, thicker.

Given its likely role as the regulator of nourishment, the next point of discussion about the natural pneuma ought to be what it nourishes. There are two – not mutually exclusive – possibilities: fleshy tissues and other pneumata. In the first case, the natural pneuma might be aiding the blood in delivering nourishment to the homoeomerous parts. Pneumatic substances change faster than any other substances, and thus the natural pneuma might help to transfer the nourishment from the liquid to the solid parts. In the second case, the natural pneuma might replenish the vital pneuma, which, in the process of turning into the finer psychic pneuma, might be, in some cases, turning too thin and scattered. Since pneumatic substances change quickly, the vital pneuma would receive the

181 And generation, see *Form. Foet.* 6, 5 Nickel (4.689K). See also Anonymous Londinensis 6.13–33 Manetti (2011: 11–12), which reports allegedly Hippocratic views. Here an analogy between 'soldier' plants, rooted in moisture and moving around seeking moisture, and humans, rooted in air, is established.

182 *San. Tu.* 6.2.11 Koch (6.386K).

183 *Thras.* 19 (57, 17–20 Helmreich=5.840K).

184 *MM* 7.7 (10.497K), see also Chapter 2.

185 See Debru (1997).

much-needed nourishment more easily from another pneumatic substance, the natural pneuma, rather than any solid part.

Although the claims about the natural pneuma are few, they do show how methodically Galen is approaching its hypothetical existence. He is clearly theorising the possible existence of this type of pneuma systematically, with a reference to the tripartition of the main physiological domains, both regarding the kind of role it would have in the body if it existed and regarding the methodological difficulties in studying the entire system to which it belongs. Thus, even his uncertainty about this type of pneuma is very much in line with how he approaches and what he claims to know of the three physiological domains. Despite the fact that Galen produced no more than a hypothetical account of the natural pneuma, his examination of its possible existence is revealing. It shows that his thinking about the functioning of the body involves a strong assumption about systematicity, modelled on the tripartition of the central physiological domains.

3.5 Concluding Remarks: On Animal Unity

As noted at the beginning of this chapter, the cardiac system is, in an important way, the hallmark of animal vitality. The key motivation for the claim is Galen's understanding of the innate heat, whose source is the heart. For all intents and purposes, its significance can be understood as the kind of homeostatic regulation of temperature.[186] The animal life is distinguished from the inanimate objects and plants by its motion. To be a living animal being means to move, both literally and figuratively. Animals are not only unrooted, but also capable of perceiving their environment and reacting to it. Animals can be moved to anger or fear or joy. All of these motions are underpinned by heat, produced by the heart. The more heat, the more motions there are. Conversely, whenever a body is chilled by either medicine or cold, arteries, nerves and muscles cease working.[187] It is for this reason that breathing is the sign of animal life too. Breath, by cooling and kindling, preserves the appropriate degree of the innate heat in all the tissues, and therefore to breathe is to be a living animal, with the heart as the centre and the ruler of the animal life.

Pneuma contributes to animal motion in more than one way: in the form of vital pneuma, it preserves the heat; in the form of the psychic pneuma, it plays a role in voluntary motion and perception of animals. Although the three main types of pneuma discussed in this chapter have

[186] A point made by Hankinson in (2003, 2008a, 2017b).

[187] *PHP* 7.7.5 de Lacy (5.703K).

different roles and activities in the body, they share some fundamental characteristics. Pneumata, even the thickest species of this genus, are the finest substances in the body. This property enables them to perform activities in accordance with their different type. The fineness allows pneumata to change by means of qualitative alteration and the inherent motion allows them to 'transmit' that change from one area or organ to another one. The differences between the types of pneuma can be spelt out in terms of the kind of properties they transmit. The natural pneuma, whose existence is only presumed, is a supplier of dry and moist nutriment. The vital pneuma, the crucial element of the cardiac system, 'transmits' thermal changes that ensure the optimal conditions for the maintenance of the innate heat. The psychic pneuma participates in the transmission of the sensory data. This is made possible by its extreme fineness, which is achieved by extensive refinement not only in the arteries but also in the ventricles of the brain, allowing this pneuma to transmit extremely fine-grained impressions. Despite being the necessary instrument of perception, the psychic pneuma is only one component of the complex process, which is explored in greater depth in Chapter 4. Before turning to the nervous system, it is worthwhile to note the significance of the cardiac system in the animal body.

Unlike plants, animals are governed by two physiological systems, and therefore they have not only the liver but also the heart as a governing part. In Galen's conceptualisation of the workings of the body, there are some parallels between the two systems these two governing organs oversee. The arteries extending from the heart are distributed throughout the body just like veins, and while the vegetative system supplies nutriment through the offshoots of the liver, the primary purpose of the cardiac system is to supply heat-regulation to the rest of the body. The two systems are not just parallel, they are also connected. As argued in Chapter 2, all the tissues are capable of absorbing and converting nutriment owing to their natural capacities, and the vegetative system helps to produce and to deliver that nutriment to the parts. Analogously, the tissues also have some internal heat, owing to the presence of the hot element in their mixtures. These are the very same mixtures that underlie the natural capacities, so both physiological systems are rooted in the same elemental composition.

However, the analogy stops when it comes to the proportions of elements in that very same composition, especially in regard to proportion heat. It is true that both systems possess some heat: Galen explicitly refers to the mild kind of heat in plants, discussed Section 2.1, contrasting it with the significantly greater heat in animals, but the animal heat makes animals a different kind of living beings. This point is first made evident by the fact that the animal heat is constantly re-supplied and tampered by breathing.

The increase of heat arrives with a further consequence: the differentiation of tissues in terms of their viscosity arising from different degrees of heat. The facts that animal bodies possess pneuma and that pneumata are divided into different types are widely discussed in Galenic scholarship, but his division of the body parts according to three different kinds of viscosity received fairly little attention. As the discussion in this chapter shows, the viscosity of tissues is very important for understanding the variety of ways in which one body part can affect another: both in terms of speed and degree.[188]

Apart from the diagnostic and therapeutic significance discussed earlier, the presence of three types of viscosity in the body has important implications for understanding animal vitality. The tripartite differentiation of tissues is only possible in higher life forms, namely in animals, because only animals possess pneuma (possibly three types of it, with slightly different activities but similar principles of performing those activities). Owing to its presence, there is significantly more motion in animal tissues and bodies. Some of that motion is breathing, which sustains the innate heat in a neat self-sufficient manner. However, the sense perception and voluntary movement that animals are endowed with are also not possible without heat-propelled motion, distributed and 'communicated' throughout the body with the help of pneuma.

In Chapter 2, it was shown that the vegetative system represents a self-sufficient system, creating unity and making the entire nutritive domain, in an important way, *one*. When it comes to the cardiac system, a high degree of self-sufficiency comes into the picture when it is considered not by itself but together with the nutritive system. This is not entirely surprising: the vegetative system can exist in isolation, as it does in plants. The cardiac system cannot exist by itself: there is no animal that is heat-regulated but does not eat and grow. At the same time, it would be wrong to think of the animal as a plant with extra cardiac activities: its mixtures are hotter and in a need of heat-regulation, unlike mixtures found in plants. The presence of the cardiac system, in other words, affects the vegetative states too, so that together they form an inter-twined and inter-connected whole. Unlike plants, animals are capable not only of nourishment and growth but also of a selection of nourishment that comes their

188 This principle also shows up in the analysis of voluntary motion, see the discussion in Chapter 4.

way by perceiving the sources of nourishment and moving towards that better nourishment.

Furthermore, rational animals can also deliberate and make choices about their nourishment. This kind of scenario involves an even greater unity, the unity of three ruling principles. The role of the psychic pneuma as an instrument of the soul hints at the connection between spirited capacities and higher cerebral functions. As argued in this chapter, the psychic pneuma behaves, in principle, like the vital one but its extensive rendering in the arteries makes it extra fine and malleable, sensitive to very fine alterations, all of which makes it most suitable for sense perception.

As Galen defines it, an organ is a part with a complete activity (as discussed in Chapter 1), and if the psychic pneuma is an organ, its complete activity must be the very fine kind of alteration required for sense perception. Within the range of parts that are called organs, the psychic pneuma seems to be comparable to the nerve rather than, for example, to the eye. The latter organ is performing its activity, seeing, owing to its own parts, the most important of which is the lens. The psychic pneuma, meanwhile, is simply an extremely viscous homoeomerous tissue that extends and is subservient to a governing part. Interestingly, the governing part it is subservient to is, technically, in charge of a different physiological system. In this respect, the psychic pneuma resembles blood: just like blood is circulated not only in veins but also arteries, so the psychic pneuma is circulated not only in arteries but also in the brain and some nerves. And if the cardiac system is the hallmark of animal life, then the nervous system is the hallmark of animal, and especially human, intelligence. The peculiar anatomy and properties of the nervous system, together with its significance for the unity of human physiology, are explored in Chapter 4.

CHAPTER 4

Perception and Voluntary Motion
The Nervous System

As noted in Chapters 2, together with a variety of explicit divisions of the body into parts discussed so far, there is another prominent, but also typically implicit, division according to the type of motion. This division is simple, consisting of only two types: involuntary and voluntary motion. The discussion in Chapters 2 and 3 focused on the physiological systems that produce involuntary motion: the vegetative and the spirited ones. However, the vital functions often involve the cooperation of different systems, at least to some extent. For example, while nutrition belongs to the vegetative domain, Galen divides the phenomenon of hunger into a physical and a psychic stage: the reaction to the lack of nutriment in tissues and the sensation of the lack via nerves (Chapter 2). Similarly, while breathing belongs to the domain of the cardiac system, according to Galen it is a matter of providential design that breathing via nose and mouth, that is respiration, obliges our will. The capacity for voluntary motion means that we are able to exercise conscious control over our own bodies. The voluntary motion is the domain of the nervous system alone, and, it is a distinguishing feature of this system, differentiating it from both the cardiac and the nutritive systems. Galen assigns it a special role when, in Book 4 of *On the Usefulness of Parts*, he cites Plato describing the liver as a wild animal, adding: 'The reasoning part of us, which is the real human, is situated in the encephalon and has as its handmaiden and servant the irascible [soul] to protect it against this wild animal. Wherefore our Creator connected these parts with offshoots [nerves, veins, arteries] and so contrived for them to heed one another.'[1] The language Galen uses here

[1] *UP* 4.13 (1.227, 10–15 Helmreich=3.309–10K) , tr. May (1968: 229), slightly altered: τὸ δὲ λογιζόμενον ὄντως ἐστὶν ἄνθρωπος, ἐν ἐγκεφάλῳ καθιδρυμένον ὑπηρέτην τέ τινα καὶ βοηθὸν ἔχον τὸν θυμὸν ἐπίκουρον ἑαυτῷ κατὰ τοῦδε τοῦ θρέμματος. ὅθεν αὐτὰ διὰ τῶν ἀποφύσεων ὁ δημιουργὸς ἡμῶν συνάψας ἐπαΐειν ἀλλήλων ἐτεχνήσατο.

closely mirrors the terminology used in his citations from Plato's *Timaeus*.[2] This claim is a philosophical background for an anatomical point. The exposition explains why the small *nervus vagus* is inserted into the liver: so that it would not be entirely without sensation (μὴ παντάπασιν ἀναίσθητον εἶναι).[3] The passages exemplify several problems concerning the role of the nervous system to be addressed in this chapter.

First, allowing that the rational soul is able to exercise some control over the irrational souls, it is reasonable to ask whether this control is manifest in the physiological domain. The case of respiration shows that it is somewhat true, but what is the full extent of this control? Is it the case, for example, that the three governing parts (as outlined in *Art of Medicine*, discussed in Chapter 1) are themselves hierarchically arranged and one of them, the nervous system, has the capacity to govern (ἄρχειν) the other two governing parts? After all, the second sentence states that the reasoning part of human beings (which is situated in the brain) is what is human, that is, it is the part distinguishing humans from other animals.[4] Second, what is at stake in the three domains having awareness of each other? Does the sensory capacity contribute to the privileged position of the nervous system and does it play any role in unifying human physiology?

Understanding the scope of the activities of the nervous system is necessary for determining its (hierarchical) relationship to the other physiological domains, and therefore this chapter begins with a discussion of the activities of the nervous system, as well as their underlying anatomy. In order to discuss these activities systematically, I will use Galen's own tripartite division of them: voluntary motion, pain and perception. A significant part of the discussion will be set against the background of his engagement with Herophilus' discoveries and theorisations of the nervous tissue. Following this discussion, the chapter ends with an argument that the role Galen assigns to the nervous system is limited by his

[2] *PHP* 6.8.68–72 de Lacy (5.580–1K). The description of the vegetative soul as θρέμμα ἄγριόν occurs in both passages (see also *Ti.* 70E). The description of the spirited part as set εἰς τὴν δορυφορικὴν οἴκησιν is found in *PHP* (coming from *Ti.* 70B), while in the previous passage, it is described as the ἐπίκουρον. Galen also appropriates this imagery in *Aff. Dig.* 6, 2–3 De Boer (5.28K), where the spirited soul is compared to an animal that can be domesticated, such as a horse or dog, while the vegetative soul is said to be like a wild animal, such as a wild boar or goat. The rational soul, thus, can 'domesticate' the spirited soul in order to make the latter its helper. The vegetative soul, however, is impervious to such efforts.

[3] The passage also mentions the arteries inserted into the liver for the sake of preserving the proper measure of heat, which, as discussed in Chapter 3, is the proper activity of the cardiac system. The presence of nerves and arteries in the liver tissue also exemplifies how the three central systems are connected anatomically, and this point is discussed in Chapter 5.

[4] *PHP* 2.6–7 de Lacy (5.262–272K); *UP* 12.4 (2.189 Helmreich=4.1K).

denial of the innate sensitivity of the nervous tissue. This point is significant not only because it is a case of rare criticism of Herophilus but also because it comes with important ramifications about the scope of the activities of nervous tissue. Moreover, the discussion of the anatomical underpinnings and the polemical issues pertaining to Galen's understanding of the nervous system shows, I argue, that its activities supplement rather than exercise control over the other two vital physiological domains, playing an important role in enabling complex organic entities to function as a single whole.

4.1 The Anatomy of the Nerves

The nervous system consists of the governing organ, the brain, and its offshoots, the nerves, following the same pattern Galen uses for the cardiac and the nutritive systems. Nerves, just like arteries and veins, are spread throughout the human body,[5] but whereas the latter receive relatively little attention, nerves are discussed extensively by Galen. Apart from the short treatise *On the Anatomy of the Nerves*, Books 8–9 in *On the Usefulness of Parts* are dedicated to both nerves and the brain (with a number of pertinent points made throughout the treatise), as well as Books 3, 8 and 9 (the latter partially surviving in Arabic) of *Anatomical Procedures*. Furthermore, some important claims and references to nerve dissections can be found in *On Doctrines of Hippocrates and Plato* Books 2 and 8, and in *On My Own Opinions*.

The prominence of the topic is reinforced by the grandiose language used to describe the nervous system. Galen describes its anatomy as 'the most beautiful thing',[6] likening nature's fashioning of the offshoots of nerves from the spinal medulla to an artist carving a relief and polishing it to make it beautiful.[7] Earlier in the same treatise, Galen implores his reader to pay more attention to the matters at hand, namely the *nervus vagus* and the *nervus hipoglossus*, than one would at the Eleusinian or the Samothracian mysteries. He adds that work on the nervous system is a mystery that he himself discovered and now practices. This proclamation is followed by more mundane claims that no other anatomist knows about these nerves, nor about the anatomy of the larynx. For these reasons, he

5 *UP* 2.19 (1.122, 20–21 Helmreich=3.166K). See also *MM* 1.6 (10.47–8K).
6 *UP* 10.14 (2.106, 26–107, 1 Helmreich=3.832K).
7 *UP* 16.11 (2.425, 17–21 Helmreich=4.330K).

complains about the errors that these doctors committed regarding the usefulness of bodily parts in question.[8]

The reader is clearly encouraged to draw two conclusions. First, the nervous system is both astoundingly complex and astoundingly well designed. Second, Galen is the supreme authority when it comes to its understanding. The more clearly the first conclusion is demonstrated, the more impressive the second conclusion appears. For this reason, it is also undoubtedly important that the nervous system is notable not only for its complexity, but also the central and fundamental role it plays in human physiology.

4.2 Herophilus

Galen's writings on nerves are profoundly indebted to the discoveries of Herophilus, and he appears to acknowledge it. During Herophilus' time, human dissection and vivisection were permitted (with restrictions) in Alexandria.[9] The relative freedom allowed him, as well as other Alexandrian doctors, including Erasistratus, to produce unparalleled work on human anatomy, especially nerves and the brain.[10] He is, to this day, sometimes called the father of neuroscience.[11] Herophilus' immense influence on Galen manifests itself in several different ways.

Galen adopted the famous Herophilean precept that one ought to start with the primary things even when they are not first in his methodology.[12] In fact, there is evidence suggesting that in certain cases he prioritised Herophilean methodology over the Aristotelian.[13] Galen presents himself as indebted to Herophilus for his work on pulse.[14] Herophilus' anatomical discoveries shaped both Galen's understanding of the body and his vocabulary. He often provides Herophilean terms for organs, such as the *calamus scriptorius* in the fourth ventricle of the brain,[15] '*parastatai*' for

[8] *UP* 7.14 (1.418–9 Helmreich=3.576K).
[9] Tertullian calls Herophilus a butcher (*De anim.* 10.4=von Staden T66), see also Celsus *Med.* 1, *prohoem.* 23–6=von Staden T63a. van Staden (1989: 139–52).
[10] Herophilus and Erasistratus did not work in isolation, of course; see Rocca (2003: 31–4).
[11] Often together with Erasistratus; see, for example, Wills (1999).
[12] *MM* 2.5 (10.107K)=von Staden T50b; see also T50a. For Herophilus' methodology, see von Staden (1989: 115–24). For Galen's engagement with Herophilus' methods, see Tieleman (1995, 2008: 58–9).
[13] Tieleman (1995: esp. 490–4).
[14] See Hankinson (2008b: 16).
[15] *AA* 9.5 (824 Garofalo=2.731K=von Staden T79). See also Rocca (2003: 160–2).

spermatic vessels or 'wine vat' for the confluence of sinuses.[16] He also often cites specifically Herophilean findings when describing peculiar features of an organ, such as the crooked neck of the uterus,[17] as well as when describing general anatomical facts, such as that certain veins (lymphatic vessels) that nourish intestines do not pass to the liver or that an artery is six times as thick as a vein.[18] The terminology introduced by the followers of Herophilus, however, does not always meet with Galen's approval.[19]

In general, unlike his fellow Alexandrian Erasistratus, Herophilus receives criticism only a handful of times. One example, discussed later in this chapter, is arguably of great importance as it shows that Galen understands the nature of the nervous tissue in a significantly different way from Herophilus, and this understanding has important implications for his conceptualisation of human nature. That disagreement is certainly a rare exception. Galen generally adopts the broad-brush understanding of the nervous system attributed to the Alexandrian doctor. Most notably, he appropriates his distinction between motor and sensory functions for theorising the activities of the nerves, although he also adds the third activity as follows:

> τρεῖς γὰρ δὴ σκοποὶ τῇ φύσει τῆς τῶν νεύρων εἰσὶ διανομῆς, ὁ μὲν αἰσθήσεως ἕνεκα τοῖς αἰσθητικοῖς ὀργάνοις, ὁ δὲ κινήσεως τοῖς κινητικοῖς, ὁ δ' εἰς τὴν τῶν λυπησόντων διάγνωσιν ἅπασι τοῖς ἄλλοις.
>
> There are three aims of the distribution of the nerves by Nature, to provide first sensitivity for the instruments of sense perception, second, motion for the instruments of motion, and third, for all the others, recognition of what will cause them pain.[20]

The first notable point in this short passage is that this is an extensive list of the purposes of the nervous system. In other parts of the very same treatise, Galen only mentions two purposes: sensation and motion.[21]

[16] On *parastatai*: *UP* 14.11 (2. 321, 9 Helmreich=4.190K). See also *UP* 14.11 (2.324, 1 Helmreich=4.193K) for the equivalent in the female anatomy. On 'wine vat': *UP* 9.6 (2.19, 7 Helmreich=3.708K); see also Longrigg (1993: 205) for Galen's adoption of Herophilean terms.

[17] *UP* 14.3 (2.290, 2–7 Helmreich=4.149K).

[18] *UP* 4.19 (1.246, 23–247, 3 Helmreich=3.335K). *UP* 6.10 (1.325, 8–10 Helmreich=3.445K).

[19] *UP* 8.11 (1.482, 22–483, 2 Helmreich=3.665K). It is not clear who these followers are. In another treatise, he is also critical of the followers of Herophilus for introducing the third kind of constitution, neutral, together with the warm and the cold, recognised by Galen (*San. Tu.* 6.2.20 Koch (6.388K)). See also Nutton (2020: 66) for criticism of the distinction between prognosis and foretelling.

[20] *UP* 5.9 (1.276, 26–277, 4 Helmreich=3.378K), tr. May (1968: 263), slightly altered. This claim is repeated more than once in this treatise, see also *UP* 14.13 (2.331, 17–21 Helmreich=4.203K).

[21] *UP* 7.14 (1.415, 9–10 Helmreich=3.571K). See also *UP* 1.16 (1.33, 5–6 Helmreich=3.45K) and *Mot. Dub.* 8.22 (158, 25–8 Nutton). Only these two activities are mentioned in the short treatise dedicated to the dissection of the nerves specifically; see *Nerv. Diss.* 1 (2.831K).

Presumably, the omission of the third element is for the sake of concision, with the tripartite description constituting the exhaustive account.[22] At the same time, this raises the question of whether there is a difference between pain and the 'sensitivity' (αἴσθησις) of the sense perception organs, which is the second important point. The third point is fairly minor, but it is worth noting that the very same treatise contains passages that describe other purposes of nerves, such as binding and structurally supporting the internal organ system.[23] This function is, presumably, marginal and unrelated to the *ousia* of the nervous system but is nonetheless an interesting detail. The structural integration of the parts of the body, which allows for a kind of multi-tasking, very much aligns with the teleological account of anatomy in *On the Usefulness of Parts*, since it supports the claim about the brilliance of the body's design.

As the seat of the rational soul, the brain and its offshoots nerves are in charge of the voluntary motion, pain and sense perception, and so it is through these activities that the rational soul manifests itself in human beings. The rationality of human beings can be inferred from the way in which they perceive their environment, and how they interact with it as a result of their perceptions.[24] Thus, the three activities of the nerves that Galen mentions show how he envisions the physiological manifestations of the higher cerebral functions.[25] In order to confirm this hypothesis, however, it is necessary to look more closely at the detailed descriptions of each of the activities of the nervous system, thereby determining how they add up to a robust account of physical manifestations of psychic activities. I start my discussion with the account of voluntary motion underpinned by the motor nerves that shows the way and the extent to which the nervous system is in control of other parts. Subsequently, I move on to discuss Galen's account of pain and sense perception, which, I argue, are conceptually similar. The discussion of the activities of the nervous tissue is rounded up with the analysis of Galen's attack on

[22] Although it could also be motivated by the fact that, from a physiological point of view, there are two kinds of nerves: motor and sensory. More detailed analyses of these nerves will be discussed later. In both cases, pain as a phenomenon presents an interesting problem for Galen, which will likewise be discussed later.

[23] *UP* 6.6 (1.315, 13 Helmreich=3.431K), where nerves are said to 'hold' the stomach.

[24] See, for example, *Prop. Plac.* 3.1 (64 Lami Garofalo).

[25] Which is not to say that it can be reduced to these activities. As discussed in the Introduction, the issue at stake here is how physiological processes enable the activities of the soul instrumentally, not whether the former constitute the latter. Human intelligence is derived from the divine intelligence; see van der Eijk (2014: 90ff.). Key here is *PA* 2.10 (655b37–656a8), where Aristotle distinguishes the humans among all animals as being able not only to live but also to live well, by virtue of having a share of the divine. See also Gotthelf (2012: 53–4).

Herophilus, which reveals the way in which he understands the limitations of the nervous tissues; this is an illuminating point, I argue, for understanding the role of the nervous system in the body as a whole.

Galen's account of voluntary, muscular motion is relatively simple. It rests on two distinctions: the difference between the motor and the sensory nerves, as well as the difference between voluntary and involuntary muscular motions of the internal organs. The argument of this chapter is tripartite, covering the following three issues: the anatomy of nerves, the voluntary and involuntary motion of the internal organs, and the range of different kinds of motion found in the human body in general. The overview of the latter helps to contextualise the nerve-derived motion and to shed some light on its significance within human bodies.

As already mentioned, Galen adopts the Herophilean division of nerves into two types: the motor and the sensory.[26] The former kind of nerves differ from their counterparts in several respects. First, they are often described by Galen as 'hard', a property that renders them especially fit for 'acting', that is, affecting muscle in such a way as to make it move.[27] In fact, the motor nerves are the reason why the body parts that move by appetition (καθ' ὁσμὴν) are capable of moving at all.[28] The size and firmness of motor nerves can vary depending on their designated activity. The motor nerves in the tongue, for example, are smaller but firmer than those of the eye muscles.[29] These properties enable them to move the tongue muscles appropriately.[30] The size of the nerves can even differ within the same part of the body. The nerves that move the upper jaw, for example, are larger than those that move the lower jaw, because the former perform a more arduous task.[31]

[26] It is worth noting that Galen's distinction is neater than the one used by Herophilus; the latter did not always distinguish between the nerves and the tendons very successfully; see von Staden (1989: 250–1, 256). Galen, meanwhile, makes a careful distinction between a nerve (only grows from the brain and the spinal medulla), a tendon (τένων) and a ligament (σύνδεσμος); see *PHP* 1.9.1–5 de Lacy (5.203–4K). It is also worth noting that even Galen's division is more of guideline than a strict distinction between kinds. This is the reason why it is also possible to find a tripartite division of nerves into soft, hard and those that are in-between. See also *AA* 11.3 (Duckworth 1962: 78).

[27] See *UP* 9.14 (2.44, 1–4 Helmreich=3.743K).

[28] *UP* 8.5 (1.459, 5–6 Helmreich=3.633K).

[29] It is worth noting that, according to Galen, the sensory nerves differ greatly from the motor nerves within the eye, owing not only to their softness, but also to their overall importance within the system, given that the 'eyes as a whole were made for the sake of the sensory nerves, and in them is lodged the whole principle of vision' *UP* 9.8 (2.25, 25–27 Helmreich=3.718K). See also *Nerv. Diss.* 2 (2.832K). The sensory tongue nerves (*geustikos*) are not described as being special (*Nerv. Diss.* 5 (2.837K)).

[30] *UP* 9.13 (2.39, 5–7 Helmreich=3.736K).

[31] *UP* 11.6 (2.128, 10–14 Helmreich=3.863K).

The same principle of correlating textural properties with activity applies to the counterpart sensory nerves, which are noted for their softness and suppleness. The optic nerves, for example, are larger and softer than any other nerves, which is why sight is the most precise of all the senses.[32] Despite various distinctions between these two types of nerve, it is important to note that the activities of the soft and hard nerves are not, in fact, mutually exclusive. They only differ in their 'roles'. The hard nerves can communicate sensations as well, but in this capacity, they are inferior to the sensory nerves.[33]

It is worth noting that there is some correlation between the location of a nerve and its firmness, although this correlation is not strong. In general, softer paired nerves tend to be closer to the brain.[34] The closer the paired nerves are to the end of the medulla, the firmer they generally are. The meeting point between the brain and the medulla constitutes the hardest part of the brain and the softest part of the medulla, thereby allowing for a kind of transition. Yet the difference in nerve tissue texture is observable not only in this part of the brain, according to Galen: the brain has both firmer and softer parts, from which emerge nerves of different textures in accordance with what is functionally necessary.[35] The priority of functional considerations explains why, despite the fact that the lower pairs tend to be firmer, the second pair of nerves inserted in the eye muscles is firmer than the third pair.

The pattern of the softer/harder parts of the brain follows the pattern of these properties in the spine. The front part of the brain is softer than the rearmost part. However, the brain is softer *tout court* than any of the nerves. Its matter is easily alterable, which means that it can readily receive impressions and process them.[36] Thus, starting with the softest part at the front of the brain, the lower the parts of the nervous system are located, the harder their texture is. The second pair of nerves makes an exception, which shows that Galen is not trying to establish a strong pattern at any cost. At the same time, it is the exception that proves the rule: the textural properties of nerves resemble the textural properties of pneumata discussed in Chapter 3. In that case too, the higher the pneuma is located, the finer it is. Generally speaking, the Galenic body is 'thick' in the bottom parts and 'fine' in the top parts. In the case of

[32] *UP* 16.3 (2.382–3, 4–5 Helmreich=4.273K).

[33] See *UP* 9.11 (2.31, 17–20 Helmreich=3.725–6K) for the claim that perfect sensation cannot be produced through hard nerves.

[34] For the claim that nerves are always paired, see *Nerv. Diss.* 5 (2.835K).

[35] *UP* 9.11 (2.31, 1–19 Helmreich=3.725–6K).

[36] *UP* 8.6 (1.461, 4–12 Helmreich=3.636K).

pneuma, this gradual change is due to the process of refinement that takes place in the arteries over a period of time.

While the textural differences in pneumata are posited theoretically, the varying degrees of softness in nerves is demonstrated by means of dissection. The latter shows that the second pair of nerves is firmer than the third, and this observation invites the theoretical explanation that the properties of the nerves depend upon their activity, and not the other way around. Here we have an interesting case of a pattern emerging that could, in principle, unify different tissues and systems of the body, and Galen eschewing such an explanation in favour of a teleological one, because of anatomical considerations. This theme is developed further in Chapter 5; for the present purposes, it is enough to note that the lower a nerve is located in the body, the more likely it is to be a motor nerve, although there are exceptions, and Galen explains them teleologically.

There is another notable point concerning nerve anatomy, that is, the presence or absence of pneuma in the nerves. This issue is not entirely straightforward. The brain ventricles contain a great quantity of pneuma,[37] which is also true of the large optic nerves. In *On the Doctrines of Hippocrates and Plato*, however, Galen clearly states that he does not believe that all the nerves contain passages like those within the optic nerve.[38] His reasoning seems to be that pneuma in the nerve is required only in certain circumstances.[39] The motivation for this becomes clear when he discusses a potential counterexample to his position: the hollow outgrowths of the spinal cord. Galen suggests that pneuma in these nerves is required in order to properly exercise the appropriate capacity. These nerves are large and hard, owing to which their alteration does not take place easily. The more solid a tissue is, the slower it is to alter qualitatively.[40] Thus, pneuma is required to supplement alterations in the nervous tissue.[41] Presumably, the same is true even for especially soft nerves that are known to contain pneuma (especially the optic nerve). Although these nerves are inherently highly pliable, the sight requires so many subtle alterations that the psychic pneuma is also needed to carry them out properly.

[37] See *UP* 8.10 (1.481, 6–10 Helmreich=3.663K). [38] *PHP* 7.4.20–1 de Lacy (5.616K).

[39] The presence of pneuma in the nerves also accounts for certain nerve pathologies; see, for example *MM* 14.7 (10.968K); when the 'spongy' nerve is filled with flatulent pneuma, it causes priapism. Pathological cases are not very informative in this case, as they, by definition, represent an unhealthy and abnormal state of affairs.

[40] This principle is explained especially clearly and succinctly in *Diff. Feb.* 2 (7.278–9K), discussed in the previous chapter.

[41] *PHP* 7.4.22–25 de Lacy (5.617K).

4.3 Voluntary and Involuntary Motion

The motor nerves, although not entirely devoid of capacity to transmit sensation, are primarily instruments of voluntary motion. We have already encountered the significant distinction between voluntary and involuntary motions in Chapter 3, in the discussion of respiration. The movement of the heart, Galen argues in Book 7 of *On the Usefulness of Parts*, is produced by nature, whereas the movement of the thorax (made up of bones, muscles and nerves) is produced by the soul; most importantly, such an arrangement is a product of design, because 'it was better for respiration to be of our own work, always subservient to the will of the animal'.[42]

The terms describing the source of motion are reminiscent of Stoic doctrine.[43] For the Stoics, the distinction between nature and the soul is underpinned by pneumatic tension. God (the active principle) pervades all inert matter (the passive principle) with different degrees of tension, thereby creating everything in the world. Lower degrees of tension result in simpler objects, such as rocks, while more complex objects (such as the rational human soul) are produced by a very high degree of tension.[44] It is, of course, not the case that these ontological states are mutually exclusive in either Stoic or Galenic texts. In the latter, the motion produced by nature is shared by humans, animals and plants. It constitutes the fundamental processes of life that maintain very basic vitality.[45] Motion that occurs by the soul produces volition, enabling humans to make choices and judgements.

Interestingly, Galen's distinction between motion on account of nature and motion on account of the soul is rather coarse. In the reports of this Stoic doctrine, especially in Philo, the Stoic distinctions appear to be more fine-grained. Most notably, they distinguish not only between animals and plants but also between the soul in general and the rational soul, the latter being present in humans alone. Galen, meanwhile, implicitly groups animals and humans together. Animals have sensory perception and are

[42] *UP* 7.9 (1.399, 15–17 Helmreich=3.549K), tr. May (1968: 351): ὅτι βέλτιον ἦν ἡμέτερον ἔργον εἶναι τὴν ἀναπνοὴν ὑπηρετοῦσαν ἀεὶ τοῦ ζῴου τῇ βουλήσει.

[43] As described in, for instance, Ps. Galen *Int.* 13.1 (45, 13–19 Petit=14.726K=*SVF* 2.716=LS 47N).

[44] Philo *Leg. alleg.* 2.22–3=*SVF* 2.458=LS 47P; Philo *Deus* 35–6=*SVF* 2.458=LS 47Q. Pneuma also becomes important at the level of more complex ontological states, for which see, for example, Hensley (2020).

[45] For Galen, these are represented by an ability to recognise nourishment and to accept what is appropriate; see *Prop. Plac.* 15.6–7 (140–2 Lami Garofalo).

able to move at will. They, therefore, seemingly share with humans the same kind of motion of the soul.

This grouping does not, however, suggest that Galen believes that human and non-human animals have the same psychic capacities. In fact, he routinely contrasts them with regard to rationality.[46] A much more likely explanation is that this coarser differentiation is sufficient for Galen's purposes and even serves them more elegantly. Medically speaking, the crucial distinction is between those muscular motions that are performed at will and those that are not. Humans are capable of the former, just like any other animal. It scarcely matters, for example, when diagnosing breathing difficulties whether the specific voluntary action is performed as a result of rational deliberation or on account of irrational impressions. In both cases, the issue at stake is an obstructed activity of the nerve tissue. If, furthermore, volition is the phenomenon that originates from the presence of nerves, then animals would not differ from humans in this regard. After all, Galen's study of the nervous system in humans was primarily – if not wholly – based on animal dissection.[47] Finally, making finer distinctions between actions that are rational and voluntary or irrational and voluntary is not just unnecessary: it also risks committing to claims regarding the ontology of psychic capacities, and Galen appears to be fairly determined to remain neutral about this issue.[48] Ultimately, his choice not to adopt the full Stoic-style classification seems not so much a missed opportunity in utilising a more sophisticated theoretical tool,[49] but a deliberate pick of the most efficient concept for distinguishing the key feature and not committing himself to anything more than he is willing to commit to.

4.3.1 Volition and Muscles

The lack of distinction between an act of a rational person and an act of an irrational animal renders the physiological account of voluntary motion

[46] See, e.g., *Aff. Dig.* 5, 2–3 De Boer (5.22–3K); although see *Protr.* 1.4 (84, 3–85, 15 Boudon=1.1–3K) for a much more careful rendering of this distinction. Here, Galen does not rule out that animals have a share of reason, while claiming that rationality *proper* is manifested in human beings alone.

[47] Salas (2020) discusses a variety of animal dissections, as well as presenting an argument proposing how Galen addressed the problem of analysing human anatomy on the basis of non-human animal dissections (see pp. 164–8); see also Rocca (2003: 67–76).

[48] *Prop. Plac.* 3.1 (64 Lami Garofalo); *Foet. Form.* 6, 34 Nickel (4.701–2K).

[49] Which is not to say that the Stoic-style unified theory would not have provided an elegant solution to a variety of problems facing Galenic psychology overall, as argued in Gill (2010).

fairly straightforward. It is simply a motion arising from the presence of the motor nerves that transmit the impulse for a wilful action from the brain. However, as a whole, a voluntary action can be a complex phenomenon. This was made evident already Chapter 1, when discussing the complete impediment of voluntary motion with the loss of a bone. The physiological account of volition, in both humans and animals, furthermore, requires the presence of muscle. Galen more than once states this quite explicitly. For instance, in Book 16 of *On the Usefulness of Parts*, dedicated to the topic of the nerves, arteries and veins, he states the following:

> πρὸς μὲν γὰρ τὴν καθ᾽ ὁρμὴν κίνησιν ἐν τοῖς ζῴοις ἡ φύσις ἓν γένος ὀργάνων κατεσκευάσατο τοὺς ὀνομαζομένους μύας. διό, καίτοι τῶν νεύρων ἁπάντων ἑκατέρας ἐχόντων τὰς δυνάμεις, λέγω δ᾽ αἴσθησίν τε καὶ κίνησιν, οὐδὲν τῶν ἄλλων μορίων, ὅσα δέχεται νεῦρα, κινεῖται προελομένων, ἀλλ᾽ αἰσθάνεται μόνον, οἷον τὸ δέρμα καὶ οἱ ὑμένες καὶ οἱ χιτῶνες καὶ ἡ ἀρτηρία καὶ ἡ φλὲψ ἔντερά τε καὶ μήτρα καὶ κύστις καὶ γαστὴρ καὶ τὰ σύμπαντα σπλάγχνα καὶ τῶν ἀδένων τὸ ἕτερον εἶδος.
>
> For voluntary motion Nature has constructed in animals one genus of instruments, called muscles. Hence, although all nerves have both capacities (I mean both sensation and motion), none of the other parts (whichsoever receive nerves) are moved deliberately, but only feel, such parts, that is as the skin, membranes, tunics, arteries and veins, intestines, the uterus, the bladder, stomach, all the viscera, and the second kind of glands.[50]

As the passage shows, presence of a nerve is not sufficient for voluntary motion. A body part may have a nerve, but if it is not present in the muscular tissue, that part will not be capable of voluntary movement.[51] Therefore, the brain, in spite of having access to the stomach via a nerve,[52] is hardly able to exercise control over it notwithstanding its ability to receive sensory data from this organ of digestion. Muscle is, therefore, a significant component of voluntary motion, although it is worth noting a few counterexamples discussed in *On Problematical Movements*.

The treatise is concerned with cases in which the source of some movement is unclear, for example, when a muscular motion occurs unprompted by a deliberate decision. The most pertinent to the current purposes is the opposite, a deliberate action that takes place without any muscles. Galen mentions various examples, including people being able to

50 *UP* 16.2 (2.380, 12–21 Helmreich=4.270K), tr. May (1968: 684), slightly altered.

51 See also *PHP* 1.10.12–13 de Lacy (5.208K) and *Mot. Dub.* 1.9–13 (124, 9–126, 2 Nutton).

52 Or, more importantly, the liver, which also has one nerve inserted into it, as the passage cited at the beginning of this chapter indicates. Both cases are discussed below.

vomit the wine they had just drunk voluntarily, but he discusses most prominently the case of the tongue expanding beyond the jaw.[53] This movement is problematic, because there is no muscle for extending the tongue in such a manner.[54] Instead, it is explained by the large arteries in the tongue that expand as they become filled with pneuma.[55] This is the first step of the argument. The second – and the crucial – step is to explain why this arterial activity corresponds to an act of volition.[56]

The upshot of Galen's explanation is a sympathetic action. He introduces this account with the example of people observing sufferers from ophthalmia and catching the illness themselves. The other examples include people seeing someone yawning, stretching or urinating and immediately feeling a desire to do the same, and children imitating adult speech. The examples are also supported with a citation from Hippocrates' *On Humours*.[57] Galen concludes that there is no reason to be surprised that, apart from being movable by muscles, the tongue itself has some power to recognise what the mind wants.[58]

The solution bears some similarity to the case of a missing stomach discussed in Chapter 1. Some actions can take place without instrumental body parts if there are other body parts that are able to perform sufficiently similar activities. Just like the nutritive system can absorb nutriment from liquids when the stomach is damaged and cannot crush food, so in this case, the arteries, when filled with pneuma, can expand, enabling the extension of the tongue beyond a jaw, even if no muscle is present. The main difference is that the former is a pathological case and the latter is not, which raises the following question. If the tongue can move without muscles, why do we need muscles in other organs? Would it not be more elegant to skip them altogether? Presumably, muscles provide a service that cannot always be replicated easily by sympathetic reactions in other tissues.

This turns out to be the case if we consider ordinary limb motion, which involves not only soft tissues but also bones and ligaments. Galen has a teleological explanation for the role that these parts play in the

[53] *Mot. Dub.* 4.2 (136, 6–7 Nutton); in the case of vomiting, he concludes that it is predominantly involuntary act brought about by natural capacities on a basis of an extensive anatomical discussion, although it can occur voluntarily too, see *Mot. Dub.* 6.8–7.1 (148, 25–152, 3 Nutton).

[54] *Mot. Dub.* 5.10–11 (144, 27–146, 2 Nutton).

[55] *Mot. Dub.* 4.25–8 (140, 23–142, 26 Nutton).

[56] See Trompeter (2018).

[57] All of these occur in a single dense passage, *Mot. Dub.* 8.15–17 (156, 27–158, 12 Nutton).

[58] The kind of *sumpatheia* at work here seems to be part-to-part transmission of affection, rather than part-to-whole transmission of ailment; see Holmes (2020: 48) for this distinction.

process of voluntary motion in *On the Usefulness of Parts*. He states that Nature is restricted by necessity in its design. Owing to this, neither ligaments nor motor nerves can be used for voluntary motion by themselves. In the case of ligaments, this is because they are not attached to the place that houses the *hēgemonikon*. More importantly, nerves cannot be used for motion by themselves because their softness renders them incapable of transporting great weight. Therefore, they move a muscle, a harder tissue, which in turn moves bones and ligaments, the hardest tissues in the body. For this reason, when some part needs only to be attached, there is a ligament; and when the part only needs sensation, there is only a nerve. In cases where there is need for both, both are present: the nerve conveying the signals from the *hēgemonikon* for motion and the ligament providing the strength needed for such a motion.[59] The same model applies to bones. In fact, later on in the treatise, Galen even remarks that damage done to the bone can result in wholesale immobility.[60] The anatomy of voluntary motion, then, consists of the nerve, the muscle, the ligament and the bone. The order of items on this list represents two overlapping points: first, 'the chain of command' in terms of the capacity for voluntary motion that is sent down from the brain. Second, the texture change in the parts involved: while softness in parts is required for the initial signal, the final motion of the limb requires strength and hardness of parts, which is achieved by means of the involvement of multiple parts with increasingly harder textures.

Muscles play in important role as 'intermediates' in both transmission of the capacity and the conversion of that signal into motion that requires strength. There is, arguably, also another reason for the significance of muscles, although it is not spelt out as explicitly. It concerns precision of motion. The body is a fairly compact structure, with many parts governed by different motions located in close proximity. In the case of respiration, for example, it is quite important that the motions of the heart and the thorax (containing the heart) are kept separate, so that an animal has some control over respiration, which is generally involuntary (and it is, of course, better for it to be so). The presence of muscles allows for the precise control of the ribcage, without affecting arteries. The muscle, thus, is not always crucial, yet often it is a fairly critical instrument for mediating voluntary motion and establishing voluntary control over body parts.

59 *UP* 12.3 (2.186 Helmreich=4.6–8K).

60 *UP* 17.2 (2.450, 16–21 Helmreich=4.364K); for the significance of the bone, see the discussion in Chapter 1.

The scheme of nerve-muscle-ligament/bone is mostly used to account for the voluntary motion of the limbs, in which case it works well. The heart, however, also seemingly meets all the criteria of an organ that is subject to voluntary motion since it is a muscle containing a nerve,[61] and it even has a bone, according to Galen's understanding.[62] Interestingly, he solves this problem by denying that the heart is a muscle in a fascinating argument. In so doing, he also explains the role of the nerve inserted into this organ and sheds some light on the interaction between the two central physiological systems.

4.3.2 *The Heart Is Not a Muscle*

In the previous passages,[63] Galen claims that the heart, as well as arteries, move involuntarily.[64] The more elaborate explanation of this view, including corroborating proof, is found in the treatise *On Anatomical Procedures*. Galen's account is clearly polemical, and, although he does not state who his opponents are, he offers a few clues.

He begins by noting that the similarity between the heart and muscular substances is an impression created by a careless glance.[65] The differences, in fact, are numerous. The activities of each of these organs attest to their differences, for the movement of the heart is involuntary and ceaseless (ἀβούλητος ... καὶ ἄπαυστος) for the duration of an animal's life. The activity of the muscles, meanwhile, is subject to the animal's impulses (ταῖς ὁρμαῖς τοῦ ζώου δουλεύουσα).[66] The activities, as Galen not only states here but also in other works,[67] are determined by the substance. This entails an interesting consequence. If two parts (μόρια) share the same substance, then they also have their activity in common, despite the fact that they are found in different animals. Galen's point is presumably that two pieces of muscle can be expected

[61] *Nerv. Diss.* 10 (2.844K). [62] Salas (2020: 145 ff.).

[63] To the modern eye, Galen might seem wrong, but the issue at stake is ultimately just a distinction of the skeletal and the cardiac types of muscles, which was observed in antiquity. Debru (1996: 103–5) shows that this claim ought to be understood against three different uses of the term μῦς in the Hippocratic corpus and argues that, ultimately, his argument is not innovative but rather built on the understanding of the cardiac tissue developed in the Hellenistic period.

[64] In *UP* 11.10 (2.140, 5–12 Helmreich=3.880K), for example, while describing the design of the tongue, Galen suggests that its brilliance is evident from the fact that it is moved voluntarily, unlike the arteries that move involuntarily (ἀβουλήτως).

[65] *Ousia* is here presumably used in the Stoic sense of *matter*. Later on in the passage, Galen discusses the differences in the *ousia* of these two organs, albeit in the sense of the Aristotelian *essence*.

[66] *AA* 7.8 (650 Garofalo=2.611K). [67] See, for example, *UP* 1.9 (1.19, 9–13 Helmreich=3.26K).

to act in the same way owing to their substance being the same, despite the fact that one might be part of a mouse and the other of a human being.[68] This part is very much in line with Galen establishing an equivalence between humans and other animals for the sake of physiological studies of motion, as discussed earlier. This, however, constitutes only the first step in the longer argument.

As the argument progresses, it becomes clear that Galen's main instrument here is the contrapositive of his principle 'activities depend on substances', and ultimately, he is interested in the differences between organs of a single body. First, he notes that the parts of an individual animal can have different activities, listing various examples of internal organs. Their differences, it is suggested, are owing to their respective substances. He then arrives at the conclusion that muscles do not have the same activity as the heart. It follows that they are not composed of the same substance either.[69] In short, the argument consists in the following *modus tollens*:[70] if the substances of two organs are the same, then their activities are the same. But the activities of the muscles and the heart are not the same. Therefore, their substances cannot be the same. In other words, the heart muscles are composed of different substances from the other muscles.

This theoretical proof is then supported by the following empirical observation.[71] When a heart and a piece of muscle are cooked and eaten, they taste different. The same is true for other organs, including the kidneys, the lungs, the liver and so on. Galen notes that they differ from one another not only in taste but also touch, appearance, hardness, softness, density and colour.[72] On the basis of this, Galen concludes that doctors who maintain that the nerves effectively determine the activity of the heart err insofar as they overlook the substance of the heart. The heart is harder than any muscle and it differs in terms of its fibre, colour and taste from other kinds of muscle, with reference to his comparison of eating a cooked heart and cooked muscle.[73]

[68] See discussion in Salas (2020: 164–5).

[69] *AA* 7.8 (650 Garofalo=2.611K): διὰ τοῦτ᾽ οὖν οὐδ᾽ οἱ μύες ἔχουσι τῇ καρδίᾳ τὴν αὐτὴν ἐνέργειαν, ὅτι μηδὲ τὴν οὐσίαν.

[70] See *Inst. Log.* 5.5 Kalbfleisch.

[71] This is not to say that everything can be shown using both methodologies. A knowledgeable doctor ought to know, for instance, which medicines were discovered through experience alone, through reason alone and through both (*MM* 14.5 (10.962K)). See van der Eijk (1997) for a seminal study of the Galenic notion of qualified experience.

[72] *AA* 7.8 (652 Garofalo=2.611–12K).

[73] *AA* 7.8 (652 Garofalo=2.612K), tr. Singer (1956: 183): ἀλλά μοι δοκοῦσιν οὐδέποτε καρδίας ἑψημένης φαγεῖν, ἢ πάντως ἔγνωσαν ἂν, ὁπόσον διαλλάττει τῶν σαρκῶν, εἰ μὴ ἄρα ἀγνοοῦσι καὶ ταῦτα, ὡς αἱ σάρκες ἅπασαι μυῶν εἰσι μόρια. 'I think they can never have eaten a cooked heart or

The second error of these doctors concerns the nature of the nerves. Here, the argument becomes less clear, with Galen beginning by remarking that his opponents are wrong insofar as they maintain that the brain is like nerves in all its parts (νομίζουσι τὸν ἐγκέφαλον ὅμοιον αὐτοῖς κατὰ πάνθ' ὑπάρχοντα τὰ μέρη), the only variation being the softness of certain nerves. Let us call this the first claim. It comes across as a point of disagreement, but in fact, these claims are all very much in line with what Galen himself maintains, as evidenced by the discussion of the anatomy of nerves up until this point.[74] It is more likely that the main point of disagreement comes in the following sentence containing the second claim. It states that, through certain nerves, the brain provides sensation to the parts below, while, through the others, it sends signals for voluntary motion. The upshot here is that Galen's opponents strictly separate the motor and sensory nerves. Taking this point to be the main issue at stake fits the polemical context, since Galen is attacking the doctors who state that the heart has no motor nerves, only sensory nerves.[75] Presumably, the position of these doctors is that the heart is a muscle and the only thing that makes its activities different (the heart beats ceaselessly and involuntarily, whereas muscles move by volition) is the absence of a motor nerve and the presence of a sensory nerve instead. This reading is further corroborated by Galen's claim that it is reasonable (εὔλογον) that all the nerves have both of these capacities. The only difference is that the soft ones are more suited to sensation while the hard ones are more suited to motion.[76] As an example, Galen names the third and sixth pairs of cranial nerves, which branch out both into muscles and other parts (μόρια). The sixth nerve-pair branches off into the heart, lungs and stomach, as well as the muscles of the larynx.

Finally, Galen adds that if the heart were a muscle and only lacked motor nerves, which would render it mobile like the other muscles, then it could neither move by volition nor receive pulsation, which must have some cause. Galen's point is apt: if the heart is like any other muscle, then it must follow the same pattern of activity. In other muscles, motor nerves

they would surely have known how much it differs from flesh, unless, of course, they do not even know that all kinds of the flesh are kinds of muscle.'

[74] He states that the brain and the nerve share the same kind of tissue in *Form. Foet.* 5, 5–6 Nickel (4.680K). See the later discussion.

[75] *AA* 7.8 (652 Garofalo=2.612K): ὅσοι δὲ διὰ τοῦτό φασι τὴν καρδίαν οὐκ ἔχειν τοῖς μυσὶ τὴν αὐτὴν ἐνέργειαν, ὅτι νεύρων οὐ μετέσχηκε κινητικῶν, ἀλλ', ὡς ἐκεῖνοι νομίζουσιν, αἰσθητικῶν, ἀθρόα πολλὰ κατὰ τὸν λόγον ἁμαρτάνουσι.

[76] This point is consistent with the description of the differences between the soft and firm nerves in *On the Usefulness of Parts*, as outlined in the section on the anatomy of nerves.

are the causes of voluntary motion. Therefore, if the heart has no motor nerve, then it should not be able to move. The motion of the heart has to be derived either from the nerves or else it is inherent in the organ. Since it cannot come from the nerves, it must be inherent. Definitive evidence that the heart has its own motion (and, to this end, does not require nerves) consists in the fact that it continues to move for a while after it is removed from the thorax.[77] This means, then, that the cardiac motion is independent of the nervous system. Indeed, as far as its motion is concerned, it can function without it.

One might be left questioning the purpose of the nerve that is found in the heart. Presumably, Galen agrees that this nerve is, to all intents and purposes, sensory. Just like the liver discussed previously, the heart lacks muscle. The brain, therefore, lacks the instrument for its voluntary movement (especially true considering that the tissue of the heart is harder than a normal muscle; possibly too hard for a soft nerve to move). Consequently, while the brain may receive sensory data from the heart, it is not able to exercise direct control over it. This has some interesting consequences for understanding the scope of the nervous system. Its role as an instrument of conscious control is greatly restricted by anatomical considerations, mainly by the presence or absence of appropriate instruments, especially muscles. The scope of the control that the nervous system has over the body can be aptly illustrated when considered in context of all the motions that the body is capable of.

4.3.3 Different Types of Movement

As well as involuntary motion, which is produced by the cardiac-respiratory system,[78] Galen describes various other kinds of bodily motions of the human being. An arm, for example, has a natural tendency to move downwards without any psychic intervention.[79] The brain itself also moves, as he notes when comparing it to the spinal medulla.[80] The pathology of nerves also presents an interesting case. Galen explains convulsions as arising from the depletion of the nerve parts (τῶν νευρωδῶν μορίων).[81] Even nerves, then, can move in an involuntary way in pathological contexts.

[77] *AA* 7.8 (654 Garofalo=2.614K). See also the anecdote in *PHP* 1.6.7 de Lacy (5.186K), which describes a dissected heart leaping from the doctor's fingers thanks to its violent palpitations.

[78] See *UP* 6.2 (1.301–2 Helmreich=3.412–13K).

[79] *UP* 13.12 (2.280, 18–19 Helmreich=4.135–6K).

[80] *UP* 13.8 (2.263, 8 Helmreich=4.112K).

[81] *MM* 12.8 (10.872K).

Bearing this in mind, the role of voluntary motion (viz. the motion deriving from the nervous system) is not as dominant as one might expect within human physiology more broadly. In the grand overview of the body as a whole, the voluntary motion enabled by the motor nerves is only one type of many types of vital bodily motions. Notably, it exercises little control on the internal processes of the body. Having said it, it is also worth noting that it would be quite incorrect to say that the voluntary motion is *on par* with downward motions of arms, pathological convulsions and so on. First, these motions are accidental, rather than essential. A part is identifiable as an arm, for example, not because it falls downward, but because it can be used for gripping, holding and similar.[82] The motion deriving from the mass of the part (or its pathological state) bears little explanatory power about the nature of that part.

The second (and related) point is that the essential feature of voluntary motion is its regulatory role. In short, the significance of this motion lies in its explanatory power rather than in its predominance. It plays a significant role in respiration, a process concerned with the regulation of the body in reference to its external environment: the intake and output of the air. More importantly, the role of the voluntary motion is significant, since it manifests the activity of the *hēgemonikon* in reference to a person's environment. The activities of the nervous system enable navigation of the outside world not only via voluntary motion but also through sensory perception. In fact, it could be argued that just as nutritive and cardiac systems regulate their respective material fluxes (nutriment and air), so the nervous system regulates its inputs and outputs: sensation and voluntary motion. The rest of this chapter is dedicated to Galen's bipartite account of its inputs: inwardly directed pain and outwardly directed sense perception, arguing that the significance of the kind of control that the nervous system is capable of becomes quite clear in these cases.

4.4 Pain and Nerves

Galen's claim that pain is an activity of the nervous system may seem strikingly insightful, given that this fact has been established by modern life sciences too.[83] This, however, would be too hasty. An entire section is

[82] The first book *On the Usefulness of Parts* is dedicated to the design of the hand, with a strong emphasis on the brilliant design enabling its many activities. See also *Trem. Palp.* 3 (7.586K) for the claim that the 'natural' downwards motion occurs when no voluntary power is present, for example, when an arm is paralysed. The downward motion is therefore not a proper motion of the part.

[83] See Ochs (2004) for an extensive study of the history of nerve functions.

dedicated to the nerves in *On My Own Opinions*, including an argument against unidentified doctors who maintain that nerves are more sensitive than flesh. It seems likely that, in this case, Galen's opponents are not identified because the view at stake is simply commonplace among physicians rather than being a doctrine of some particular medical school. He explains what medical phenomenon motivates 'many doctors' and why that view is wrong. He argues that the nerves are no more sensitive than ordinary flesh.

He begins by stating that the foremost sensitive body part is where the *hēgemonikon* is located, whence the nerves connect to the rest of the body. Every part of the body to which nervous impulses flow is thereby rendered sensitive (αἰσθητικός). The capacity running through the nerves[84] causes the nerves to be sensitive but, importantly, no more sensitive than any flesh. Galen provides a proof of this based on what can be seen through vivisection. Having exposed both the nerve and flesh, he finds that an animal complains more following the stimulation of the latter, while stimulating the former does not agitate the animal to the same extent.[85]

Subsequently, Galen explains the reason why many doctors suppose that the nerves are more sensitive than ordinary flesh. It is owing to their connection to the *hēgemonikon*, as well as the dangers attending nerve inflammation. Although Galen does not explain this position very clearly, it seems that the sensitivity of the nerves is here inferred from a therapeutic phenomenon. The inflammation of the nerves is a more dangerous condition than the inflammation of the flesh since it affects offshoots of the *hēgemonikon*. Thus, nerves must be more sensitive than flesh. Dissection reveals that this conclusion is erroneous, according to Galen, owing to the fact that the condition of a patient does not worsen when an inflamed nerve is severed. He also recounts cases in which doctors did sever the nerve only to find that their patient had not realised this. In other cases, the surgeon accidentally severed the nerve during venesection, but this did not result in the patient experiencing more pain.[86] Galen's commitment to the view that flesh is as sensitive as nerves raises two questions. First, what is the nature of the phenomenon of pain? Second, how can nerves be less sensitive to pain than flesh while having the sensibility for pain as one of their three activities?

One might claim that, although Galen names pain as one of the three activities of the nervous system in *On the Usefulness of Parts*, he does not do

[84] The word for 'channel' here is ὀχετός, not the Herophilean πόρος.
[85] *Prop. Plac.* 6.2 (82 Lami Garofalo). [86] *Prop. Plac.* 6.3 (82 Lami Garofalo).

so consistently. However, for the sake of charity, it is important to note that this inconsistency is probably owing to the vague relationship between the sensation of pain and sense perception (that is to say, sensation) in general. Thus, it would not be unreasonable, in certain contexts, to subsume pain under the category of 'sensation' since it is, after all, one form of sensation. The question regarding whether (and how) pain differs from sensation in general is the third and final issue to be considered in this section.

4.4.1 The Causes of Pain

Galen mentions pain and palliative care regularly in various medical texts, building on the preceding tradition.[87] However, unlike the description of voluntary motion, which is always said to be lost when the nerve is ligated, his descriptions of the origins of pain are not consistent. He names various causes of pain, so much so that different treatises come across as propounding disparate accounts. For instance, in his commentary on Hippocrates' *On the Nature of Man*, Galen states that both pain and health are caused by the four humours: pain arises when one of the humours is either present to excess, or deficient or is separated in the body and not combined with the others.[88]

In Book 12 of *On the Therapeutic Method*, Galen provides a different and extensive account of pain and its aetiology. Ultimately, there are two primary origins of pain. It occurs either by the dissolution of unity or on account of change.[89] Galen proceeds to remark that change that produces pain cannot be gradual but sudden,[90] adding that this type of pain must originate from *dyskrasia*. He notes that he is not talking about external injuries here.[91] The following exposition of causes provides a clear picture of how the dissolution of continuity can occur internally:

> καὶ πρῶτόν γε θεασώμεθα τίνος εἶναι χρὴ φύσεως ὃ διαιρήσει τὴν συνέχειαν. ἀναγκαῖον οὖν ἤτοι ῥῆξιν ἢ θλάσιν ἢ διάβρωσιν εἶναι τὴν διάθεσιν ἐν τῷ διαιρεῖσθαι τὸ συνεχές. ἀλλ᾽ ἡ μὲν ῥῆξις ἐκ τάσεώς τινος, ἡ

[87] An extensive discussion of the dependence on the earlier tradition in King (2018).
[88] *HNH* 2.1 (15.113K); see also 1.6 (15.38K).
[89] It is also worth noting that Galen says that it is not necessary to know whether pain is produced owing to the loss of continuity or change in order to discover what will cure it. It is sufficient to be aware that what rapidly heats or cools produces pain in bodies that are capable of sensation (*MM* 12.7 (10.854K)).
[90] *MM* 12.7 (10.853K): ἀναγκαῖον ἀθρόαν τε ἅμα καὶ βιαίαν γίνεσθαι τὴν μεταβολήν, εἰ μέλλει τις ὀδύνη γενήσεσθαι.
[91] *MM* 12.7 (10.854K).

δὲ θλάσις ἐκ βάρους, ἡ δὲ διάβρωσις ἐκ δακνώδους γίνεται ποιότητος. ὅταν οὖν ἔξωθεν μὲν μηδὲν ᾖ τὸ τεῖνον ἢ βαρῦνον ἢ δάκνον, ἐξ ἑαυτοῦ δέ τι πάσχῃ τούτων τὸ σῶμα, παντί που δῆλον ὡς ἡ μὲν τάσις ὑπό τινος ἔνδον οὐσίας πολλῆς διατεινούσης τὸ περιέχον αὐτὴν σῶμα γίνοιτ' ἂν ἢ ἀμέτρου ξηρότητος, ἡ δὲ θλάσις ἔξωθεν ἐπιπεπτωκυίας οὐσίας σκληρᾶς ἢ μεγάλης ἢ βαρείας ἢ συναμφοτέρων, ἡ δὲ δῆξις ὑπὸ χυμοῦ δακνώδη φύσιν ἔχοντος· ἐπισκεπτέον οὖν ἡμῖν ἐν ταῖς σφοδραῖς ὀδύναις ἤτοι χυμὸν πολὺν ἢ πνεῦμα διέξοδον οὐκ ἔχον, ἢ βαρὺν ὄγκον, ἢ δακνῶδες ὑγρὸν ἢ διάθεσιν ξηράν· ἔτι δὲ πρὸς τούτοις, ὡς ἐν ἀρχῇ διῄρηται, τὸ θερμαῖνον ἰσχυρῶς ἢ ψῦχον. ὧν πάλιν αὐτῶν τὰς αἰτίας ἢ ἐν τῷ πνεύματι θετέον ἢ ἐν τοῖς ὑγροῖς ἢ ἐν τοῖς στερεοῖς· ὅ τι γὰρ ἂν αὐτῶν ἰσχυρῶς ψυχθὲν ἢ ὑποθερμανθὲν ψαύῃ τῶν πλησιαζόντων, ὀδυνηρὸν αὐτοῖς γίγνεται.

First, let us look into what the nature of that which will divide continuity must be. It is, of necessity, a rupture, contusion or erosion – that is, a condition in which a continuity is divided. But rupture arises from some tension, contusion from a weighing down and erosion from a biting quality. Therefore, when there is nothing external stretching, weighing down or biting and yet, of itself, the body suffers one of these, it is surely clear to everyone that tension arises when the body is stretched significantly by some large substance which it contains within, or by excessive dryness; contusion arises when a hard, large, or heavy substance, or all of these together, has impinged on it from without; gnawing arises due to a humour which has a biting nature. What we must consider, then, in severe pains is either abundant humour, or pneuma not having a path out, or a heavy mass, or a biting fluid, or a dry condition. Over and above these are severe heating or cooling, as I distinguished at the start. We must, in turn, establish the causes of these same things, either in the pneuma, or in the fluids, or in the solid [parts] because, if one of those that has been strongly cooled or heated touches the parts adjacent, it generates pain in them.[92]

This extensive aetiology of pain includes not only the bodily humours but also obstructed pneuma, heavy masses, biting fluid, a drying condition and severe heating and cooling.[93] The causes of these conditions, according to Galen, are to be found respectively in the pneuma, bodily fluids and solid parts.[94] When these are cooled or heated excessively, they make contact with adjacent parts, generating pain. Extremes of temperature presumably affect the size of certain masses. A heated tissue expands (becoming finer and more loose-textured), owing to which it takes up more space than usual. The ultimate cause of the phenomenon of pain in

92 *MM* 12.7 (10.855–6K), tr. Johnston and Horsley (2011: 291).

93 It is worth noting that the shorthand explanation for how humours cause pain only mentions 'abundance', unlike in *HNH* 2.59 (15.113K) cited earlier.

94 For a discussion of these three kinds of substances as foundational to physiology, Section 3.2.3.

this case is the touching of two parts that would not touch under normal circumstances. Thus, pathological touching originates from excessive heating or cooling.[95] It is also worth noting that these explanations are therapeutically relevant. Given that Galen advocates for an 'opposites-heal-opposites' methodology,[96] knowing that pain is caused by, for instance, heating, is indispensable to its treatment. There is, arguably, no inherent inconsistency between the causes of pain, as described in the passages of *On the Therapeutic Method*, and the commentary on Hippocrates' *On the Nature of Man*. The former therapeutic treatise provides an exhaustive account, while in the commentary, Galen only mentions the part of the phenomenon of pain that is contextually relevant.

The second cause of pain, namely *change*, is discussed briefly in *On the Therapeutic Method*, but a more elaborate treatment of this topic can be found in a different treatise, the commentary on Hippocrates' *On Elements*. At the beginning of this treatise, Galen presents an elaborate discussion of the phenomenon in a polemical context, thereby clarifying not only why change is one of the two causes of pain but also what is at stake in his theorisation about this phenomenon.

4.4.2 *Pain Requires Plurality: The Concept of an Element*

The notion of the element is crucial to Galen's argument. The very first sentence of this treatise presents a working definition: an element is the least of the thing of which it is an element.[97] Galen then qualifies this claim, stating that elements are not the smallest perceptible parts, owing to which sense perception is not a judge of elements. Although it brings to mind the empiricist method, which relies solely on sense perception,[98] this part of the definition rules out treating the limbs and organs as elements in general. Galen's argument consists in a kind of *reductio ad absurdum*, reminiscent of one of the Pyrrhonian Modes.[99] He notes that animals with keen vision, such as eagles, would be able to discern different (and presumably, finer) elements than those that humans are capable of

[95] An interesting illustration is the cases when pain does not occur thanks to the brilliance of human body design. Take, for example, the way in which tunic does not produce pain by touching the lens due to soft, spongy material, *UP* 10.4 (2.69, 11–14H=3.778–9K).

[96] *MM* 11.12 (10.771K).

[97] *Hipp. Elem.* 1.1 de Lacy (1.413K), tr. de Lacy (1996: 57). See also *PHP* 8.2.2–3 de Lacy (5.661K).

[98] To be precise, experience acquired through sense perception; see *MM* 1.2 (10.122K); Frede (1987: 250).

[99] See Sextus Empiricus *PH* 1.49; 1.64. See Frede (1987) for a discussion of the relationship between Empiricism and Pyrrhonism.

perceiving. The sceptical argument excludes there being a ground for empirical knowledge in general, but Galen does not subscribe to such a view. Instead, he uses the same kind of argumentative tactic to effectively eliminate the empirical position in this particular case.

'Element' does not, therefore, stand for a limb, nor any discernible part. It denotes a fundamental *constitutive* part, which is discoverable by means of reason. This leads to the question of whether the element is singular or plural in kind and, in case of the latter, what these kinds are (in addition to some related issues). For this, Galen turns to Hippocrates and his proof that the elements are plural:[100] 'I say that if man were one thing he would never feel pain, for there would be nothing that would cause him pain if he were one.'[101]

Galen uses this proof against his target, that is, those who maintain that there is a singular kind of element. To be precise, the target here is atomism. Their fundamental particles are the single type of material accounting for the world's construction. Galen cites the famous saying of Democritus that properties such as colour or sweetness are merely 'by convention', whereas, in reality, there are only atoms and void.[102] It is worth noting, however, that Galen's target is most likely not only the atomists in general, but the medical atomists in particular, especially Asclepiades of Bithynia and his followers.[103] Although at the beginning of the treatise Galen names Democritus and Epicurus as atomists,[104] the very same argument is levelled in other works directly against Asclepiades. Despite Galen's phrasing, there are some significant differences between such atomists as Epicurus or Democritus and the medical atomists. They not only differ in terms of the issues in which they were interested, but also in terms of their respective theories of atomic particles. As Galen notes in *On the Constitution of the Art of Medicine*, the *anarmos* particle (posited by Asclepiades) is fragile but it is not the cause of pain when it is broken,

[100] Loosely speaking, of course. See Leith (2014) for the discussion of a confluence of influences, showing that Galen takes the Hippocratic argument aimed at monists and meshes it with the Peripatetic argument against atomists.

[101] *Hipp. Elem.* 2.3 de Lacy (1.415K), tr. de Lacy (1996: 59). This claim comes from Hippocrates' *On the Nature of Man* (*Nat. Hom.* 2.3 (168, 4–5 Jouanna= Littré 6.35–6)). See also Galen's *HNH* 1.1 (15.21K) and *CAM* 7, 6–9 Fortuna (1.247–8K).

[102] *Hipp. Elem.* 2.12 de Lacy (1.417K).

[103] Nutton (2012a: 173) explains that Asclepiades can be seen as the doctor whose work marks the arrival of Greek medicine in Rome. He was a celebrated doctor with many followers (see 170–3), which may have made him an especially clear rival to Galen. Later in the treatise, Galen also attacks the Pneumatists, although then the issue at stake is the nature of elements; see Kupreeva (2014: 184–9).

[104] *Hipp. Elem.* 2.6 de Lacy (1.416K).

because it is not capable of being affected.[105] Galen repeats this argument in *On the Constitution of the Art of Medicine*. If the element composing flesh is not capable of being affected, sensation would not be possible; but there is sensation, therefore the element must be capable of being affected.[106] He then remarks that this argument overturns the hypothesis of atoms – *anarma* and *minina* – clearly referring to Asclepiades.[107] Likewise in *On the Therapeutic Method*, the inability of atomic particles to be affected is said to be the fatal shortcoming of the account of pain posited by those who subscribe to such a view. Galen then refers his readers to his *On the Opinions of Asclepiades*, suggesting that Asclepiades and his school are the targets of his critique.[108]

It is also possible that Galen addresses the followers of Asclepiades more generally given the phrasing in a passage from *On the Therapeutic Method*, which suggests that his opponents admit to their theory's shortcomings. He explains that those who subscribe to the view that the body is composed of atoms correctly claim that it is impossible to find the condition from which pain results.[109] This may indicate that Galen's opponents were certain contemporary followers of Asclepiades who publicly conceded their point by the time that Galen composed *On the Therapeutic Method*.

Galen's argument against these doctors and philosophers goes as follows: the atomists posit a single unit as the 'element', but this unit is such that it is unable to be affected. At this point, an atomist, of course, could retort that an aggregate of atoms produces the phenomenon of sensation. Therefore, a substantial part of Galen's attack is focused on showing that such aggregates would not be able to generate the phenomenon of sensation either.[110] He does so by theoretical means, that is, logic,[111] while occasionally also invoking appeals to empirical data.[112] The upshot of his argument is that, if one atom is not able to be affected, then neither will two atoms put together, and so forth.[113] Galen's refutation here follows the account of an element that he provides at the beginning of the treatise. Elements are primary parts of an object, but they are not ontologically

105 *CAM* 7, 13 Fortuna (1.249K). On the fragility of Asclepiades' particles, see Vallance (1990: 24–43).

106 See Caston (1997: 352–3).

107 *CAM* 7, 9 Fortuna (1.248K).

108 *MM* 12.7 (10.852–3K).

109 *MM* 12.7 (10.852K).

110 It has been argued in the scholarship that this argument is also found before Galen, in Plutarch *Adv. Col.* 1112B–C; 1113E; see Gemelli Marciano (2007: 259). See also the discussion in Leith (2014: 222–4).

111 See *Hipp. Elem.* 2.22 de Lacy (1.420K).

112 *Hipp. Elem.* 2.38 de Lacy (1.423K).

113 *Hipp. Elem.* 2.24–40 de Lacy (1.420–4K).

distinct. As Galen later states in the treatise, especially in his discussion of the differences between the principle and the element, an element is entirely homogenous with the object that it composes.[114] If an atom is an element of an animal (on Galen's definition of an element), then it must share the properties of the animal.[115]

Thus, Galen rejects elemental 'monism' because it cannot account for the change indicated by the phenomenon of pain. To be more precise, this leads to the conclusion that the phenomenon of pain requires two conditions: (1) qualitative alteration;[116] and (2) sensation.[117] These are discussed more extensively later on in the treatise, but the discussion of pain as such is not prolonged beyond the first proof, viz. that there are many elements. Galen later arrives at the conclusion that a mixture of the four elements is a likely candidate for explaining qualitative change and sensation,[118] which is likewise the phenomenon underlying pain.

4.4.3 *Pain as a Phenomenon and a Sensation*

Sensation, which includes pain and sense perception in general, is a phenomenon of the tissues, that is, the homoeomerous parts. It is worth remembering that the other cause of pain discussed earlier, namely the

114 *Hipp. Elem.* 6.39 de Lacy (1.470K). The principle is not entirely homogenous with the object of which it is a principle. The elements, meanwhile, are entirely homogenous: ἐν τούτῳ γὰρ δὴ καὶ διήνεγκεν ἀρχὴ στοιχείου, τῷ τὰς μὲν ἀρχὰς οὐκ ἐξ ἀνάγκης ὁμογενεῖς εἶναι τοῖς πράγμασιν, ὧν ὑπάρχουσιν ἀρχαί, τὰ δὲ στοιχεῖα πάντως ὁμογενῆ. An element, then, must be the smallest part of the thing of which it is an element, but it also has to be recognisable as a part (however small) of that object.

115 A somewhat strange consequence of this claim is that Galen's argument does not suggest that the world *per se* is not composed of atoms. It merely shows that atoms are not elements. To use Galen's own terminology, atoms cannot be elements, but his argument does not rule out the possibility that atoms could be principles. Thus, the elements of the human body could be composed of atoms, but atoms themselves cannot be the elements.

116 Galen is adopting and adapting the Aristotelian notion of alteration here. For a discussion of his innovations, see Kupreeva (2014).

117 *Hipp. Elem.* 2.18–20 de Lacy (1.419–20K), tr. de Lacy (1996: 63): τὸ γὰρ ἀλγῆσον χρὴ δήπου δύο ταῦτα ἔχειν ἐξ ἀνάγκης, ἀλλοιωτόν τε καὶ αἰσθητικὸν ὑπάρχειν. εἴτε γὰρ μηδέποτε μηδεμίαν ἀλλοίωσιν ἐπιδέχοιτο, φυλάξει διαπαντὸς ἣν εἶχεν ἐξ ἀρχῆς κατάστασιν· οὐ φυλάττει δέ γε τὸ ἀλγοῦν· εἴτε δέ γε μεταβάλλει, καθάπερ οἱ λίθοι τε καὶ τὰ ξύλα θερμαινόμενα τε καὶ ψυχόμενα καὶ διαιρούμενα, μὴ παρείη δὲ αὐτῷ τις αἴσθησις σύμφυτος, οὐκ αἰσθήσεται τῆς ἀμφ' αὐτὸ γενομένης διαθέσεως, ὥσπερ οὐδ' οἱ λίθοι. 'Surely something that is to feel pain must necessarily meet these two requirements: it must be capable of change and capable of sensation. If it never undergoes any change, it will retain at all times the state in which it was at the beginning; but what feels pain does not retain it; and if it changes its state, as stones and wood do when being heated and chilled and split, but no sensation is by nature present in it, it will not perceive the occurrence of the condition that is affecting it, just as stones do not.' See also *Hipp. Elem.* 2.41 de Lacy (1.424K).

118 *Hipp. Elem.* 3.18 de Lacy (1.430–1K).

dissolution of unity, also originates in these parts. To answer the first question raised at the beginning of this section, the nature of pain is such that it has its grounds in the properties of tissues, including flesh. This point is in line with Galen's argument that flesh is even more pain-sensitive than nerves. At the same time, this leads to the question of whether these views are also compatible with the claim that pain is one of the three purposes in distributing the nerves throughout the body, as Galen states in *On the Usefulness of Parts*.

There are two ways of approaching this problem. First, one could take this as a genuine inconsistency that indicates a change in Galen's views. Indeed, given his long and prolific career, this is entirely possible. It is, nonetheless, hard to prove. Thus, it would be best to resort to this conclusion when all the other possibilities have been explored and excluded. The second option, however, would be to consider the contextual differences, after which we can determine whether the differences between the two claims are merely apparent.

Most of the discussions in *On My Own Opinions* are polemical, and the treatise could reasonably be described as a collection of clarifications. As Galen explains at the beginning of the treatise, there are people who misunderstood his works (and thereby, we may presume, criticised him unduly), much of the treatise is therefore intended as a corrective to those errors through the clarification and reiteration of his actual position. In some sections, the debate at stake is very clear. The section on nerves, however, is less explicit, and primarily describes dissections, concluding that nerves are not more sensitive than flesh. Arguably, Galen's way of framing the discussion at the beginning of the section offers hints about the broader debate.

The section begins with the claim that the most sensitive part of the body is that which hosts the *hēgemonikon*, and from it flows the capacity of sensation to the rest of the body by means of nerves.[119] Given that the rest of the section shows the nerves to be no more sensitive than flesh, the position under attack here is that the nerves are inherently sensitive and have the capacity for sensation in themselves. This theory is later discussed in greater detail. For current purposes, the salient claim here is not that the nerves are generally less sensitive than flesh, but rather that the nerve tissues are not inherently imbued with sensitivity. They only obtain this capacity from their connection to the brain, and this claim is supported by

[119] *Prop. Plac.* 6.1 (80 Lami Garofalo): Πρῶτον μὲν γὰρ αἰσθητικὸν ἐδείξαμεν εἶναι τὸ μόριον, ὡς καὶ τοῖς παλαιοῖς ἔδοξεν εἶναι, <ἐν> ᾧι τὸ τῆς ψυχῆς ἡγεμονικόν ἐστιν.

dissections that reveal the nerves are not more sensitive than flesh. Thus, the most important claim here very much coheres with Galen's position in *On the Usefulness of Parts*.

On the Usefulness of Parts repeatedly describes the nerves as being necessary for sensation. In describing the muscles of the hand in Book 1, for instance, Galen explicitly states that sensation is not inherent in the flesh: nerves have to extend from the brain to render this prehensile instrument sensitive.[120] Sensitivity therefore arises from the connection to the brain by means of nerves. This leads to the following picture of the phenomenon of pain with regard to the relationship between the brain, nerves and flesh.

A change in tissues (whether this is qualitative or consists in a change in unity) constitutes the phenomenon of pain. Nevertheless, it is only through a connection with nerves that sensations such as pain can be actually *felt*. In other words, there can be no sensation of pain without the nerves, regardless of the sensitivity of the flesh. A loss of sensation at the ligature of a nerve is an established claim in Galenic corpus,[121] but the discussion of the sensitivity of flesh suggests that what does the heavy lifting on this model is the very distribution of the nerves within the structure of the body, not any innate properties of the nerve tissue. This is a potentially significant insight in understanding the systematicity of Galenic physiology.

Before moving onto the final activity of the nervous system, viz. sense perception, there is still one remaining question to be addressed: the relationship between pain and sensation. These activities are evidently related, but perhaps the reason why Galen separates them is that pain is a distinct kind of sensation. First, unlike sense perception, pain is not continuously present. Its presence signifies some kind of disorder. Second, and more importantly, pain is internally directed. As argued in the discussion of the causes of pain, pain indicates that some pathological event is taking place in the tissues. It is an inwardly directed perception of a pathological state within the body.[122] Given Galen's understanding of the body as, to a certain extent, a self-regulating system,[123] pain affords a valuable tool for the coordination of body parts with a view to health.

[120] *UP* 1.18 (1.44, 18 Helmreich=3.61K).
[121] *Form. Foet.* 5, 2–3 Nickel (4.679K); *PHP* 2.6.6 de Lacy (5.263–4K). See also Ierodiakonou (2022: 221–3).
[122] See *PHP* 7.6.33–6 de Lacy (5.636–7K), where Galen makes his claim while commenting on Hippocrates (*Aph.* 2.6 (4.470 Littré)). See also *Mot. Dub.* 8.21–2 (158, 21–9 Nutton).
[123] See van der Eijk (2017: 237–9).

4.5 Internal Perception and External Sense Perception

The concept of pain as internally directed sense perception neatly captures all of Galen's claims about pain. However, it is important to note that pain is not the only example of such a perception. This chapter began with his claim that the three governing parts are also connected by their offshoots so that they might heed (ἐπαΐειν) each other, followed by the claim that the *nervus vagus* is inserted into the liver so that it would not be entirely without sensation. My discussion of the role that the nerves play in perception will start with the inward-directed perception before moving on to the discussion of the sense perception and the problems of the nature of the nervous tissue.

As well as describing the nerve in the liver as serving a sensory purpose, Galen makes similar claims about the reproductive organs and the stomach;[124] the heart too contains nerves, the significance of which was discussed earlier in this chapter. These organs lack muscles, owing to which nerves are not able to move them. In these cases, nerves only serve the purpose of sensation; and so, his claim about the purpose of the *nervus vagus* in the liver is consistent with his anatomical understanding that for a nerve to exercise control via voluntary motion, an instrument is required. The sensory role of the nerves in these organs, however, cannot be extensive, because only a small number of nerves are present. In the case of the liver, for example, Galen states that a single, small nerve renders the liver barely sensitive at all.[125] This claim reflects ordinary experience. The nerve in the liver simply cannot produce the same sensitivity as, for instance, the optic nerve, because animals see their environment with great precision, which is not the case with the liver. It is barely possible to feel what one's liver is doing. Internally directed perception, therefore, is quite distinct from that which is directed externally. The physiological process underpinning both of them might be the same, but their purposes subtly differ, meaning they are not univocal.

Galen acknowledges the limitations of the sensory role of these nerves when he states that internal organs receive some share of nerves in order that they might not be completely plant-like. However, the liver and heart receive nerves because they are the sources of certain capacities (διότι καὶ αὐτὰ δυνάμεών τινων ὑπάρχουσιν ἀρχαί).[126] In either case, the stakes are

[124] Both female and male reproductive organs; see *UP* 14.13 (2.331, 22–5 Helmreich=4.203K). *UP* 16.5 (2.394, 18–24 Helmreich=4.289K).

[125] *UP* 4.13 (1.226, 2–5 Helmreich=3.308K).

[126] *UP* 6.18 (1.365, 8–9 Helmreich=3.501K).

low: these nerves only need to make the organs more sensitive than the simplest form of organic life. The claim raises two questions. First, why is such a limited role sufficient for the healthy functioning of the body? Second, how can the presence of a nerve elevate an organ from being merely plant-like?

The second question can be answered easily by referring to the case discussed earlier in this work. The kind of 'perception', described as *γνωρίζειν* by Galen, is possessed by plants and bodily tissues has been discussed in Chapter 2. There, I argued that this perception is binary, in the sense that it consists of two reactions: these kinds of entities can only accept or reject material presented to them. The same chapter also presented a discussion of the phenomenon of hunger. Galen divided it into two stages, the physical and the psychic. The physical stage consists of tissues drawing nutriment from the veins and emptying them, prompting the veins to draw from the stomach, which in turn uses food as a remedy. This action does not produce the sensation of hunger by itself. Hunger arises when the stomach perceives the drawing of veins, which leads to the proper sensory perception of hunger. Galen divides the whole process into five parts as follows: 'First there is the emptying; second is the physical appetite of the emptied parts; next is the sucking of the stomach; next is the sensation of this; last of all there is the psychical appetite of this.'[127]

While the text does not include an explicit reference to the nerves, the fifth and final stage must be enabled by the presence of the nerve in the stomach, not least because, elsewhere, Galen notes that perception in organs such as the stomach is grounded in the presence of a nerve.[128] His distinction between nature and soul makes it clear at what point sensation is produced, and thereby when the nervous system comes into play.[129] Lack of nourishment leads the venous tissues to exercise their attractive powers.[130] This leads them to draw from the stomach. The following step involves sensation in the stomach, as denoted by the word αἴσθησις. Both language and conceptual apparatus suggests that this is where the nervous system comes into play. The stomach's sense perception must be owing to the presence of a nerve that sends a signal to the brain, from which results what Galen calls the psychic appetite. Thus, the origin

[127] *Symp. Caus.* 1.7.3 (7.130–1K), tr. Johnston (2006: 227): κένωσις μὲν πρώτη, δευτέρα δὲ ὄρεξις ἡ φυσικὴ τῶν κενωθέντων μορίων, εἶτα ἡ μύζησις τῆς κοιλίας, εἶτα ἡ ταύτης αἴσθησις, εἶτα ἡ ὄρεξις αὐτῆς ἡ ψυχικὴ ἁπασῶν ὑστάτη. This passage is cited in full in Chapter 2.

[128] Stated explicitly in *UP* 4.7 (1.203, 3–9 Helmreich=3.277K).

[129] See *UP* 7.9 (1.399 Helmreich=3.549K), cited and discussed earlier.

[130] See *Nat. Fac.* 2.6–7 (178 Helmreich=2.106K).

of sensation is the point at which physical appetite changes into a psychic one. The former is the change within the tissues, caused by a lack of nourishment. It turns into the latter when a nerve in the stomach registers the changes in its tissue and sends this signal to the brain, which results in a desire for food (and not just – it is worth noting – awareness of lack).

This passage answers the question of how the presence of the nerve makes an organ not entirely plant-like: the nerve allows a psychic sensation of hunger to be produced, thus involving an organ into animalian sense perception. This is an important point. The tissues of an organ can be plant-like in nature, but when put into combination with animal-like organs, the organ is regarded as more animalian just by virtue of the whole to which it belongs. The combination of parts has an impact on the nature of the parts themselves.

This passage also provides an answer to the first question. Only one small nerve is sufficient, because the nerves in these organs only need to register a single kind of phenomenon. Once the brain is informed of the lack of nutriment in the form of appetite, appropriate signals can be sent by means of other sensory and motor nerves. It is also worth noting that such an arrangement keeps the two physiological systems quite distinct: the nerve system is only informed of the state that the nutritive system is in; and while the former can make decisions about supplying or withdrawing food, it cannot exercise any direct control on the latter.

So far, my discussion concerned the instrumental parts, especially the stomach. Can the same explanation be used for the other two governing parts that have nerves inserted in them? Galen himself notes, insofar as the liver is the seat of the nutritive soul, it ought not to require a nerve,[131] but then goes on to explain that the three seats of the souls need to heed each other in the passage cited at the beginning of this chapter. He calls this a philosophical explanation. However, for the sake of making it clear to everyone, it is sufficient to say that the nerve is present in order that the liver is not entirely insensible.

In the explanation obvious to everyone, the liver does not differ from a stomach, insofar as its nerve renders it sensitive. Its special role, then, is primarily to be explained philosophically. Arguably, the liver is distinguished from other internal organs by being the central part in which the desire for bodily pleasure (arising from the vegetative soul) is located.[132] Notably, the stomach only begins to request food as a response to the drawing sensation that comes when veins are emptied of nourishment.

[131] *UP* 4.13 (1.226, 15–18 Helmreich=3.308–9K). [132] *Aff. Dig.* 6.1–2 De Boer (5.27K).

The liver, meanwhile, desires pleasure. This desire might lead to the emptying of veins, which would thereby cause incessant hunger. If left unchecked, the vegetative soul, which is like a wild beast,[133] would render someone completely helpless to their appetites. It is possible to avoid this owing to the presence of the nerve in the liver. However, given that there are no muscles in the liver, this organ cannot be controlled by means of voluntary motion.

Since the nerve of the liver has only sensory powers, perception of the liver's activities must be the means by which the rational part can exercise control over the vegetative. This answer is suggested in a passage from *The Diagnosis and Cure of the Soul's Passions*. Having compared the spirited soul to an animal that can be domesticated, and the vegetative soul to a wild, untameable animal, Galen goes on to say that, although the latter cannot be trained, it can nonetheless be subjected to chastisement (ἡ κόλασις). The more the vegetative soul indulges in its characteristic pleasures, the stronger it grows and *vice versa*. In the latter case, the vegetative soul ends up following the reasoning part because it is small and weak, rather than owing to obedience.[134] The rational part is able to exercise power over the vegetative part indirectly, namely by employing the resources within its power to prevent the expansion of the activities of this soul.

Under normal circumstances, the nerve of the liver simply helps to regulate the intake of nourishment, which is vital for the maintenance of life. This nerve sends a signal to the brain that nutrition is lacking. Subsequently, a voluntary signal can be sent from the brain via the nerves to the other organs to act appropriately. A person might, for example, decide to have a meal. Alternatively, they might refrain from eating because their doctor temporarily prohibits it. It is crucial that the rational part is alert when decisions like these are made. If it is complacent and grants the vegetative soul its desires, then the latter grows in power and becomes unruly. Thus, interestingly, the mere awareness of the activities of the vegetative soul is the key tool of the rational soul to exercise power over the lower irrational soul. This issue, however, is a concern for moral philosophers, not physicians.

Indeed, from a physiological perspective, it is sufficient to note that the perception of the liver's activities allows the nervous system to level responses by enlisting other organs under its control. Without such neural

[133] See the discussion at the beginning of this chapter.

[134] *Aff. Dig.* 6.4 De Boer (5.28K). This point has repercussions for the understanding of weakness as illness; see the discussion in Hankison (2014).

connections, there would be no way for the two internal organs to communicate and maintain life by way of adequate nourishment. This likely explains why organs lacking muscle contain some nerves for the sake of internal sensation.

4.5.1 Sense Perception

Sense perception in the conventional sense, that is, externally directed perception, is a complex phenomenon. This is not only because it involves objects external to the perceiver (thereby raising the epistemological question of the relationship between the agent and the world), but also because it is far from clear which organs are involved internally. Perhaps unsurprisingly, ancient medicine is preoccupied with the latter point. The most unorthodox position is taken up by Asclepiades of Bithynia, who denied the existence of the *hēgemonikon*, stating controversially that all psychic activity is sensory in origin.[135] Arguably, Asclepiades effectively challenged the need for a centralising mechanism that receives the signals of sense perception and, in return, sends out signals for volition. Most ancient physicians posited the existence of such a mechanism, some identifying it with the brain, others with the heart. Regardless of whether they were 'cardiocentrists' or 'encephalocentrists', however, these doctors had to explain the relationship between the sensory and vital organs.

Galen is acutely aware of these issues, as reflected in his discussion of sense perception. The role of the nerves is central to his account, although their role is far from straightforward. For the sake of brevity, this chapter focuses on Galen's discussion of sight as a representative account of all kinds of sense perception. The main reason for this is that Galen often uses eyesight as an example in his therapeutic works, and as a result, there are abundant textual resources. The sensory nerves are central instruments to sense perception, and as mentioned earlier, Galen typically describes them as being especially soft. For this reason, they are receptive to being acted upon and thus receive an impression.[136] The example of a sensory nerve *par excellence* is the optic nerve. This pair of nerves is larger and softer than any others. Owing to this, sight is the most precise of all the senses.[137]

[135] Caelius Aurelianus 1.14.115; Sextus Empiricus *M* 7.1.202.
[136] *UP* 8.5 (1.458, 26–459, 2 Helmreich=3.633K).
[137] *UP* 16.3 (2.383, 4–5 Helmreich=4.273K).

The problem of the parts of the eye and the role each of them plays in eyesight was discussed in Chapter 1. To reiterate briefly, there are seemingly two parts of the eye with identical activities. Galen generally claims that the most important part of the eye is the lens, which is (properly speaking) the part responsible for sight.[138] It is a homoeomerous part capable of being altered by external colours, thereby enabling an animal to see.[139] The optic nerves, however, are also special organs of sight, not only owing to their special attributes (such as their size, softness and the presence of channels for pneuma), but also owing to the fact that the severance of the nerve completely deprives the organ of sensation. For this reason, when determining a diagnosis, the loss of sight indicates a nerve injury.[140] Sight is damaged when either of these two parts is injured.[141] Chapter 1 presented an argument, using the example of the optic nerve, that the parthood ought to be understood functionally and therefore the boundaries of an organ can be relative. More importantly for the current purposes, the argument pointed out that Galen makes a distinction between registering sensation in the lens and properly perceiving it by means of the nerve connection to the brain.[142]

This conclusion is reinforced by the understanding of the overall function of the sensory nerves developed in this chapter. There is a parallel between the way in which Galen conceptualises external sense perception on the one hand, and pain and inward-directed perception on the other hand. The role of the lens is comparable to the role of the stomach: Galen named the sensations in the latter 'physical' until the alteration in the tissues was registered by the nerve, at which point it became psychic. The

138 *Inst. Od.* 3, 6 Kollesch (2.864K); *Symp. Caus.* 1.2.1 (7.86K). For Galen's account of vision, see *PHP* 7.5.5–7 de Lacy (5.619K) and Ierodiakonou (2014); Ierodiakonou (2022) discusses the philosophical background of this theory.

139 *MM* 1.6 (10.48–9K). See also *Plat. Tim.* Fr. 22–3 (Larrain). It is quite telling that, although sight can be impeded by various illnesses and injuries affecting the supporting parts, the proper illnesses of sight are said to be those deriving from the *dyskrasia* of the lens.

140 *UP* 10.8 (2.82 Helmreich=3.798K) describes a case in which one of a person's eyes is more prominent than the other. Since the person could still see, Galen inferred that the nerve was stretched. Had this person lost sight, Galen would have inferred that the nerve was injured as well.

141 Galen says so explicitly in *Symp. Caus.* 1.2.1 (7.86K): Οἷον ἐν ὀφθαλμῷ τὸ μὲν πρῶτον ὄργανον αἰσθητικόν ἐστιν τὸ κρυσταλλοειδὲς, ἐδείχθη γὰρ τοῦτο μόνον ὑπὸ χρωμάτων ἀλλοιούμενον· ἡ δὲ αἰσθητικὴ δύναμις, ἡ ἐξ ἐγκεφάλου παραγινομένη διὰ τοῦ καθήκοντος εἰς αὐτὸν νεύρου· τὰ δ' εἰς ὑπηρεσίαν αὐτοῦ γεγονότα σύμπαντά ἐστι τὰ ἄλλα τὰ κατὰ τὸν ὀφθαλμὸν μόρια. καὶ τοίνυν ἤτοι κακῶς, ἢ οὐδ' ὅλως ὄψεται τὸ ζῶον, ἑνός γέ τινος ἐκ τῶν εἰρημένων βεβλαμμένου.

142 He states this explicitly in his argument *PHP* 7.6.31 de Lacy (5.636K), noting that 'perception, then, is not alteration, as some say, but discernment of alteration' (οὔκουν ἀλλοίωσίς ἐστιν ἡ αἴσθησις, ὥς ἔνιοί φασιν, ἀλλα διάγνωσις ἀλλοιώσεως), tr. de Lacy (1978–84: 469).

same must be true in the case of the former, even if we do not get a description with the exact same terms. By virtue of its mixture, the lens processes pneuma, however, as with all homoeomerous tissues, it merely alters in the presence of an external impression. Visual perception takes place when qualitative changes in the lens affect the optic nerve, which in turn carries this signal to the brain. Both alterations in the lens and in the stomach do not produce sensory perception until they are registered by their nerves inserted in these organs.

Although this point clarifies the relationship between the nerve and other tissues, Galen's understanding of the very nature of the nervous tissue needs to be analysed still further. He states that it is the nerve tissue that provides visual capacity, even if it is not able to convert external impressions on its own, owing to which it requires a lens. One might read this as a claim that perception occurs in the nerve tissue. Such a commitment would have far-reaching ramifications. Were this the case, Galen would be stating that rationality can be grounded in the activities of the nerve tissue, which not only raises the question of how he accounts for it, but also suggests a possibility that Galen might be (in spite of his praising the design of Nature) a closet physicalist, in the sense that he was implicitly committed to the view that psychic properties can be fully and sufficiently accounted for by means of the properties and activities of the nerve tissue. This would extend beyond sense perception and include accounting for intelligence in the form of rational, deliberate actions. The issue at stake here is actually rather simple: it is the inherent sensitivity of the nerve tissue, by virtue of which a signal can be produced. If the nerve tissue can be shown, according to Galen, to have inherent properties that allow them to perform the constitutive activities of sense perception or voluntary motion, then this would count as the foundation for a physicalist stance.

4.6 The Inherent Sensitivity of the Nervous Tissue

Arguably, one crucial piece of evidence for settling this issue can be found in Galen's criticism of Herophilus' account of nerve sensitivity. In *On Tremor, Palpitation, Spasm and Rigor*, Galen attacks Praxagoras and Herophilus for their views regarding the extent of the activities of the nerve tissue:

> πεπονθὼς δὲ τόπος εἷς οὐδείς ἐστιν ἐξ ἀνάγκης ἐν τρόμοις, καὶ μέμφομαί γε ἐνταῦθα Πραξαγόρᾳ καὶ Ἡροφίλῳ, τῷ μὲν ἀρτηριῶν πάθος εἰπόντι τὸν

τρόμον, Ἡροφίλῳ δὲ φιλοτιμουμένῳ δεῖξαι περὶ τὸ νευρῶδες αὐτὸ γένος ἀεὶ συνιστάμενον. ὁ μὲν οὖν Πραξαγόρας πόρρω τοῦ ἀληθοῦς ἥκει· ὁ δὲ Ἡρόφιλος ἠπατήθη τὸ τῆς δυνάμεως πάθος ἀναφέρων τοῖς ὀργάνοις. ὅτι μὲν γὰρ τὸ νευρῶδες γένος, οὐ τὸ ἀρτηριῶδες, ὑπηρετεῖ ταῖς κατὰ προαίρεσιν κινήσεσιν, ὀρθῶς ἐγίνωσκεν· ὅτι δὲ οὐκ αὐτὸ τὸ σῶμα τῶν νεύρων αἴτιον κινήσεως, ἀλλὰ τοῦτο μὲν ὄργανον, ἡ κινοῦσα δ᾽ αἰτία ἡ διήκουσα δύναμις διὰ τῶν νεύρων ἐστὶν, ἐνταῦθα μέμφομαι αὐτῷ μὴ διορίσαντι δύναμίν τε καὶ ὄργανον. εἰ γὰρ διώρισεν, εὐθὺς ἂν ἔγνω διότι βλαβήσεται τοὖργον οὐκ ὀργάνων μόνων, ἀλλὰ καὶ δυνάμεων πάθει. ἐπὶ μὲν οὖν τῶν τεθνεώτων οὐδὲν οὔτε τὰ νεῦρα πέπονθεν οὔθ᾽ οἱ μύες, ὅσα πάθη πάσχειν αὐτὰ νομίζουσιν Ἡρόφιλός τε καὶ Πραξαγόρας· ἀπολέλοιπε δ᾽ αὐτῶν πᾶσα κίνησις εὐθὺς ἅμα τῇ ψυχῇ, μύες δὲ καὶ νεῦρα ταύτης ὄργανα. οὔκουν μυὸς οὐδὲ νεύρου τὸ κινεῖν, ἀλλὰ ψυχῆς. οὐδὲ γὰρ αὐλῶν ἔργον ἡ αὔλησις, οὐδὲ κιθάρας ἡ κιθάρισις· ἀλλ᾽ αὔλησις μὲν ἔργον αὐλητοῦ δι᾽ ὀργάνων αὐλῶν, κιθάρισις δὲ τοῦ μουσικοῦ, τὸ δ᾽ ὄργανον ἡ κιθάρα. διαφθαρήσεται δὲ καὶ αὔλημα καὶ κιθάρισις πολλάκις μὲν διὰ τοὺς τῶν ἔργων δημιουργούς, ἔσθ᾽ ὅτε δὲ διὰ τὴν τῶν ὀργάνων οἷς χρῶνται βλάβην. οὕτω δὲ καὶ κινήσεως ἐν τῷ ζώῳ τῆς κατὰ προαίρεσιν ὁ μὲν οὖν δημιουργὸς καὶ τεχνίτης ἡ διοικοῦσα τὸ ζῶόν ἐστι δύναμις, τὰ δὲ ὄργανα νεῦρα καὶ μύες.

There is necessarily no one affected place in tremors, and here I find fault with Praxagoras and Herophilus – with the former for saying that tremor is an affection of the arteries, with Herophilus for being so eager to show that tremor is always associated with the nerves. Praxagoras is further from the truth; but Herophilus erred in attributing to the organs [i.e., instruments] an illness that is actually of the motive capacity. He understood correctly that it is the nerves, not the arteries, which serve the voluntary motions. But since the body of the nerves is not itself the cause of motion, but is only the instrument, and since the cause of motion is the motive capacity moving through the nerves, I find fault with him for not having distinguished capacity from instrument. For if he had made such a distinction, he would have straightaway recognised that actions will suffer not only because of affections of the instruments, but also because of affections of the body's capacities. Thus, in dead men neither nerves or muscles experience anything such as Herophilus and Praxagoras think they experience, yet every motion has left them the instant the soul does, and muscles and nerves are instruments of the soul. Hence motion does not come from the muscle or nerve, but from the soul. Just so, pipe-playing is not an activity of pipes, nor lyre-playing of the lyre; pipe-playing is an activity of the pipe-player with the pipes as instruments, and lyre-playing that of the musician, the lyre being the instrument. Often the playing of the pipe or lyre is brought to a bad end because of the craftsmen of these activities, and sometimes because of damage to the instruments which they use. Similarly, the craftsman and artificer of voluntary motion in animal life is the capacity governing the animal, while the instruments are the nerves and muscles.[143]

For the purposes of this chapter, I am going to concentrate on Galen's attack on Herophilus, putting to one side his comments about Praxagoras.[144] His criticism incorporates two key claims: the first being conceptual, the other, anatomical. With regard to the former, these doctors mistake an instrument for a capacity. Galen illustrates this error with the analogy of a musician and a musical instrument. An injury to an instrument might prevent a certain activity, namely playing, but one would be making a conceptual error in assuming that the activity is caused by the instrument. While Galen's point seems apt in principle, nothing in his description suggests that the Alexandrian anatomist used the language of an instrument and a craftsman.[145] From what he reports, Herophilus' point was primarily a matter of anatomical observation.

Here, it seems fairly clear that, on Galen's account, Herophilus argued that the nerves are composed of inherently sensitive tissue. This would explain Galen's statement that, in the case of the deceased, nerves and muscles do not suffer the affection that these two doctors claim they do. Although no concrete example is given, it seems likely that Herophilus performed a dissection on a recently deceased body, thereby finding that nerves remain sensitive after death. His experimentation revealed that pinching a nerve can result in a degree of muscular movement.[146] Notably, in some other works, Galen presents a *diaeresis* of opinions of those who maintain that the nerves are sensitive, and those who claim that they get their sensitivity from another organ, namely the brain.

[143] Galen *Trem. Palp.* 5 (7.605–6K), tr. Sider and McVaugh (1979: 194–5), slightly altered. See also von Staden (1989: 255–7).

[144] For an in-depth study of Praxagoras' views, and the sources for those views, see Lewis (2017).

[145] See the discussion of the notion of the *demiurge* in Chapter 3.

[146] For comparison, Praxagoras, who is also attacked in this passage, argued that arteries pulsate when ligated; see Lewis (2017: 242–6). There are two questions following this point. First, one might wonder why Galen did not repeat Herophilus' experiment in order to try to obtain the same result. A brief remark in his discussion of the problems pertaining to the muscular motion (see also the discussion in the Introduction) shows that he may have. While discussing the lack of awareness of the nerves that move our bodies while alive, he notes that these nerves 'even in a dead body, when activated manually, do not appear to draw in the muscles in the way that the muscles do the bones and joints', *Form. Foet.* 6, 11 Nickel (4.691K), tr. Singer (1997: 196). This remark suggests that Galen did attempt to produce a dissection that resembled Herophilus', but without success. Second, one might also wonder whether Galen failed to take into account the case of an animal continuing to move shortly after decapitation. The answer to the latter question is quite easy: Galen ascribed to the nerves voluntary motion *alone*. The erratic motion of an animal's body can be explained by other means, not by the functioning of the nervous system, according to his theoretical framework.

At the beginning of *On Problematical Movements*, for example, particularly in a generic description of the work of anatomists, it is clearly stated that, in terms of motion in the nerves, the central question is whether their activity is owing to their own nature or whether another part provided them with this activity.[147] This shows that both were viable options for an anatomist to consider in Galen's time. In *On the Formation of the Embryo*, while discussing paralysis, Galen mentions that knowing whether the parts themselves are endowed with perception and voluntary motion, or whether this capacity flows from the brain (or the heart), constitutes the first step in deciding upon the right treatment.[148] This preoccupation can moreover be found outside of Galen's texts. For example, in a passage in *On the Anatomy of the Parts of the Body* (an anonymous treatise attributed to Rufus of Ephesus), Herophilus and Erasistratus (by contrast with Asclepiades) putatively maintain that the nerves are *aisthētika*.[149]

Thus, it is clear that Galen and Herophilus adopt different positions. Although Galen routinely reiterates that one of the primary activities of the nervous system is sensation, the nerves themselves are not inherently capable of sensation. Rather, they enjoy this ability by virtue of being connected to the brain. It is not uncommon to find explicit examples in the Galenic corpus of the relationship between sensation and the brain.[150] He claims that parts unconnected to the brain lack sensation,[151] in some places even stating that 'the source of sensation and of all the nerves is in the *encephalon*',[152] thereby indicating that not just all the other parts but the nerves themselves depend on the brain for their sensitivity. This is often supported by demonstration. The ligature of a nerve will result in the loss of sensation below the cut, but the part above the cut will retain sensation and the ability to move voluntarily, provided it is connected to the brain.[153]

Galen's stance has significant consequences. Since he does not subscribe to the view held by Herophilus, which attributes some sensitivity to the nerve tissue itself, there is no way of providing a reductive account that would explain the activities of rationality (especially sensation and voluntary movement) in physicalist terms. One might consider the possibility that, while the nerves are simply channel-like organs, the brain itself is

[147] *Mot. Dub.* 1.11 (124, 21–4 Nutton). [148] For instance, see *Foet. Form.* 4, 5 Nickel (4.676K).
[149] Rufus of Ephesus *Anat.* 73 (184–5 Daremberg Ruelle). [150] *MM* 6.4 (10.409K).
[151] *MM* 6.4 (10.409K).
[152] *UP* 3.11 (1.178, 3–4 Helmreich=3.242K), tr. May (1968: 191): αἰσθήσεως ἀρχὴ καὶ νεύρων ἁπάντων ἐν ἐγκεφάλῳ.
[153] As in, for instance, *Foet. Form.* 6, 26 Nickel (4.697K).

different. Yet Galen explicitly denies this. In *On the Formation of the Embryo*, he sets out to examine whether the substance of bodies (σωμάτων ἡ οὐσία) is the same throughout or manifold.[154] He immediately adds that the brain and nerves share a tissue type:

> ἡ μὲν γὰρ τοῦ νωτιαίου τε καὶ τῶν νεύρων ἡ αὐτὴ κατὰ πάντ' ἐστὶ ἐγκεφάλῳ, καθάπερ γε καὶ ἡ τῶν περιεχόντων αὐτὰ σκεπασμάτων τῇ τῶν περιεχουσῶν μηνίγγων τὸν ἐγκέφαλον·
>
> Now the substance of the spinal cord and the nerves is in every respect the same as that of the brain, just as that of the casements which contain them is the same as that of the membranes which contain the brain.[155]

Consequently, if the tissues of the nerves are not able to carry out certain activities merely by virtue of their inherent properties, nor will the brain. It then follows that, for the higher cerebral functions to take place, there must either be a further precondition or some crucial piece of physiological knowledge is missing, although we do not know what that might be.[156] There is an interesting consequence worth noting here. Given the data of Galenic physiology, it is not possible for him to give a comprehensive aetiological account of all the activities that the nervous system participates in and even governs with the bottom-up explanation. This observation is consistent with Galen's repeated disavowal of any knowledge of the soul's substance.[157] There is a clear correlation between the activities of the soul and the activities of the nervous system, although the latter cannot account for the full range of the former and thus cannot be identified as its substance.[158]

[154] Here, substance is meant in the Stoic, rather than the Aristotelian, sense.

[155] *Foet. Form.* 5, 5 Nickel (4.680K), tr. Singer (1997: 190).

[156] One might wonder whether psychic pneuma may be able to play the missing role. This issue is discussed in Chapter 5. However, it is worth noting even here that Galen describes pneuma as an instrument of the rational soul, not to be identified with the substance of the latter (see Hankinson 2006: 235–6 and Rocca 2003: 196–8).

[157] *Foet. Form.* 6, 34 Nickel (4.701–2K); *Prop. Plac.* 3.5 (68 Lami Garofalo); 7.1–2 (86 Lami Garofalo).

[158] The question of the exact relationship between the two is complex, and Galen's treatise on this topic (*The Capacities of the Soul Follow the Mixtures of the Body*) is not as straightforward as one might hope (see the extensive discussion in Singer (2013: 337ff., esp. 357–9) and Jouanna (2009: 196ff.)). The problem lies in the terminology, especially the verb *hepesthai*, which can have different meanings (Hankinson 2006: 243–3). When Galen discusses this term in his *Institutio Logica* (4.7 Kalbfleisch), he uses it to denote a consequent in a hypothetical proposition, adding that this relationship occurs in many ways and is the task of the theory of proof to investigate. Therefore, encountering this verb in Galen means that we are faced with the relationship that can be put into a hypothetical proposition, if p, then q. This only allows for a logical relation between an antecedent and a consequent, but of course, the really interesting question here is whether there

Such a physiological account of the nervous system aligns with Platonist commitments, although it is not motivated by them. Ultimately, Galen's hesitation in committing to a physicalist explanation of rational activities might be owing not so much to personal faith or commitments to Platonism (although these are no doubt relevant factors too), but very likely the impossibility of finding clear and sound grounds for the claim that rational activities can be reduced to physical substances or processes. The fact that an injury of certain nerves affects sense perception shows that there is a connection between nerve tissue and the *hēgemonikon*. Yet Galen only has enough evidence to render the nervous system necessary for higher cerebral functions. His rejection of Herophilus' conclusion prevents him from taking the nervous system to provide a sufficient condition of higher cerebral functions.

Galen's denial of the results of Herophilus' dissection has far-reaching consequences. While it explains Galen's *aporia* with regard to the substance of the soul, it leads to a further question: why does Galen reject the results of Herophilus' dissection? There are at least two possible motivations: the methods of dissection, and his theory of homoeomerous tissues. In certain aforementioned passages, Galen presents his own dissections, thereby demonstrating that nerves lose their capacity once severed from the brain. He calls these demonstrations, a term used for scientifically established pieces of knowledge.[159] He may have genuinely thought that Herophilus' dissection was not scientific enough, given the dismissive tone he assumes. A pertinent consideration for him may be the fact that, in principle, there are several different types of motions in bodies – voluntary motion being only one of them,[160] and it could be argued that it is less than clear that the motion described by Herophilus is indeed voluntary

is also something like a metaphysical relation. It has been argued recently that the relationship between the mixtures and the capacities of the soul ought to be read metaphysically, as a claim about the constitution of capacities (Marechal 2019: 10–12), but without an attempt to rule out other possible readings. Also, as Singer (2013: 358–9) points out, the view of strong dependency must come with substantial caveats in any case.

159 The main treatise on this topic, *On Demonstration*, is not extant, but Galen refers to this method in his other works; see Havrda (2015). On the notion of demonstration, see Hankinson (2009: 208–14). For applications of demonstration for understanding the nervous system, including the brain, see Rocca (2003: 50–8).

160 There are, for example, involuntary motions of the heart, the motions caused by natural capacities (attraction and expulsion), 'natural' tendencies for downward movement (*UP* 13.12 (2.280, 17–19 Helmreich=4.135–6K); see also *UP* 11.6 (2.128, 13–15 Helmreich=3.863K)), as well as various pathological motions (*MM* 12.8 (10.872K)). The entire *Trem. Palp.* presents an in-depth study of these movements.

and not some other, posthumous bodily reaction.[161] Galen might have been genuinely concerned that Herophilus' observation is not in accordance with investigating the substance of the matter,[162] but rather an accidental property. This must remain a somewhat speculative reading, however, because Galen does not provide us with a more elaborate critique of Herophilus' experiment.

Second, Herophilus' results cannot be supported by the Galenic understanding of the homoeomerous tissues. In terms of constitution, the nerves are typical homoeomerous tissues containing four properties. By virtue of the specific combination of these properties, nerve tissues are endowed with their peculiar capacities.[163] The most pertinent capacity of the nerve tissue is the alterative one, since it enables the transmission of the signals of voluntary motion and perception. In his commentary on Hippocrates' *On Elements*, while criticising atomistic accounts of sense perception, Galen clearly makes the alterative capacity necessary for perception.[164] It is not, however, limited to perception. The very same alterative capacity plays a crucial role in the absorption of nutriment, as discussed in Chapter 2.

In an elaborate discussion of natural capacities in *On the Natural Capacities*, Galen shows that the tissues endowed with them are limited in their capacity to generate: they can increase in mass something that already exists, in other words, they cause growth, but they cannot generate something entirely new. Genesis requires the shaping capacity, which is, as Galen says, present at the conception of an embryo,[165] but distinct from the alterative, attractive, repulsive and retentive capacities, which enable the embryo to develop after the conception.

Given that the nervous tissue is, according to Galen, a typical homoeomerous body, the same limitations must apply to its activities too. As such, it is endowed with natural capacities, primarily the alterative capacity. Nonetheless, this alterative capacity, while being absolutely instrumental to rationality, is not itself rational. This tissue can accept/reject/alter/retain in response to objects presented to it externally, but it cannot do something deliberatively, viz. in order to achieve a result. In this

161 Putative support for such a reading can be found in *PHP* 1.5.13 de Lacy (5.184K), where, having given several examples involving dead animals, Galen calls these examples superfluous. It is not clear whether he simply means to say that he has given too many examples or that the examples involving dead animals are not very effective, owing to which it is superfluous to include them. However, the fact that (in the very next sentence) he claims that he is now returning to the living indicates the likelihood of the latter.

162 See Frede (1987: 279–300); Tieleman (2008).

163 *Nat. Fac.* 1.3 (106 Helmreich=2.7–8 K).

164 *Hipp. Elem.* 1.2 de Lacy (1.419–20K) and 1.3 de Lacy (1.430–1K).

165 See the discussion in Chapter 2.

respect, an informative passage comes from *On Problematical Movements*. Here, the natural capacities in organs are described as acting for themselves alone, not out of foresight for the body as a whole, viz. the stomach does not digest food for the body as a whole, nor does the liver make the blood for the body as a whole.[166] These activities do serve a purpose for the body as a whole, but this purpose does not originate in the organs themselves. The stomach and the liver lack intent. The same must be true of the nerve tissue. The activities motivated by intentions are done by the shaping capacity, which Galen does not locate in any tissue, precisely because tissues are too ergonomically primitive to do anything quite so sophisticated. Galen's understanding of the fundamental constitution of human bodies is, paradoxically, so reductive that it leaves no way to account for the mind in physicalist terms.[167]

4.7 Concluding Remarks: The Self-sensing, Self-moving Unity of Parts

In many respects, it is no wonder that the nerves receive significantly more attention from Galen than any of the other offshoots from the ruling parts. Building on the crucial discoveries of Herophilus, he attempts to systematise the activities of the nervous system as tripartite: the motor nerves are responsible for voluntary motion, the sensory ones for pain and sense perception. Although Galen's discussions of nerves tend to be more elaborate and extensive than the discussions of veins or arteries, his theorisation of the nervous tissues follows a pattern found in his accounts of the other systems too. The texture and location of the sensory nerves in comparison to the motor ones correspond to the texture and location of the psychic pneuma in comparison to the vital one. Similarly, the activities of the nerves are dependent on instrumental parts as follows: even the relatively sturdy motor nerves are too soft to move hard bones. Therefore, muscles are needed, creating a chain of motion: soft nerve moves slightly harder tissue of a muscle which, in turn, moves even harder tissue of a bone. The scheme resembles Galen's division of tissues according to their density in Chapter 3, only in that case, the issue at stake was alterative change (heating) rather than kinetic. The Galenic body is, thus, textured: the density of tissues explains how different bodily parts affect each other.

[166] *Mot. Dub.* 4.32–3 (142, 16–25 Nutton).
[167] See also the discussion of the scholarship on this issue in the Introduction.

The nervous system has two key activities: perception and voluntary motion. Both of them have important implications for the unity of the body in distinct ways. Beginning with the former, consider the distinction between the psychic and the physical part of the phenomenon of hunger, discussed in this chapter and Chapter 1. The physical part consists of a series of one tissue drawing from another tissue due to lack of nutriment. When the nerve 'senses' this lack in the stomach, it is not because the stomach drew from the nerve; it is a new kind of relationship between the tissues that starts the psychic stage of the hunger phenomenon. The sensory nerves register and transmit change in their own way, not by being affected in the same way that the suffering tissue or organ is being affected. The nervous system enables the body to perceive its parts as parts, to differentiate sensation and the perception of sensation. This differentiation reveals the significance of the second activity of the nervous system, voluntary motion, for the physiological unity.

Voluntary motion is in particular concerned with control, as noted at the beginning of the chapter. The ensuing discussion has shown, however, that the nerves have direct control over other parts only in a relatively small way. The nervous system exercises control only over the body parts with muscles that partake in voluntary motion. The majority of internal bodily motions do not fall under the jurisdiction of the nervous system at all. The nerves do reach all of the large organs, but the nerves inserted in such parts as the stomach or even the liver are sensory. At the same time, this sensory connection does allow it to exercise some control indirectly. By 'sensing', for example, hunger, the brain can direct the body to seek food and eat; it can also refuse to seek food despite the urge from the nutritive system. The extent of the control that the nervous system has over the cardiac and the nutritive systems amounts only to this: the capacity to deny (some of) the influx of matter these systems control.

At the same time, the phenomenon that constitutes denial to certain appetites on a psychological level also constitutes a mechanism for protecting vitality on the physiological level: to hold the breath in smoke,[168] to take medicine when needed and similar. Similarly, pain, the perception of damage in the tissues, also ultimately serves the purpose of self-protection of the body. Other tissues in the body, such as flesh, would have a fairly solipsistic existence without the presence of nerves, which could also

[168] An example used in *UP* 6.2 (1.302, 10–15 Helmreich=3.414K).

endanger life. Awareness of the damage to tissues is necessary in order to take an action to avoid or rectify the damage. The nervous system, therefore, enables the body to act in a more unified manner: not merely to be drawn or repulsed (in both vegetative and spirited senses) but also to have a sensation of oneself as a whole composed of different parts, to act with intention with an aim of self-reservation.

Ultimately, the nervous system does not seem to have a privileged governing status in comparison to the other two physiological domains. It is true that its capacities are more complex, and its role as the seat of the rational soul inevitably ties it closely to human identity. However, as a physiological governing part (ἀρχή), the brain is *on par* with the heart and the liver. In a way, the genuine tripartition of the physiological domains raises a more significant challenge to the bodily unity than any other type of division. How the three form a single unified whole that can be genuinely called one? Chapter 5 addresses this problem and examines in greater detail how Galen adopts and adapts this Platonic model as well as what devices he uses for unifying the body.

CHAPTER 5

Tripartition
Putting the Body Back Together

Each of the preceding chapters addressed the question of systematic unity. The emerging picture shows that every physiological system not only acts in a unified, self-sustaining way, they also work together to enable the animal to function as a multipart yet self-sustaining compound, forming a unified whole. While the physiological cohesion of activities is clear enough, the philosophical motivation and framing of Galen's project warrants further discussion. If there is one model for theorising bodily functions that is genuinely crucial for Galen, it is undoubtedly tripartition. His commitment to this model is not only stated outright – by positing three governing parts and three souls – but also reflected in his tendency to seek out and theorise three types even when there is only clear evidence for two. For example, his considerations about the possible existence of the natural pneuma clearly originate from the idea that if the cardiac and the nervous systems each have their pneuma, then the nutritive system might have too. Similarly, the standard division of motion into voluntary and involuntary is sometimes accompanied by a note that there is the third type, located in veins and unnoticeable.[1] Presumably, Galen's interest in finding tripartitions is motivated by his engagement with Platonist tradition and commitment to the tripartition of the soul.

However, his adoption of the Platonic model comes with a distinct set of problems and challenges. Some of them are a matter of consistent application of the model. For example, while generally sticking to the three-systems model, Galen sometimes names the fourth ruling principle, the reproductive system, and it is not entirely clear how the reproductive system ought to be accommodated with tripartition. More importantly, the Platonic model is motivated by the need to account for the psychological conflict of desires, emotions and thoughts. An important example of such conflict is the problem of *akrasia*, the failing of the will to choose

[1] For instance, *Trem. Palp.* 2 (7.585K).

the better action. In Plato, this problem presupposes a complex multipart soul, and it does not arise when working with a simple model of the soul.[2] By locating each of the souls in a part of the body,[3] Plato also implies physiological dependencies and, potentially, conflicts, but leaves them vague. Galen, meanwhile, is keen on elaborating these dependencies,[4] but he faces a problem.[5] If the souls can have conflicting desires,[6] and these desires have physiological manifestations (which either constitute the desires, like in the two lower souls, or enable them instrumentally),[7] then there must be some evidence of conflict on the physiological level too. There is, however, little grounds for a genuine conflict in Galen's description of physical interaction between soul domains, and this problem is well known in Galenic scholarship.[8] This study also found hardly any evidence of tension among central physiological systems. Even when certain activities are partially taken over by another system, it is not

[2] This is pointed out in Shields (2007: 61); on the psychological conflict in Plato, see also Kamtekar (2017: 144–57). Although *akrasia* is most prominently problematised by Aristotle (see Destrée 2007), the Stoic account of moral weakness is an important alternative owing to their commitment to unitary psychology. They argued that passions and inclinations are judgements in their own right. Galen reports this view, citing Chrysippus, polemically in *PHP* 4.5.13–23 de Lacy (5.394–6K). For more on Stoic account, see Gourinat (2007), Joyce (1995) and Sorabji (2000: 56–61).

[3] *Ti.* 69E–70E; it is worth noting that this passage not only talks about the locations (the head, the thorax and below the midriff) but also the separation of these areas by the neck and the diaphragm.

[4] In *PHP* 6.8.57 de Lacy (5.577K), he claims that while Plato talks of 'the soul', Hippocrates talks of body parts, and such descriptions are appropriate to their respective disciplines, even if, ultimately, they speak of the same thing.

[5] Notably, Galen says he follows Plato who maintains that his account is 'reasonable' and 'probable'. At the same time, Galen talks about proofs that there are three forms of the soul (*PHP* 9.9.6–7 de Lacy (5.793K)); on Galen's approach to the plausible arguments of Plato's, see Tieleman (1996: 55–65, 2022: 145–6).

[6] Although deliberation (see Schiefsky 2012: 348) and voluntary action is the domain of the rational soul, strong emotions can also trigger action; Galen talks of, for example, anger in this way in *PHP* 6.1.17–18 de Lacy (5.510K); see Singer (2017).

[7] In *QAM* 2 (33, 10–16 Müller=4.768–9K), Galen argues that one can infer that the souls have different substances on the basis of the differences in their activities (ἐνεργεῖαι) and affections (πάθη). His main argument amounts to the claim that if the activities and affections are different, then the capacities must be so as well. The capacities of the two lower souls are completely reducible to the properties of their material constitution, as argued in Havrda (2017); the hunger sensation discussed in Chapters 2 (the 'physical' part of the process) is an illustration of how this theorisation manifests in a physiological process. Body parts as instruments to the rational have been discussed in Chapters 3 and 4.

[8] The seminal article in this case is Mansfeld (1991: esp. 138–45). As Mansfeld rightly points out, Galen's tripartition is fairly inelegant when it comes to accounting for the physical underpinnings of the inner conflict. Schiefsky (2012) and Trompeter (2018) address this problem to some extent, although Mansfeld's point largely still stands; see also Tieleman (2003b). The extensive study in Gill (2010: see esp. 103–24) addresses the problematic aspects of Galen's psychological tripartition constructively; the analysis results in the argument that the unitary model of psychology would have fitted Galen's anatomical data and psychological commitments better.

described as a struggle but as an arrangement that benefits the whole body.

I would argue that Galen's approach to the tripartition can be made clearer by carefully delineating psychological and physiological aspects of this model. Ultimately, both of them are manifest in the same single whole: a human being. However, this whole can be studied in different ways, and, in fact, Galen does so. While putting an emphasis on the cohesion of the different soul domains in the passages discussed in this study so far, he does discuss the conflict of the souls explicitly in his psychological works, such as *On Character Traits* or *The Diagnosis and Treatment of the Affections and Errors Peculiar to Each Person's Soul.* He talks extensively of moral excellence or failure in terms of the hierarchy of the souls: ideally, the rational soul reigns with its helper the spirited soul, while the lowest soul is subdued.[9] When the latter grows strong, moral problems ensue.

However, despite having physiological manifestations, these problems are not physiological inasmuch as they do not pose a threat to vitality. Physiological and psychological enquiries concern themselves with different questions. In the case of the former, it is the question of what must be done to keep a person alive, or, in Callimachean terms, to postpone death. A morally good person is as susceptible to death when deprived of breath as a morally bad person. All body parts are necessary for vitality, and they have to work together to preserve it (this theme will be developed further in this chapter). From a physiological point of view, the tripartition is a unifying mechanism that enables the body to be a living *one*. In the case of moral psychology, the key concern is the relationship between these parts, especially in terms of their hierarchical arrangement. Psychological enquiry presupposes the physiological unity (the three domains are in place and working so as to keep the person alive), further asking what roles the three souls and their respective domains *ought to* have within that functioning system. In short, the physiology of tripartition presupposes cooperative existence (maintaining life), the psychology of tripartition presupposes a potential for conflict (determining how that life ought to be lived).[10] Some

[9] *Morb.* 1, 28, 10–15 Kr. Cf. *Republic* 9.580D–581C, see Schiefsky (2012: 336). See also *Morb.* 2, 39, 20–40, 5 Kr., together with Hankinson (1993: 203–4) for the explanation of how the spirited soul aids the rational soul. Galen compares the two lower souls to domesticated and wild animals in *Aff. Dig.* 1.5.11–6.2 De Boer (5.27–28K); see also *Morb.* 1, 27, 19–20 Kr.; *PHP* 6.2.14 de Lacy (5.518K).

[10] An important point is that Galen does not import the notion of psychological conflict *tout court* from Plato. As Kaufman (2017) shows, in Galenic tripartition, the desires of the three domains are irreplaceable and therefore, it is not possible to have a rational desire of, for instance, food.

aspects of this conflict can have physical manifestations in physiological systems,[11] but the study of such manifestations is very different from the study of vital functions.

Although physiological unity emerged from the discussion so far, it is important to note that it is not clear how Galen theorises it. After all, however cooperative the three governing organs might be, they are still three in number. How do they form *one*? This chapter is dedicated to investigating theoretical devices that Galen employs to account for the unity of tripartition. It especially focuses on two notions: the form and the cohesive cause, examining how each of them can help to understanding the unitary nature of tripartition.

Starting with the discussion of how the central systems are connected anatomically, the chapter investigates Galen's understanding of the unity of the body via two concepts: the form and the cohesive cause. The living body, according to Galen, is different from non-living entities because it 'flows together', and the material flux is governed by the form. The ensuing discussion shows how he adopts this fairly standard Aristotelian solution to his purposes. The form, while significant when accounting for the substantial identity of a living being, does not provide as fine-grained understanding of unity as one might like in the realm of vital functions. I argue that the notion of a cohesive cause is, in several ways, better at capturing all the key features that Galen often assigns to unified vitality.

5.1 The Anatomy of the Three Soul Domains

In order for bodily parts to be in conflict with each other, they need to come into contact with each other in some way. The connection between the three central physiological systems can be either anatomical or functional. A few connections of the former type were already mentioned in the course of this work, but it is worthwhile revisiting those findings because previous chapters made no comment on the overall interconnectedness of these systems. Furthermore, the anatomical connection between the central organs presents a small but interesting anatomical problem.

The liver, whose main activity is the final step of the conversion of food into blood, is also responsible for sending out the nutriment into the rest of the body via the veins, as shown in Chapter 2. The blood, however, flows not only in the veins but also in the arteries. This is an important point for Galen, as he is engaged in prominent polemics on this question with

[11] For instance, anger, for which see Singer (2017) and Trompeter (2018).

Erasistratus' followers.[12] How does blood get into the arteries that are connected to the heart and not the liver? The most compact answer can be found in *On the Natural Capacities*, in one of the few cases where he employs the mechanistic explanation. Galen outlines two ways of attraction: the mechanistic type, primarily affecting the finer portions of matter, and the attraction-by-appropriateness-of-quality type, which attracts the heavier matter too. As hollow organs, the heart and the arteries first attract the finer matter mechanistically via diastole,[13] and their coats attract nourishment into themselves.[14] The diastolic attraction is responsible for pushing blood from the right heart ventricle, delivered there by vena cava, to the left ventricle through many small perforations in the septum dividing them. From this ventricle, the blood moves out from the heart to the arteries.[15]

As the arteries dilate, they continue drawing fine material into themselves. The arteries just under the skin draw in air,[16] whereas the arteries deeper in the body draw in the finer parts of blood.[17] In both cases, it is the finer parts of the matter that percolate into arteries mechanically, via *horror vacui*.[18] An undoubtedly relevant anatomical fact here is that veins and arteries are typically co-present in muscles so that where there is a vein, there is also an artery, although this is not universally true.[19]

Arteries, as mentioned earlier, are a part of the cardiac, or the innate heat, system, as they spring from the heart, the seat of the spirited soul. Through the arteries flows not only the blood but also the vital pneuma, which reached the heart via the pulmonary vein.[20] While in the arteries, the vital pneuma is gradually refined until it becomes the psychic

[12] *Ven. Sect. Er.* 3 (11.153–4K). The entirely of *Whether Blood Is Naturally Contained in the Arteries* is dedicated to the attack on Erasistratus and his followers, including the femoral artery experiment (*Art. Sang.* 8.4 (178 Furley and Wilkie=4.733–4K)). See Salas (2020, chapters 6 and 7) for the argument that the latter was appropriate from Erasistratus himself by Galen.

[13] This claim does not contradict his extensive rejection of the Erasistratean account of cardiac motion via the *horror vacui* principle in *Whether Blood Is Naturally Contained in the Arteries*. The problem with Erasistratus' explanation is that the mechanical motion of matter is supposed to be the fundamental case of the physiological process. For Galen, the mechanistic explanation is acceptable only as long as it is understood that the mechanical type of motion is ultimately explainable in reference to the peculiar properties and innate capacities of the heart and the arterial tissues (see Section 4.3.2). See Adamson (2014: 202–4).

[14] *Nat. Fac.* 3.15 (251, 5–20 Helmreich=2.206–7K).

[15] *Nat. Fac.* 3.15 (251, 27–252, 3 Helmreich=2.207–8K).

[16] This theory has been discussed in Chapter 3.

[17] *Nat. Fac.* 3.14 (249–50 Helmreich=2.205–6K).

[18] See *Nat. Fac.* 3. 15 (Helmreich 253, 17–19=2.210K).

[19] *AA* 13.8 (Duckworth 1962: 168). In *AA* 13.10 (Duckworth 1962: 177–80), Galen provides a list of un-paired blood vessels.

[20] The movement of pneuma and blood in reference to the left ventricle of the heart is, however, not outlined clearly and consistently enough by Galen, see Harris (1973: 336–7).

pneuma.[21] The process of refinement reaches an especially important stage in the *rete mirabile*, the plexus under the brain, and in the ventricles of the brain. Although Galen never makes this comparison explicitly, the conversion of the vital pneuma into the psychic pneuma resembles the conversion of food into blood. In both cases, the process consists of long, gradual conversion. In addition to this, both contain the special final stage, associated with a certain organ, constituting the crucial step in the conversion. Both organs, the liver and the brain, are the rulers of their respective systems.

Once the psychic pneuma is refined in the ventricles of the brain, the seat of the rational soul, it is sent from there via the nerves to the limbs and organs for the purposes of voluntary motion and perception.[22] As this sketch shows, the three systems governed by the three souls are anatomically distinct. At no point are the seats and their offshoots directly connected, viz. at no point does an artery turn into a nerve or a vein. The body is, thus, primarily composed of the three discrete systems. Instead, they are linked by overlapping offshoots, which are either co-present in such tissues as muscle or are inserted into organs, for example, the nerve present in the liver. The significance of the latter is that the seats can be 'aware' of each other by overlapping connections. At the same time, their fundamental differences remain intact, so that no system can directly affect any of the other ones.[23]

Anatomically speaking, the human body is a collection of discrete parts intertwined together. This way of thinking about the body is problematic from the physiological and philosophical points of view. If each of the three physiological systems operate effectively independently, with mere awareness of the other two as if neighbours, an animal body would be just a collection of parts, with almost incidental unity. Galen consistently claims that the tradition he follows theorises the animal body as flowing together (almost always ascribed to Hippocrates),[24] typically in opposition

[21] See Chapter 3 for a detailed account. [22] This process is discussed in detail in Chapter 4.

[23] This is the case even if we take into account that the offshoots of the seats of the souls branch into each other, e.g., in *UP* 16.3 (2.385, 22–25 Helmreich=4.276K), the nerves go to the heart because all the capacities governing the human must be connected. See also *UP* 6.18 (1.365, 1–13 Helmreich=3.501K).

[24] *Nat Fac.* 1.12 (122, 6–9 Helmreich=2.29K); 3.13 (238, 4–7 Helmreich=2.189K); 3.13 (243, 10–13 Helmreich=2.196K); *Us. Puls.* 2.5 (202 Furley and Wilkie=5.157K); *Diff. Feb.* 13 (7.379K); *Trem. Palp.* 6 (7.616K); *Caus. Puls.* 2.12 (9.88K); *MM* 1.2 (10.16K). Although variations of the verb συρρέω do appear in the Hippocratic corpus, the conjunction of adjectives σύμπνοος and σύρροος (as used by Galen) does not seem to appear in this corpus at all; see Holmes (2015) for a more thorough discussion of the 'hippocratisation' of *sumpatheia*.

to the mechanistic theorists. Thus, he implies that it is his rivals who make the body a collection of discrete parts, whereas his own position, among other advantages, shows that the body is unified. It could be argued that Galen's language implies a kind of sympathetic reaction,[25] and such a reaction does not require more than the kind of anatomical cohesion described earlier. As long as parts can 'perceive' each other, we can talk about the body as unified. However, there is arguably much more at stake here. The governing parts each controls distinct material flux, and all of these flows affect health and vitality if disrupted. In Section 5.2, I examine how Galen theorises the unification of these material flows.

5.2 The Material Flux

Each of the three central systems has a distinct process, characterised by various inflows and outflows from the body. The vegetative soul oversees the intake nutriment and the discard of excrement, while the spirited soul oversees the inflow and outflow of pneuma. Even the rational soul is dealing with the inflow of sensory perceptions via appropriate sense organs, and it has an output in the shape of voluntary actions, although this is a more metaphorical 'flow'. From the physiological point of view, the three soul domains together constitute a single central manager of the material flux. The significance of this flux cannot be overestimated, as Galen's discussion at the beginning of *On Hygiene* shows.

In order to underline the importance of the medical area of hygiene, Galen discusses two ways in which life can come to an end. The first is the natural devastation of the tissues by means of the ever-drying of mixtures. To illustrate this process, he describes the way in which mixtures of the tissues change throughout one's lifetime. He starts with the conception of an embryo from blood and seed, stating that moistness is the crucial property at first. As the embryo develops, the heat inherent in the seed and the blood starts to play an increasingly significant role, first by generating the solidity in the embryo by drying it out, and then, as the drying continues, by giving rough shapes to the organs. Further down the line, it refines organs into their best states. However, the drying process does not stop with birth and even childhood. It continues into old age, and gradually

[25] Galen does use the term for different phenomena, as argued by Brooke Holmes; in this case, the issue at stake would be the kind of *sumpatheia* that denotes the body suffering together, for which Galen credits the Stoics (*MM* 1.2 (10.16K)), but only as adherents to the originally Hippocratic idea (Holmes 2015: 62); see also Holmes (2020).

the drying capacity turns from constructive to destructive, inevitably leading to the death of the body.[26] Galen compares old age to the drying of the plants and calls it the eventual destruction of any generated living organism, adding that in animals another type of destruction is possible.

The second way in which life can come to an end is 'a flowing away of their whole substance brought about by the innate heat'.[27] Having noted that it is impossible to escape the former, while it is possible to avoid the latter with proper care, Galen writes that the latter usually comes about when people try to amend inevitable harms. He explains that all the substances need to be replenished by eating and breathing, and then continues:

> Ἐπειδὴ γὰρ ἀπορρεῖ μὲν ἁπάντων τῶν ζῴων ὁσημέραι πολὺ μέρος τῆς οὐσίας διὰ τὴν ἔμφυτον θερμότητα, δεόμεθα δὲ ὑπὲρ τοῦ τὴν συμμετρίαν αὐτῆς διαφυλάττεσθαι σιτίων τε καὶ πομάτων, ἀναπνοῆς τε καὶ σφυγμῶν, ἐξ ἀνάγκης ἀκολουθήσει τοῖσδε περιττωμάτων γένεσις. εἰ μὲν γάρ, οἷόνπερ ἦν τὸ κενωθέν, ἕτερον ἀκριβῶς τοιοῦτον εἴχομεν αὐτῷ προσφῦσαι δι' ὅλου, κάλλιστον ἂν ἦν τοῦτο καὶ ὑγιεινότατον. ἐπεὶ δὲ τὸ μὲν ἀπορρέον ἑκάστου τῶν μορίων τοιοῦτον τὴν φύσιν ἐστίν, οἷόνπερ αὐτὸ τὸ μόριον, οὐδὲν δὲ τῶν ἐσθιομένων ἢ πινομένων ἀκριβῶς ἐστι τοιοῦτον, ἀναγκαῖον ἐγένετο τῇ φύσει προμεταβάλλειν τε καὶ προπέττειν αὐτὰ καὶ ὡς ἔνι μάλιστα προπαρασκευάζειν ὅμοια τῷ θρεψομένῳ σώματι. κἀν τούτῳ τὸ μὴ κατεργασθὲν ἀκριβῶς μηδ' ἐξομοιωθὲν οὔτε προσφύεται τῷ σώματι καὶ περιττὸν ὂν ἀλᾶται κατὰ τὰς ἔνδον εὐρυχωρίας.
>
> Since a great part of the substance of all animals flows away every day due to the innate heat, we need food, drink, respiration and pulses for preserving the balance of this substance, but the creation of superfluities will inevitably follow from these things. If we were able to replace precisely what has been emptied out with something else and assimilate this completely, it would be the best and most healthy situation. However, since what flows away from each of the parts is the same in nature as the part itself, whereas nothing that is eaten or drunk is exactly this sort of thing, it naturally becomes necessary to change and digest these things beforehand, and as far as possible to prepare them beforehand to be like the body that will be nourished. And in this, what is not entirely prevailed upon or assimilated is not incorporated into the body, but passes into the internal spaces (cavities) as superfluity.[28]

[26] *San Tu.*1.2.4–10 Koch (6.4–5K). See also *Marc.* 3 (7.676K).

[27] *San. Tu.* 1.2.11 Koch (6.6K), tr. Johnston (2018: 9): τῆς ὅλης αὐτῶν οὐσίας ἡ ῥύσις ἐκ τῆς ἐμφύτου θερμότητος ἀποτελουμένη. Presumably, one such case is discussed at *MM* 9.10 (10.637–8K), where Galen accounts for witnessing two men dying due to incorrectly performed phlebotomies. He also notes other cases where patients' whole mixtures were made colder by phlebotomy and became impossible to fix.

[28] *San. Tu.* 1.3.1–4 Koch (6.7–8K), tr. Johnston (2018: 11–13).

Having offered this explanation, Galen notes that Nature provides animals with appropriate organs for discarding superfluities, and then concludes that there are two objectives (*skopoi*) in regard to the healthy regimen: the replenishment of substance and the separation of superfluities. In fact, making sure that the flux is proportionate (*summetrōs*) and not damaged in some way is the fundamental point of medicine. Galen emphasises this point by noting that all medical traditions agree that health is a balance, whether the balance of the four qualities or corpuscles and pores or atoms or homoiomeres or anhomoiomeres or any other primary element. Everyone agrees that the balance of the primary elements enables healthy functioning,[29] and if there is a difference in activities, that means there is a difference in balance (συμμετρία).[30] The constant flux of matter into and out of the body, as well as its balance, is mentioned numerous times in not only therapeutic but also more philosophical works of Galen,[31] so it is a crucial part of his conception of the human body.

This naturally raises the question of what constitutes this *summetria*? Much can be glimpsed from the discussions so far. The inflows and outflows of matter into the body are governed by the main vital processes that are carried out by the three systems: the vegetative, the cardiac and the nervous. It is worth noting that Galen's description of the governance of the material flux also motivates his classification of the brain, the heart and the liver as the special kind of parts, the governing parts, discussed in Chapter 1. The three ruling organs govern the healthy ways of interacting with and processing the material external to the body; they determine how the body can exist in the external world. Such an interpretation also explains Galen's interest in adopting the Platonic tripartite model for physiological, not only psychological, purposes. The tripartition is a useful tool for modelling the physiological material flux that underscores animal

[29] This is a strikingly peaceful depiction of the rival theories by Galen. It is very rare for him to talk of common ground with figures such as Asclepiades of Bithynia, whose *poroi* and *onkoi* he generally fiercely criticizes; see *Nat. Fac.* 1.13 (129 Helmreich=2.39K) for the criticism of the details of Asclepiadean flux system, especially regarding the *peritomata*. Arguably, Galen's keenness on finding commonalities is motivated by the methodological principle to start from what is agreed by everyone (*MM* 1.5 (10.42K)).

[30] *San. Tu.* 1.5.11–13 Koch (6.15K): συμμετρία γὰρ δή τις ἡ ὑγεία κατὰ πάσας ἐστὶ τὰς αἱρέσεις, ἀλλὰ καθ' ἡμᾶς μὲν ὑγροῦ καὶ ξηροῦ καὶ θερμοῦ καὶ ψυχροῦ, κατ' ἄλλους δὲ ὄγκων καὶ πόρων, κατ' ἄλλους δὲ ἀτόμων ἢ ἀνάρμων ἢ ἀμερῶν ἢ ὁμοιομερῶν ἢ ἀνομοιομερῶν ἢ ὅτου δὴ τῶν πρώτων στοιχείων, ἀλλὰ κατὰ πάντας γε διὰ τὴν συμμετρίαν αὐτῶν ἐνεργοῦμεν τοῖς μορίοις. εἴπερ οὖν διαφόρως ἐνεργοῦμεν, διάφορός ἐστι καὶ ἡ καθ' ἕκαστον συμμετρία τῶν στοιχείων, ἥπερ ἦν ἡ ὑγεία. See also *PHP* 5.3.15–21 de Lacy (5.448–51K).

[31] For the therapeutic, *Ars. Med.* 28.6 (361, 14–16 Boudon=1.381K), where healing is described as restoring *summetria*. *Form. Foet.* 5, 16 Nickel (4.684K).

life. When it comes to organising the physiological processes, no other manner of dividing the body plays as important a role as tripartition, since it helps to identify the principal parts and, subsequently, to define the rest in reference to them. The key feature that is of special interest is not the conflict, but the combined management of the material flux that is necessary for the animal's (healthy) existence in the external world. The ideas about the material flux are an important background and motivation for understanding Galen's adoption of the tripartition, but they are also relevant for interpreting his ideas about the unity of the body.

5.2.1 The Persistence through Material Change

Material flux presents a number of problems that all the ancient theorists of the body, whether medical or philosophical, had to address. Most of them concern the persistence of identity through change. The inflow and outflow of matter means that the material constitution of the animal is ever changing; this raises a more philosophical question of how the animal can retain the identity through such change? A very similar question can be phrased in more medical terms: how does the intake of material allow for the growth (or any other change) of the animal? Galen engages extensively with the latter question, partly owing to polemical concerns, but the kind of answer he provides borrows from the debates concerned with the former.

In the treatise *On the Natural Capacities*, Galen distinguishes three central activities of nature in animals: genesis, growth and nutrition.[32] When explaining the growth, Galen uses the rival Erasistratean theory as a foil for elaborating his own. The crucial component of growth, the aspect that distinguishes Nature's actions from human craftsmanship, is the ability to expand in all directions rather than simply increase the amount of matter. This is an oft-repeated condition in this treatise, and it is first introduced with the anecdote about a game popular among children in Ionia and elsewhere. The children take the bladders of pigs, fill them with air and run them on the ashes near the fire. The ashes warm the bladder and allow it to expand, and children sing certain songs encouraging the bladder to expand. Once it distends, they blow more air into the bladder and repeat the process. Galen notes that as the bladder grows in size, its substance is getting thinner. This is the type of 'growth' that humans can bring about. If the children were able to nourish the bladder as it extends,

[32] *Nat. Fac.* 1.5 (108, 6–7 Helmreich=2.10K).

then it would be genuine growth, just like the one Nature performs.[33] Then he adds that 'thus Nature alone has the power to expand a body in all directions so that it remains unruptured and preserves completely its previous form'.[34] Although the term for form here is ἰδέα, the form is clearly embodied; it is also the condition that allows for the persistence of identity through material expansion.[35]

Galen's ideas about the grounds for identity appear to be inspired by Aristotelian works, especially the argument that the change by growth is governed by form in *On Generation and Corruption*.[36] When discussing the conditions for the change of *polis*, Aristotle also concludes that such a change occurs not when inhabitants change (the body of citizens is constantly changing through birth and death) but when the form (εἶδος) of governance changes.[37] In the Hellenistic period, the problem is that persistence through material change comes to the forefront of metaphysics, producing complex accounts,[38] but Galen seems to be opting for a fairly straightforward approach to the problem, similar to what can be found in Aristotelian texts.[39] Later in this treatise, however, Galen comes back to

[33] See *Nat. Fac.* 1.7 (113, 9–19 Helmreich=2.17–18K).

[34] *Nat. Fac.* 1.7 (114, 1–3 Helmreich=2.18K), tr. Brock (1916: 179). μόνης οὖν τῆς φύσεως τὸ πάντη διιστάναι συνεχὲς ἑαυτῷ μένον ἔτι καὶ τὴν ἀρχαίαν ἅπασαν ἰδέαν φυλάττον τὸ σῶμα.

[35] Possibly relevant background here is the problem of artefact form. The question of whether there are artefact forms or only forms of living things is an important problem in philosophy from the Classical period. There is, broadly speaking, some consensus in the scholarship that, despite the fact that Plato uses a bed for illustrating the arguments about the form (*R.* 10.597A–D), Platonists are not committed to the view that artefacts have forms, as Aristotle reports in *Metaph.* 1.9 (991b3–6) (for the analysis of this particular text, see Broadie (2007)). Since the form is the ultimate unity (for an extensive discussion of platonic mereology see Harte (2002)), the artefacts possess a lesser degree of unity than the natural entities. There is a degree of similarity between Plato and Aristotle in this respect (discussed in Koslicki 2008, chapter 6). Aristotle too maintains that the ultimate unity is the substance (*Metaph.* 5.6 (1016b15)); the artefacts are not included among the things that have substance; this problem is tackled in Broadie (2007) and Katayama (1999); see also Shields (2008: 129) for the claim that living entities are proper substances. See *Metaph.* 5.6 (1016a4) for the claim that natural entities are more continuous than artefacts. By the Hellenistic period, the problem of unity becomes a topic of discussion in its own right. Especially notable is the Stoic distinction, reported by Sextus Empiricus (*M* 9.78–9) between unified entities (plants and animals), collected entities held by a goal (chains, ships) and entities that are simply grouped together (armies, choruses). Regardless of the details and the context, these philosophers generally take the body to be possessed of the kind of unity that is not possible in artefacts.

[36] *GC* 1.5 (321a30ff.); although the Aristotelian term for the form here is εἶδος.

[37] *Pol.* 3.3 (1276a34–b13).

[38] Most notably, in the form of the Growing Argument, see Lewis (1995) and Sedley (1982); see also Čelkytė (2020a).

[39] This also might be partly due to the fact that Hellenistic philosophers were materialists; the Stoics, for example, assume a reductive nominalist position about the form (Syrianus *in. Metaph.* 105, 21–5=LS 30H), thus depriving the concept of any significant causal role. In Epicureanism, some of the explanatory roles of the forms are relegated to preconceptions (Diog. Laert. 10.33=LS 17E), others rendered superfluous by alternative cosmology (Lucretius *DRN* 5.156–234=LS 13F).

this problem and introduces some surprising elements to this, originally simple, answer.

When attacking the account of growth put forth by Erasistratus, he references the anecdote about the children playing with a bladder, thus making a connection with his previous remarks. He complains that Erasistratus thinks that animals grow like webs, ropes, sacks, baskets: by adding to their edges the same type of material from which they are composed.[40] Galen's report might be uncharitable here, but presumably, Erasistratus' view must have amounted to the claim that food is broken down in the digestive system and then distributed throughout the body, with particles of food being added to the existing tissues.[41] This process, Galen argues, is generation, not growth. For a basket to really grow, it would have to become larger after all of its parts are already shaped and completed. Thus 'growth concerns that which has already been completed in respect to its form, but the process by which that which is still becoming attains its form is named not growth but genesis. That which is, grows, while that which is not, becomes.'[42]

The last sentence, contrasting being and becoming, invokes the famous Platonic binary in ontology.[43] In this context, however, Galen uses it to differentiate between natural entities and artefacts, in the process of refuting Erasistratus. Both artefacts and natural entities have their respective forms. They also both undergo genesis, that is, at some point, they become. The key difference between natural entities and artefacts is the way in which the addition of matter affects them. The addition of matter to artefacts changes their form; thus, they only become, going from non-existence to becoming. However, natural entities are capable of growth; the addition of matter does not affect their form that is already existing, τὸ ὄν, and continues to exist through material change. Implicitly, Galen

In short, the forms do not feature prominently in the Hellenistic debates. By Galen's time, the form was back in fashion with the rise of Middle Platonist tradition (see Boys-Stones 2018: 1–23); counter-intuitively, this 'old-fashioned' approach was also very much in line with current trends.

40 *Nat. Fac.* 2.3 (164, 12–15 Helmreich=2.87K): [Ἐρασίστρατος] ἀλλ' οὕτως αὐξάνεσθαι τὰ ζῷα νομίζει καθάπερ τινὰ κρησέραν ἢ σειρὰν ἢ σάκκον ἢ τάλαρον, ὧν ἑκάστῳ κατὰ τὸ πέρας ἐπιπλεκομένων ὁμοίων ἑτέρων τοῖς ἐξ ἀρχῆς αὐτὰ συντιθεῖσιν ἡ πρόσθεσις γίγνεται.

41 Celsus *Med.* 1, *prohoem.* 20 reports the Erasistratean view that food is crushed in the stomach (*et duce alii Erasistrato teri cibum in ventre contendunt*).

42 *Nat. Fac.* 2.3 (165, 2–6 Helmreich=2.88K): τοῦ μὲν γὰρ ἤδη συμπεπληρωμένου κατὰ τὸ εἶδος ἡ αὔξησις, τοῦ δ' ἔτι γιγνομένου ἡ εἰς τὸ εἶδος ὁδὸς οὐκ αὔξησις ἀλλὰ γένεσις ὀνομάζεται· αὐξάνεται μὲν γὰρ τὸ ὄν, γίγνεται δὲ τὸ οὐκ ὄν. See also *Ars. Med.* 33.2 (371, 7–9 Boudon =1.390–1K), conveying a similar thought with different terminology: τῶν μὲν οὖν ἔτι αὐξανομένων οἷον τε τὸ σχῆμα τῶν πλείστων μορίων ἐπανορθώσασθαι, τῶν δ' ηὐξημένων οὐκέτι.

43 For example, in *Ti.* 27D–28A.

establishes a difference between the natural forms τὸ ὄν, capable of persisting through material change, and the forms of artefacts that always undergo 'becoming' when such change occurs.[44] This move helps to show that the Erasistratean account does not sufficiently explain the complexity of organic entities, whereas the accounts positing the innate capacities do.[45]

Form, thus, appears to play the crucial role in establishing the identity. The forms of natural entities in particular are key for explaining what 'holds' the body together through material change and what unifies it. Given the significant role that the form plays in explanations of vital functions, it would be reasonable to expect that Galen considers forms to be the fundamental building blocks of animal metaphysics. However, that this is not entirely the case.

5.2.2 *The Form as a Cause*

The notion of the form is central in ancient philosophy and it is important for medicine too, as far as Galen is concerned. In medicine, however, this notion comes with a distinct set of problems, and Galen discusses them in Book 6 of *On the Usefulness of Parts*. His discussion takes place in a very specific polemical context. He attacks Asclepiades of Bithynia for rejecting the final and the efficient cause as the most important in medical explanations and positing what Galen calls a formal cause in their stead. At first sight, this position might seem to be inconsistent with the claims he makes in *On the Natural Capacities*, where he himself uses the notion of the form to reject mechanistic medicine, but a closer look at the context reveals that there is no inconsistency as such. The discussion in *On the Usefulness of Parts* is more nuanced and very helpful when it comes to understanding the role that the form plays in an animal constitution.

Book 6 is dedicated to the exposition of the instruments of pneuma, viz. the cardiac system and the organs adjacent to it. Having given his account of the functioning of this system, Galen launches an attack on Asclepiades regarding his explanation of the properties of pulmonary vessels.[46] This piece of Galenic polemic is rather elaborate, and therefore it is worth

[44] See also the discussion of the problem with artefacts in Chapter 1.

[45] Owing to the fact that they show how organic entities can turn external material into themselves by attracting what benefits (retaining it and altering it) and rejecting what harms; see *Nat. Fac.* 2.3 (159 Helmreich=2.80K); see also the discussion in Chapter 2.

[46] *UP* 6.12 (1.338 Helmreich=3.464K)ff.

breaking it down into steps. He starts with the claim that the final cause was called the first cause by Plato. He offers an illustration to support this by inviting his readers to imagine asking someone why they came to a market. A sensible answer would be to say that the purpose is to buy something or to meet someone and it would be ridiculous to reply with 'because I have two healthy legs capable of doing it'. This, it is implied, is what Asclepiades effectively commits to, although no particular details are given just yet. Galen only adds that the person offering this type of an explanation 'has, perhaps, given one cause, but not the real, first one; on the contrary, his is an instrumental cause, one without which [an action cannot be performed], or rather, one that is not [really] a cause'.[47]

Plato, Galen contends, was right about the causes, and there were several of them. He proceeds to list five: the final, the efficient, the material, the instrumental and then the formal. The way in which Galen introduces the latter is remarkable because he adds a comment 'if you wish' (εἰ βούλει), as if the inclusion of this cause on the list was optional.[48] The reason for this phrasing is explained soon thereafter when he starts his attack on mechanistic doctors. Before he launches this attack, however, he notes that all good natural philosophers take into account all of these causes. And if anyone asked him why the artery in the lungs is veinous and the vein arterial, Galen would give the first and true cause, namely, because it is better so.[49] It might strike one as an unsatisfying answer, but he does, in fact, provide a more elaborate explanation later in the text, but this comes after his attack on the rival mechanistic medical accounts, represented by Erasistratus and Asclepiades.

He covers the Erasistratean account very briefly and then moves on to what appears to be his main target, viz. Asclepiades' explanation of why arteries are veinous and veins are arterial in the lungs.[50] This critique starts with the claim that Asclepiades passes the first two causes: the one derived from the providence of the creator (this cause ought to be first), and the

[47] *UP* 6.12 (1.339, 7–10 Helmreich=3.464–5K), tr. May (1968): εἴρηκε μὲν γάρ τινα καὶ οὗτος ἴσως αἰτίαν, ἀλλ' οὐ τὴν ὄντως αἰτίαν οὐδὲ τὴν πρώτην, ἀλλ' ὀργανικήν τέ τινα καὶ ὧν οὐκ ἄνευ, μᾶλλον οὐκ αἰτίαν.

[48] *UP* 6.12 (1.339, 15–16 Helmreich=3.465K). It is also worth noting that Galen suggests that both the formal and the instrumental causes are of low significance. This might be due to the way in which Galen envisions the sequence of causes, as argued in Hankinson (1994: 1770–1).

[49] Galen especially draws from the Aristotelian tradition here; see Hankinson (1994: 1768–9).

[50] Erasistratus reportedly maintained that, in the lungs, the vein is arterial because it originates from the part of the heart where most arteries originate from and it is inserted into the 'blood' ventricle of the heart. The artery, meanwhile, is veinous because it originates from the same part where most veins originate from and it is inserted into the ventricle of 'pneuma'. *UP* 6.12 (1.339–40 Helmreich=3.465–6K).

material cause (this cause ought to be second). Instead, Galen concentrates on the least important one that he calls consequential and contingent and compares it to a counterfeit drachma.[51] Notably, this classification of causes differs from the one just given. What seems like an efficient one, 'from the providence of the creator' (ἐκ προνοίας τοῦ δημιουργοῦ) comes in first, rather than second. The material cause comes in second rather than third. More importantly, Galen's classification implies that there are only three causes. Given that the first cause, 'from the providence of the creator', could be read as a teleological cause, it seems that he collapses the first two causes into one here. This reading is confirmed here, when Galen contrasts and compares Asclepiades' and his own accounts. First, he cites Asclepiades:

> διότι γάρ, φησίν, ἐν τῷ πνεύμονι μόνῳ τῶν ἁπάντων ὀργάνων αἱ μὲν ἀρτηρίαι διπλῆν κινοῦνται κίνησιν, ἥν τ' οἴκοθεν ἔχουσιν ἐκ τῆς σφετέρας αὐτῶν οὐσίας, σφύζουσαι δηλονότι, καὶ ἣν ἐκ τοῦ τῆς ἀναπνοῆς ἔργου, σειομένου διὰ παντὸς τοῦ πνεύμονος, ἐπικτῶνται, διὰ τοῦθ' ὑπερπονοῦσαι καταλεπτύνονται, τῶν ἐν τοῖς ἄλλοις μορίοις ἀρτηριῶν αὐτάρκως κινουμένων τὴν οἰκείαν κίνησιν οὖσαν μίαν καὶ διὰ τοῦτ' εὐτραφῶν τε καὶ ἰσχυρῶν γιγνομένων. αἱ δ' αὖ φλέβες, φησίν, αἱ μὲν καθ' ὅλον τὸ ζῷον ἀκίνητοι μένουσαι δίκην ἀνδραπόδου τινὸς ἀργοῦ καὶ ἀγυμνάστου, δικαίως ἀτροφοῦσιν· αἱ δὲ κατὰ τὸν πνεύμονα τὴν τοῦ σπλάγχνου κίνησιν ἐπικτησάμεναι παχύνονται παραπλησίως τοῖς τὰ μέτρια γυμναζομένοις.
>
> 'Now of all the instruments', he says, 'the lung is the only one in which the arteries have two motions, one of which is proper to them and derived from their own substance, that is, the pulse; the other they acquire from the act of respiration, since the lung is always in motion. For this reason the arteries of the lung labor excessively and grow very thin, whereas in the other parts of the body they move moderately with only their one proper motion and thus become very well nourished and strong. The veins throughout the body, on the other hand', he continues 'remain without motion and so logically waste away like a lazy slave that takes no exercise, but those in the lung acquire the motion of this viscus and so grow strong like persons who exercise moderately'.[52]

Galen is quite generous with his citations here, and they appear to be quite good illustrations of Asclepiades' explanation of the differences in the anatomy of pulmonary vessels. Excessive activity wears a vessel down, and therefore the arteries, which are moved both by means of the pulse and the

[51] *UP* 6.13 (1.340, 11 Helmreich=3.466K).
[52] *UP* 6.13 (1.340, 15–341, 3 Helmreich=3.467K), tr. May (1968: 309).

lung-induced motion, grow thinner in the lungs than elsewhere in the body. The veins, by contrast, are strengthened by the lung-induced motion, because they do not have an innate motion and this amount of activity allows them to grow more robust than elsewhere in a body. In short, pulmonary arteries suffer from overexertion while pulmonary veins get a healthy amount of exercise.

In what sense is Asclepiades, an advocate of the mechanistic understanding of physiology, positing the form? Presumably, the answer lies in the fact that, in Asclepiades' account of the pulmonary arteries, the primary cause is the motion of the lungs. It is this motion that, in combination with their innate movement, wears out arteries and makes them thin, inducing motion to normally non-moving veins, thus making them thicker. In order to explain the anatomy of these vessels, it is necessary to refer to their location in the body. The form, then, amounts to the structure of the body.[53]

Galen first refutes the cited view with some anatomical observations,[54] before moving on to the more philosophical point. His own position is summarised in a single sentence as follows: 'there is an Intelligence ordering and arranging all these things, not merely corpuscles combining with one another automatically'.[55] Soon thereafter, he explains what this commitment means in this particular case. Although he uses the model of five causes, the final cause is clearly the most important, and terms referring to it are scattered throughout the passage, as Galen explains the shape of the vessels, their anatomical positions, constitution and so on.[56]

He also explains that the five-cause classification is not different from the three-cause model he uses earlier. The causes, it seems, can be classified

[53] The reason why this kind of explanation is like 'a counterfeit drachma', as Galen calls it, is that the structural properties of bodies are just imprints of the design that originally comes from the designing creator. Although they themselves exhibit rational functioning and, to some extent, rational working of an animal body can be explained in terms of them, they are counterfeit causes, because they simply replicate the design coming from the real cause, the creator. See also *CC* 8.6 Lyons, where Galen says that the structure of the arteries and the heart are instrumental causes of the pulse, like a lead bar propping a statue upright.

[54] In *UP* 6.13 (1.341–2 Helmreich=3.468–9K), he argues that Asclepiades is ignorant of dissection and completely misses the fact that the veins and arteries are peculiar in the lung not merely in terms of their thickness but also in a number of tunics. Asclepiades' theory is, Galen maintains, inconsistent with a number of other phenomena observable in the human body. If it was true, people who suffer from the condition affecting the eye, phthisis, would have fewer tunics in their eyes, whereas those with excellent vision would have more than normal.

[55] *UP* 6.13 (1.342, 13–15 Helmreich=3.469K), tr. May (1968: 310): νοῦς ἐστὶν ὁ πάντα διατάττων ταῦτα καὶ κοσμῶν, οὐκ ὄγκοι σωμάτων αὐτομάτως ἀλλήλοις περιπλεκόμενοι.

[56] *UP* 6.13 (1.343–4 Helmreich=3.470–1K).

either in a three-fold or in a five-fold manner. The final and the efficient causes are equivalent to the cause 'from the demiurge'. It is worth noting that Galen might not be doing anything very outlandish here. The Middle Platonist philosophers, some of whom were Galen's contemporaries and teachers,[57] appear to have combined the final with the efficient cause into the cause that is derived from the creator.[58] This first group of causes, equivalent to the cause from the creator, uses material and instrumental causes in order to confer form. This indicates that the formal is the third-tier cause. The material and the instrumental causes, meanwhile, are the second-tier causes. Thus, a robust hierarchy emerges from the grouping of the five causes into the three categories.

It is not hard to surmise why Galen does this. By setting the causes in a hierarchy, he can show that physicalist accounts, such as Asclepiades', fail to produce the full picture. At first sight, this is not the most defeating of moves. After all, Galen simply appears to accuse Asclepiades of not subscribing to the kind of theory that he is subscribing to. This, however, would only be the case if all five causes were on equal footing. The Galenic introduction of the three-dimensional hierarchy is a clever move because it undermines the explanatory power of the formal cause by making it merely tertiary. This means that its existence presupposes the existence of the second-level causes, the instrumental and the material, and *a fortiori*, the first-level causes 'from the creator'. The formal cause is, thus, derivative and an explanation built on the basis of it is missing some key elements an explanation ought to have.

5.2.3 Galenic Forms

Before moving on to further discussion, it is worth noting that Galen's understanding of the form here is striking. In claiming that the form is something tertiary and dependent on other causes, he is much closer to his contemporary Middle Platonists than the revered ancients, Plato and Aristotle.[59] The tenet stating that no one produces or creates the form is

[57] Galen studied with Albinus (*Lib. Prop.* 2.1 (140, 16 Boudon–Millot=19.16–17K)).

[58] The efficient and the final causes are discussed together (and in opposition to Anaxagoras, just like Galen does in *On the Usefulness of Parts*) in Plutarch *Def. Orac.* 435E=Boys-Stones 3H. See also Aëtius *Plac.* 1.11.1–2 Mansfeld and Runia=Boys-Stones 3B.

[59] This point is closely related to the reading of Galen's notion of the demiurge, also influenced by the Middle Platonist tradition; for this interpretation, see Rocca (2017) and the discussion in Chapter 2.

fundamental in Aristotelian metaphysics,[60] and Galen goes in the opposite direction. His position could be in line with the view that the forms are products of the creator, to be more precise, the forms are in the mind of the creator. Plotinus spells out such a view fairly elaborately in his *Enneads*,[61] although given the fact that he did not conceptualise the creator as providential,[62] Galen might be closer to the Middle Platonist tradition.[63] These later Platonists appropriated the innovations of the Hellenistic philosophers, in this case, the Stoics and their notion of cause as a creator,[64] but interpreted these innovations as already present in Platonic dialogues. As a result, the Middle Platonists take the ultimate cause to be the designing creator and also retain the Platonic notion of the forms, locating them in the mind of the creator.[65] This makes the forms instruments of the creator. The contemporary Platonist influence, therefore, could explain why Galen finds it quite natural to collapse the causes and make the formal cause merely tertiary, a consequence of the work of the primary cause.

The issue at stake is more than the adoption of the current philosophical trends in this text. Arguably, the more interesting here is the fact that Galen applies these issues to the medical context. Galen's downgrading of the formal cause is in sync with an oft-repeated principle in his therapeutics: it is the purpose (*chreia*) that determines the significance of an organ as well as the required therapeutic approach. In *On the Therapeutic Method*, while discussing the diseases of magnitude and number, Galen acknowledges that vagueness can arise when doctors use the phrase 'in accordance with nature'. He notes that it is not up to us to choose primarily what is in accordance with nature but only secondarily and contingently. In the case of a person born with six fingers or four fingers, it would be inappropriate and the opposite of the actions of nature to change this (presumably, by means of surgery) rather than preserve them as they are, even if these cases were many. He ends up with the warning about a false conflict, based on

60 Aristotle *Metaph.* 8.3 (1043b14).

61 *En.* 5.5.1–2, see also 3.9.1, which is a comment on Plato's *Timaeus.*

62 See esp. *En.* 6.7.128–32. See also Chiaradonna (2015).

63 Atticus Fr.28.1–7=Proclus *On the Timaeus* i.393.31–394.8=Boys-Stones 6O; Atticus Fr. 13=Proclus *On the Timaeus* i.366.9–13=Boys-Stones 6P; see also Boys-Stones (2018: 151).

64 For providential creator in Middle Platonism, see Atticus Fr. 3=Boys-Stones 11A; although the problem is also combining the Aristotelian and the Platonic accounts too; see Boys-Stones (2018: 323–8). See Sedley (2005: 134–8) for a discussion of how Platonic, Aristotelian and Stoic accounts of causes are whittled down into a single system in Seneca, in a manner emblematic of the first-century Platonists. For the crucial development of the notion of demiurge, see Opsomer (2005).

65 Alcinous *Didask.* 9.1–4=Boys-Stones 5E.

merely verbal disagreement, that might arise if one doctor urges the excision of everything contrary to nature while another one speaks of the harm to the activities.[66] Galen is firmly in the latter category. The same position is reiterated in *Thrasybulus*, where, after raising the question of whether each body part is needed for its constitution or for its activity, he argues: 'Surely everyone would agree in not wanting any part unable to perform its activity – eyes unable to see, for example, a nose unable to smell, legs unable to walk, or, in general, any part which either does not perform its activity at all or performs it badly.'[67] Subsequently, he provides a parallel with artefacts. When we need a house, a shoe and so on, we need them in a complete state. These claims echo the position in *On the Usefulness of Parts*: the structure serves the design (or purpose), and it has primarily an instrumental function. Taken by itself, the form is not very relevant therapeutically. The failures in form do not necessarily impede health and 'fixing' the form might also not result in the improvement of health *per se*; for example, removing the sixth finger yields no graspable benefits to health.[68]

This brings us back to the question of the form as the solution to the problem of the constant flux of matter. The form that unifies the physiological activities of the three soul domains is itself not a cause but only an instrument of unification. The real cause is the designing creator. For the current purposes, the pertinent question is not so much the designer but the contents of the form this designer imposes on the body so that the three soul domains form functional unity. It is clear that the form here is a particular structure and interconnections of the body parts, but is it possible to find a scheme in accordance with which all these very different parts are joined into unity? Arguably, there is an affirmative answer in the Galenic texts discussing the notion of cohesive causes.

[66] *MM* 15.14 (10.991–2K).

[67] *Thras.* 11 (45, 15–20 Helmreich=5.823K), tr. Singer (1997: 61, slightly altered): ἐμοὶ μὲν πάντες δοκοῦσιν οὐδ᾽ ἂν ὅλως θελῆσαι μόριον ἔχειν οὐδὲν ἀργὸν ἔργου τινός, οὔτ᾽ οὖν ὀφθαλμοὺς μὴ βλέποντας οὔτε ῥῖνας ὀσμᾶσθαι μὴ δυναμένας οὔτε σκέλη μὴ βαδίζοντα οὔτ᾽ ἄλλο τῶν πάντων οὐδὲν ἢ μηδ᾽ ὅλως ἐνεργοῦν ἢ κακῶς ἐνεργοῦν. See also the discussion of the seeming inferiority (and functional excellence) of female reproductive system in Section 4.1.

[68] See also *UP* 6.9 (1.323, 9–13 Helmreich=3.443K), in the context of criticising Aristotle regarding the claim that the heart has the number of ventricles in accordance with its size, so that larger animals have more, smaller fewer: 'Nature pays no attention to the large or small size of the body when she varies the form (τὴν ἰδέαν) of instruments; on the contrary, her guide in construction is the difference of action, and she measures the actions themselves in turn by their principal usefulness', tr. May (1968: 295).

5.3 The Cohesive Cause

The notion of the cohesive cause is associated with the Stoic thought.[69] Although cognate language and concepts predate this Hellenistic philosophical school,[70] their conceptualisation become dominant, and it is primarily the Stoic understanding of the cohesive cause that Galen engages with. The key features of this concept are as follows. A cohesive cause can be found in structures with several discrete parts; it cannot be present in, for example, homoeomerous parts.[71] While cohesive causes help to unify discrete entities, they do not generate a new entity but rather a phenomenon, something in the becoming. Such a phenomenon is observable, although it is not possible to pin it down to a specific entity as it is grounded in a combination or a structure of several things. The cohesive cause has three elements: the purpose (the most important of them all), the capacities and the supporting organs. When combined, they produce a distinctly recognisable phenomenon that does not have an independent existence as a separate entity. Galen uses pulse to explain his understanding of cohesive causes as follows:

> People have seen it [pulse] in the arteries and the heart, never failing throughout the life span, and for that reason they have thought of it as something that exists. But, in fact, it is not extant in the same way as are the arteries, the heart, and the other parts of the body. It is only to be found in the state of coming into being, as no single part of it has any permanence. Admittedly its parts may be thought of by some as permanent, but that is because these people are unable to make the mental distinction between what comes into existence and what is extant. For the former resembles running water and the latter water is still. You find the same thing in rivers, particularly when they are seen from a distance. For then their water seems to be standing still, though in fact no single part of it really is. But as the general form of the water always remains fixed in the flowing stream, it often seems to us that its water is still and not flowing. The same thing applies to the pulse. What there is of it that has already come into existence and been finished with does not exist nor does what is about to come into existence. In fact, its only extant part is what lies beneath the fingers at the moment that it actually does so, though even this has no absolute existence but one that is found only in generation. For no single one of its parts is permanent, but each one passes away when once it has come into being or, put more comprehensively, at the time when it comes into being.

69 The seminal work is in Frede (1987: 140–50); see also the discussions in Bobzien (1998) and Hankinson (1998).

70 See Coughlin (2020).

71 This is stated explicitly in *CC* 9.1 Lyons.

> As for the causes of its generation, these I have shown to be three in number, that is, the useful purpose because of which we need this, the animal force from which it is generated and the structure of the arteries and of the heart which serves as an instrument for it. There is no harm in calling these things, if you choose, cohesive causes for the generation of the pulse, as I myself have often done for clarity and conciseness in my book *On the Pulse*, though this is not an actual but, rather, a metaphorical use of the terms. A parallel here is the use of lead in some statues that lean forwards. Where the body of one of these statues is not firmly attached to its feet, it will fall on its face, but if it is secured with lead it will stand upright. For, though the natural inclination peculiar to it will still remain as it was, the lead will check, hold, and draw it backwards. It follows that the lead is a cause only of some form of generation and not of absolute existence. But since what is generated here remains for its whole span in a self-consistent state, those who see it first imagine that it is a single determining thing, though it is neither, in fact, determinate nor any form of existence at all, but rather generation that takes place in a quantity of determinate matter through a single cause.[72]

In these passages, Galen attempts a painstaking definition of an elusive point: the ontological status of a phenomenon that is only 'in becoming'. In a Platonic framework, the entire physical world is in the realm of becoming, but Galen is focusing on phenomena that are ephemeral. They do not merely undergo change like all the other corporeal entities, they are *constituted* and defined by change. These are things in becoming *par excellence*. The comparison with the river, a well-used trope in philosophy and medicine,[73] is illuminating. From afar, a river seems to stand still, because its form remains the same, however, the water keeps on flowing and no part of it is fixed and stable. Galen does not seem to deny the existence of the river as a stable entity *per se*, only to point out that within that stable entity, circumscribed by its form, there is constant coming into being.

Pulse is one of these comings-into-being and it has three causes. It is noteworthy that the causes mentioned are the same as the causes of respiration in other works,[74] they are: the purpose, the capacity and the supporting organs or anatomical structure. In this passage, Galen adds that the three elements constituting these phenomena can only be described as

[72] *CC* 8.6–8 Lyons, tr. Lyons from Arabic (1969: 67).

[73] Apart from the fragments of Heraclitus (DK 22B12; 22B49a; 22B91), see Plato *Ti.* 43A; Sextus Empiricus *M* 8.6–7; see also Lucretius *DRN* 1.225–37 where literal rivers are discussed analogously to the physiological material flux.

[74] *Diff. Puls.* 4.2 (8.714K). *Caus. Resp.* 2 (240 Furley and Wilkie=4.465–6K).

cohesive causes metaphorically. The significance of this note is made clear in another analogy, this time with a lead rod that supports a leaning statue so that it may stand upright. The rod in this scenario is responsible for certain properties of the statue, but it is not the cause of its absolute existence. As the final sentence emphasises, the rod as the cohesive cause is responsible for some generation in the statue.

Galen clearly wants to draw attention to the fact that he does not consider the cohesive cause a full cause of something. In doing so, he presumably wishes to distance himself from materialist accounts of physiology. An example of such an account could very well be the Stoics themselves who assigned a significant generative role to the cohesive cause, identifying it with pneuma. Michael Frede noted that this cause is 'the Stoic analogue of an Aristotelian form.'[75] Galen is tacitly emphasising that materialist account of a physiological phenomenon does not amount to a materialist account of human existence. This reading can be supported further by a brief remark he makes on the cohesive cause in his *Against Julian*.

In the context of criticising Asclepiades' vague use of the term 'abundance', he turns to unidentified contemporary doctors who misuse the notion of the cohesive cause. Noting that somewhere else he explained that the notion is Stoic in origin, he goes on to point out that doctors misunderstand and misapply it. Interestingly, he states that, wishing to avoid quibbling about terminology, he often adopts this use of the term too, referring not to what there is *per se*, but what is acquired by means of becoming.[76] This remark not only lends support to the reading suggesting that Galen used the notion of the cohesive cause to explain 'in becoming' bodily phenomena but also that such use was likely not original. At the same time, it must be noted that, without further evidence, it is neither clear how prevalent this practice was, nor is it conclusive that Galen adopted the use of the term exactly, without his own modifications.

Despite the question of originality, the concept of the cohesive cause seems to have much explanatory potential with Galenic physiological framework. This potential depends on the question of how widely and how productively this concept could be applied. Would it be possible to use this model of 'in becoming' or 'in generation' unity for accounting for vitality in an animal as a whole? The focus on vitality is key here: it is quite

[75] Frede (1987: 145); for more on Stoic materialism and the role of the cohesive cause, see Hankinson (1998: 239–41).

[76] *Adv. Jul.* 6.13 Wenkebach (17a.279–80K).

clear that Galen does not wish to account for the entire human existence by means of the cohesive cause. He denies this explicitly in *Against Julian* and somewhat less directly in *On Cohesive Causes* when he states that a lead rod supporting a leaning statue is not cause of the statue as such. Accounting for the human as a whole as something 'in becoming' would mean committing to a materialist understanding of the soul, and it would potentially amount to denying that humans have a persisting essential identity. It is clear that humans, just like the river in the previously cited passage, have a form and substantial existence. The question of using the notion of the cohesive cause more broadly only concerns the physiological aspect of this existence or, to be more precise, the totality of vital processes in a human. If pulse and respiration individually can be accounted for by means of the cohesive cause, can this concept also be used to explain how blood flow and respiration, in combination with other activities, cause someone to be alive?

Galen does not make such a claim explicitly, but arguably, there are some grounds for supposing so. It has been shown by Philip de Lacy that Galen uses the more general concept of συνέχεια to talk about a variety of manifestations of continuity in the body as 'events in time or extensions in space'.[77] The notion of cohesive cause, as defined by Galen, captures all the key points for conceptualising human vitality. First, the *telos* of the overall functioning is the activities of the rational soul or to be more precise, the rational life,[78] as he states in *On the Usefulness of Parts*.[79] The purpose is imparted by the designing creator (although not a proper part at all but something reflected in the arrangement and structure of the whole body) would be the most important aspect of understanding the life of an organism.[80] Another part of the cohesive cause is an instrumental one, which, in the case of overall vitality, includes all the organs and their

[77] De Lacy (1979: 369); the cohesive cause is briefly discussed on p. 366.

[78] The activities are the important factors; see *MM* 10.9 (10.643K).

[79] See, for example, *UP* 1.2 (1.1, 13 Helmreich=3.2K). This text only refers to the soul in general terms, so one might argue that rationality is not the only concern in view of which humans are constructed, but it is worth noting that in other corresponding passages, Galen clearly means the rational soul that distinguishes humans from, for example, apes that are very similar in all the other respects *UP* 3.16 (1.194 Helmreich=3.264K). He is echoing the Aristotelian position that the soul is superior to the body in, for example, *Pol.* 1.5 (1254a34–b6). The idea that the final cause lays the foundation for scientific explanations and therefore has a certain priority over the other causes is also Aristotelian. See, for example, *PA* 1.1 (639b12–20). The argument states that the final cause is prior because the end goal determines what other causes are involved. In this way, a doctor can tell what is needed to achieve health, and a builder can tell what is needed to build a house.

[80] Galen's commitment to the view that everything in the world is arranged only in the best way possible is unwavering; see the extensive discussion in Hankinson (1989).

parts. Finally, cohesive cause also includes the capacity. Arguably, the three soul domains fit the role as capacities, and in Section 5.3.1 is dedicated to examining closer the evidence for approaching them as capacities for life, so that life itself, in the sense of an ongoing process from birth to death, can be accounted for within the theoretical framework of cohesive causes.

5.3.1 The Three Soul Domains as a Single Vital Capacity

The importance of preserving the capacities in the three soul domains, and thus, their activities, is often emphasised in the discussion of fevers. For example, in Book 9 of *On the Therapeutic Method*, Galen discusses ephemeral fevers. These are quite complex illnesses because they are not generated by a single localised condition, unlike, for example, a heatstroke, in case of which a doctor must only treat the condition of the head. In order to treat the ephemeral fevers successfully, it is necessary to understand the primary capacities governing the body as a whole. Having noted that he explained that there are three governing capacities in his *On the Doctrines of Hippocrates and Plato*, Galen goes on to reiterate that each is distributed throughout the body from a source; Plato, furthermore, called them 'souls'.[81] Then he gives a brief description of each of these capacities as follows:

> ἔστι δ᾽ ἡ μέν τις αὐτῶν εἰς τὸ τρέφεσθαι τὸ ζῶον ἀναγκαία καὶ κοινὴ πρὸς τὰ φυτά, τὴν μὲν οἷον πηγὴν ἔχουσα τὸ ἧπαρ, ὀχετοὺς δ᾽ ἐξ αὐτῆς εἰς ὅλον τὸ σῶμα διασπειρομένους τὰς φλέβας· ἣν εἴτ᾽ ἐπιθυμητικὴν, εἴτε φυσικὴν, εἴτε θρεπτικὴν ὀνομάζοις, οὐδὲν διοίσει, καθάπερ οὐδὲ εἰ ψυχὴν ἢ δύναμιν. ἑτέρα ζοις, οὐδὲν διοίσει, καθάπερ οὐδὲ εἰ ψυχὴν ἢ δύναμιν. ἑτέρα δ᾽ οὐ μόνον ὡς φυτοῖς ἡμῖν ἢ ζῶσιν, ἀλλὰ καὶ ὡς ζώοις ὑπάρχουσα ψυχὴ, κατὰ τὴν καρδίαν ἵδρυται πηγή τις οὖσα καὶ ἥδε τῆς ἐμφύτου θερμασίας· ὀχετοὶ δὲ καὶ ταύτης τῆς πηγῆς αἱ ἀρτηρίαι, καλουμένης καὶ αὐτῆς ὀνόμασι πολλοῖς· καὶ γὰρ δύναμις ζωτικὴ καὶ δύναμις θυμοειδὴς καὶ ψυχὴ ζωτικὴ καὶ ψυχὴ θυμοειδὴς ὀνομάζεται. τρίτη δ᾽ ἐν ἐγκεφάλῳ καθίδρυται ψυχὴ λογικὴ, τῶν κατὰ προαίρεσιν ἐνεργειῶν ἅμα ταῖς αἰσθήσεσιν ἐξηγουμένη, χρῆται δὲ μορίοις καὶ ἥδε καθάπερ ὀχετοῖς τισι τοῖς νεύροις, αἴσθησίν τε καὶ κίνησιν ἐπιπέμπουσα δι᾽ αὐτῶν τῷ ζώῳ παντί. τὸ μὲν δὴ ταύτας φυλάττειν τὰς δυνάμεις οὐδὲν ἄλλο ἐστὶν ἢ τὸ φυλάττειν τὴν ζωήν· ἐδείχθη γὰρ ὅπως ἀπολομένης ἡστινοσοῦν ἐξ αὐτῶν μιᾶς ἀναγκαῖόν ἐστι καὶ τὰς λοιπὰς συναπόλλυσθαι.

One of them, essential to nourishing the organism and in common with plants, is the liver which is as it were the fount, and the veins are the

[81] Thus making it clear that he thinks of the Platonic tripartition as a physiological phenomenon too.

> conduits distributing from this to the whole body. Whether you call this 'appetitive', or 'physical' or 'nourishing' will make no difference, just as it makes no difference if you call it 'soul' or 'capacity'. Another, which is not only in plants and animals but also in us as living creatures, is a soul seated in the heart, and this is also a source of the innate heat. The arteries are the conduits of this fount which is called by many names, for it is termed vital capacity or passionate capacity or vital soul or passionate soul. The third, which is the rational soul, is seated in the brain and governs the activities of volition along with those of sensation. This uses parts including certain nerves as conduits, sending via these sensation and movement to the whole organism. Certainly to preserve these capacities is nothing other than to preserve life. For it was shown that, if there is a destruction of any one of these whatsoever, of necessity those remaining are destroyed with it.[82]

This passage sets out the familiar picture of the physiological activities of the three organs acting as the seats of the souls and their respective offshoots. For current purposes, it is important in two respects: the terminology it employs and the way the relationship between the three souls is conceptualised. Regarding the former, Galen remarkably equates the terms 'the soul' and 'a capacity' in this context. In describing the three souls domains, he does not refer to the properties of the souls but their activities, putting an emphasis on what purposes they accomplish in the body. There are comparative cases in Galenic corpus, where he talks about the three domains in terms of vital activities, referring to these domains as capacities.[83] The claim that the terms the 'soul' and the 'capacity' are interchangeable,[84] presumably, clarifies for the reader that there is nothing else at stake here but the physiological activities described.

Second, the key point comes towards the end of the passage, Galen states that the preservation of all three of them is necessary for the functioning of the human body.[85] The last sentence indicates that the

[82] *MM* 9.10 (10.635–6K), tr. Johnston and Horsley (2011: 503–5), slightly altered. See also *Mot. Dub.* 1.19 (126, 18–22 Nutton).

[83] For example, *Cur. Rat. Ven. Sect.* 6 (11.268–9K), tr. Brain (1986: 76), slightly altered: 'The capacities in the nerves, and in their origin, the brain, are assessed by the state of the deliberative activities, and those in the arteries and heart by the pulse, while by the good or poor state of nutrition and by the good colour or pallor of the complexion the decision is made concerning the third capacity, the nutritive, which I have shown to proceed from the liver.'

[84] Donini (2008: 187) argues that calling the souls capacities (as opposed to parts or forms of the soul as Galen does in *PHP*) presupposes the Aristotelian picture of different capacities predicated on a single substrate. Such a reading is supported by *QAM* 2 (33, 10–25 Müller=4.769K). In this particular passage, however, the Aristotelian language is applied to a clearly tripartite picture of the soul that presupposes the three capacities to be derived from three substances.

[85] See also *UP* 14.1 (2.284, 20–285, 6 Helmreich=4.142–3K), where Galen says that nature has three aims when constructing the parts of an animal. The first aim is the preservation of life itself and for

souls do not merely act as an instrument for each other, their existence is genuinely co-dependent. As the discussions in Chapters 1 and 3 showed, the loss of a necessary instrument, such as a leg bone or the psychic pneuma, destroys the activity. However, once the instrument is restored, the activity can be resumed.[86] This is not the case for the physiological domains of the three souls. Galen states here that damage to one capacity necessarily co-destroys the other two.

Claims to the same effect can be found in Galen's other works. In *On the Usefulness of Parts*, for example, he divides all the human parts into three groups in accordance to their usefulness or purpose: for life itself, for living well and for reproduction. He calls the first one the most crucial as vitality itself depends on it, and makes it clear that the heart is one such organ, as it is the cornerstone of the innate heat system.[87] The same idea is presented more elaborately in *On the Formation of the Embryo*. He starts with the importance of the cardiac system, but then he goes on to explain that the other two systems have a similar role in maintaining life:

> ἡ γοῦν καρδία – ταύτην γὰρ μόνην ἔνιοι διοικεῖν βούλονται τὸ ζῷον – ἐπειδὰν στερηθῇ τῆς ἀναπνοῆς, αὐτή τε παύεται κινουμένη, καὶ σὺν αὐτῇ τὸ πᾶν ζῷον ἀπόλλυται. στερίσκεται δὲ τῆς ἀναπνοῆς οὐ μόνον τοῖς ἀπαγξαμένοις ἢ διὰ φλεγμονὴν τῶν περὶ τὸν λάρυγγα μορίων φραχθέντος τοῦ πόρου τῆς εἰσπνοῆς, ἀλλὰ καὶ τῶν κινούντων τὸν θώρακα νεύρων κακωθέντων ἤτοι διὰ τομῆς ἢ θλάσεως ἢ βρόχου, ὧν ἁπάντων ἐστὶν ὁ νωτιαῖος ἀρχὴ καθάπερ ἐγκέφαλος ἐκείνου. ὥσπερ οὖν ὁ ἐγκέφαλος εἰς τὴν διαμονὴν τῇ καρδίᾳ χρήσιμος ὑπάρχει διὰ νεύρων τὸν θώρακα κινῶν, οὗ διαστελλομένου μὲν εἰσπνοὴ γίγνεται, συστελλομένου δ' ἐκπνοή, κατὰ τὸν αὐτὸν τρόπον ἐγκεφάλῳ παρέχει τινὰ χρείαν ἡ καρδία καὶ τούτοις ἀμφοτέροις τὸ ἧπαρ.

> The heart, then (which some believe to be alone responsible for the management of the animal), when deprived of breath, ceases its motion, and with it the whole animal dies. Such deprivation of breath takes place not just in cases of strangulation, or where the channel of breathing is blocked by inflammation of the parts around the larynx, but also through damage to the nerves which move the chest (by incision, compression, or ligature), the spinal cord being the source of all these nerves, and the brain in turn of it. Thus, the brain is of importance to the heart in order for the latter to sustain itself: it moves the chest by nerves, and it is by diastalsis of the chest that inhalation takes place; by

this purpose, the brain, heart and liver are constructed. The other two aims are the better life and procreation for the sake of which sensory organs and reproductive organs are constructed, respectively.

86 *PHP* 7.3.27 de Lacy (5.608K).

87 *UP* 6.7 (1.318, 16 Helmreich=3.436K).

> systalsis, exhalation. And, in the same way, the heart provides a service to the brain, and the liver to both of these.[88]

The relationship between the cardiac and the nervous systems in the case of respiration has already been discussed in Chapter 3. The way in which the cardiac system is dependent on the nervous system for healthy respiration is quite clear. Damage to the nerves would prevent the 'cooling' cycle of the innate heat to take place, thus creating the risk of overheating the tissues, which in turn leads to mutilation of the organs and a risk of death. It is not only the damage to the nervous system that might trigger the chain of destruction. Inflammation of parts around the larynx, for example, would prevent respiration, triggering the overheating of various organs, including those belonging to the nervous system.

Galen does not spell out the details of the ways in which the vegetative system is also involved in this co-dependency, but these are fairly obvious. The lack of nutriment devastates the body in an easily observable way, eventually stopping the activities of the other two central systems. And although he does not state this in so many words, the vegetative system is dependent on the latter too. The regulation of heat ensures the normal functioning of all the parts necessary for nutrition. The nerves control not only the mastication but also the muscular motions around the oesophagus. Serious damage to each of the systems, therefore, poses a direct risk to the other two systems.

The co-dependency arises partly from the fact that each of the souls has a very specific and limited scope. The nerves are only in control of the voluntary motion, the pneumatic system only regulates the innate heat, while the vegetative soul is limited to overseeing the nourishment and the growth of tissues. None of them has a means of compensating, even temporarily, for the activities of the other two. The same is true of necessary instruments, the parts that carry out distinct proper activities. However, there is more at stake when it comes to the central systems. They are not merely instrumentally necessary for each other; the damage to one system, as the first sentence indicates, results in the dissipation of the other two, in other words, the death of the animal as a whole. Activity-stopping damage to one necessarily constitutes a vital threat to them all. Such co-dependency ties the respective systems governed by each of the souls into a single whole. From the functional point of view, the three is one! The three

[88] *Form. Foet.* 5, 17–18 Nickel (4.685K), tr. Singer (1997: 192–3, slightly altered). See Also *Mot. Dub.* 1.19 (126, 18–22 Nutton).

governing parts differ from all the other parts in the body not only owing to their capacity to govern but also owing to the profound relationship they share with each other: the three form, in an important sense, a unity. They co-depend on each other, and life-preservation requires the three of them to function as one living entity.

The profound interconnectedness of the three systems sheds light on the seeming inconsistency in Galen's claims when, in some works, he mentions three, while in others, he writes of four governing systems. This point deserves to be addressed in greater detail.

5.4 The Reproductive System as the Fourth Principle

The system sometimes called the fourth ἀρχή is reproductive, with testicles (both masculine and feminine) as its governing part.[89] Galen's description of the reproductive system follows the pattern of other systems: it has a ruling organ, it has offshoots,[90] its activities are not affections, in the sense that the seed is not produced by another system, rendering it an independent system. Furthermore, the seed even contains pneuma.[91] The existence of the seminal pneuma might seem like an indication of a distinct activity. The tripartition of pneumata, as argued in Chapter 3, maps onto the tripartition of the governing parts. In support of this view, it could be pointed out that the seminal pneuma plays a distinct formative role in the development of the embryo. According to Galen, an embryo is produced from the mixture of seeds coming from both the mother and father, as well as blood. Warm arterial blood is, in combination with the substance of the seed, the matter from which warm inner organs are formed.[92]

In Chapter 2, the passage describing the generation of the spinal medulla was cited in the discussion of the generative capacities of the tissues.[93] The passage is primarily preoccupied with explaining the generation of two types of tissues: bone and brain tissues that form crucial parts of the spine. It also accounts for the way in which the spinal bone is

[89] See, for example, *Sem.* 1.15.26 de Lacy (4.569K). *Ars. Med.* 5.2 (287, 2 Boudon=1.319K); *MMG* 2.4 (11.97K).

[90] Spermatic ducts (τα σπερματικά αγγεία), mentioned in *Ars. Med.* 5.2 (287, 4 Boudon =1.319K).

[91] In *UP* 14.9 (2.315, 19–24 Helmreich=4.183K), Galen presents an argument for this point. He claims that it is evident from the fact that the seed is foam-like and shrinks in the open air, presumably due to the fact that the pneuma contained in it is dispersed. The understanding of the seed as foam-like comes from Hippocratic texts, see Hankinson (2017b: 245). The seed is not the only source of pneuma in the embryo. Pneuma is also supplied by the arteries descending from the womb, see *Sem.* 1.8.1 de Lacy (4.539K).

[92] *Sem.* 1.8.1–4 de Lacy (4.539K).

[93] *Sem.* 1.8.6–7 de Lacy (4.540K); see Section 2.4.

formed around the spinal medulla.[94] Most striking here is the description of the seminal pneuma as self-moving; however, such a description does not necessarily differentiate it from other types. Its motion downwards for self-preservation is parallel to the motion of the innate heat downwards for nourishment. The motion directed this way, it is worth remembering, kindles and preserves the heat, whereas the motion upwards scatters and quenches it. The vital pneuma, regulating the heat in the body as a whole by 'carrying' heat and cold to the solids and fluids in the body (which themselves move very little, see Section 3.2.3), also moves in the same pattern. And, in fact, in another passage of *On Seed*, Galen explicitly identifies the seminal pneuma as the vital pneuma.[95]

The significance of the seminal pneuma in conception lies in its location rather than in its special properties. In his attack on the Aristotelian claim that the matter of seed is not used for the formation of the material parts of an embryo,[96] Galen explicitly calls the seminal pneuma an instrument rather than the agent of generation, when he rhetorically asks Aristotle 'τί δώσεις ὄργανον τῇ φύσει τούτου βέλτιον' in reference to the shaping of cavities and moulding of matter. The claim that it is an instrument by means of which some parts of the matter are inflated, widened and aerated is repeated throughout the treatise, often referring to the elemental properties of air and fire,[97] comparing the hot and pliable matter of pneuma to cheese or clay.[98] In a way, the seminal pneuma is the vital pneuma that gains a formative role because it finds itself in the right place at the right time.[99]

Just as the seminal pneuma is not distinctive enough to form a separate type of pneumata, so the reproductive system does not play a significant

94 *Sem.* 1.8.10 de Lacy (4.541K).

95 *Sem.* 1.5.18–20 de Lacy (4.531–2K), tr. de Lacy (1992: 83): οὐδὲ γὰρ οὐδ' ὅτι πλῆρές ἐστι τοῦ πνεύματος τοῦ ζωτικοῦ, τοῦτο λέληθέ σε.

96 *Sem.* 1.5.11 de Lacy (4.530K).

97 *Sem.* 2.5.55–60 de Lacy (4.637–8K), tr. de Lacy (1992: 193): χρῆται μὲν ὀργάνοις ἡ φύσις εἰς τὴν τῶν μορίων δημιουργίαν καὶ μάλιστα τῶν ἐχόντων κοιλίας ἀέρι τε καὶ πυρί. καὶ γὰρ εὐρῦναι καὶ διαφυσῆσαι καὶ παρατεῖναι καὶ ξηρᾶναι καὶ κρατῦναι τὰ σώματα τούτων ἔργον ἐστίν· 'Nature uses as instruments for the fashioning of the parts, especially the parts that have hollows, air and fire. It is their function to broaden, aerate, stretch, dry, and strengthen the bodies.' Later in this passage, Galen also explains how body parts may be undeveloped, using the example of the eyes of a mole. The example is presumably inspired by Aristotle *HA* 1.9, discussed in Chapter 1. According to Galen, underdeveloped mole's eyes are due to the nature of the animal running out of strength to send pneuma forcefully enough to send the eyes outwards.

98 *Sem.* 2.5.30–5 de Lacy (4.632–3K).

99 The very same properties of pneuma produce pathological effects equally well. For example, the cause of palpitations is thick and vaporous pneuma collecting in a cavity that is too small and has no outlet. Galen calls this a complete explanation and adds that no other element constituting the body (of which there are three, following Hippocrates, solids, fluids and pneumata) would be able to move very quickly and easily throughout the whole body. *Trem. Palp.* 5 (7.596–7K).

enough role to make it one of the vital systems. The loss of reproductive capacity does not constitute a threat to vitality, even if it does cause considerable damage to the body.[100] The body can very well keep on functioning without it. Presumably, this is why in his classification of all the parts in *On the Usefulness of Parts*, he puts reproduction in a category separate from the parts necessary for life itself or good life. The understanding of reproduction *qua* independent system is important for therapeutic purposes (so that pertinent illnesses can be treated via the reproductive organs), but it is not a system that a doctor has to take into account when treating patients with life-threatening conditions, such as certain fevers.[101]

5.5 Concluding Remarks: A Living Body as a Unified Whole

In as far as Galen himself does not describe vitality as constituted of a cohesive cause and does not identify tripartition as the 'capacity' element in his definition of these causes in his extant works, this reading is somewhat speculative. However, it is nonetheless true that he uses the notion of a cohesive cause to theorise and reflect on vital processes. If we have to find a theoretical device in his works by means of which a Galenic thinker could conceptualise the vital unity and explain what makes a living, breathing, moving organism one, the cohesive cause would have to be, at the very least, a serious contender. If such phenomena as pulse and respiration can be accounted for with a reference to a cohesive cause, then it is reasonable to argue that this notion could apply on a larger scale, to the vitality of a living being as a whole.

The discussion of the cohesive cause also helps to show the way in which the tripartite physiological domains are 'one'. The three souls together constitute the single capacity vitality: the ability to eat, breathe and perceive/move voluntarily constitutes, in a distinctly Galenic sense, the form of animate life. This point builds on the reading presented at the end of Chapter 3 namely, that the presence of one system affects another: the vegetative system as it is present in animals could not be separated and exist in isolation *qua* plant. The presence of these physiological domains affects each other in profound ways, forming a single inseparable unity:

100 Galen argues against the excision of testicles and the subsequent damage to the body as a whole in *Sem.* 1.15.37–43 de Lacy (4.37–43).

101 As in *MM* 9.10 (10.635–8K); and, in fact, even in *Sem.* 1.15.49 de Lacy (4.574K), he talks of the heart as the source of living and the testicles as the source of living well.

vitality. Building on this point, this chapter has shown that the significance of this tripartite capacity is closely tied to the way in which Galen accounts for the significance of the instruments, such as a bone or the psychic pneuma.[102] In both cases, the functional aspect of parts plays the key explanatory role. The only difference is in what is at stake. The loss of an instrument can be restored, but the loss of even one of the vital processes that constitute vitality inevitably leads to the end of life, since they are functionally one, forming a single unified manifestation of vitality.

[102] Arguably, a fairly direct statement to this effect can be found in *UP* 17.2 (2.450, 6–16 Helmreich=4.363–4K). Walking is impeded when the main agents of motion, the nerves and muscles, are destroyed, but it is also destroyed when the supportive parts, the bones, are broken. See also the discussion in Chapter 1.

Conclusions

> Οἰκοδόμοι ἐκ διαφόρων σύμφορον ἐργάζονται, τὰ μὲν ξηρὰ ὑγραίνοντες, τὰ δὲ ὑγρὰ ξηραίνοντες, τὰ μὲν ὅλα διαιρέοντες, τὰ δὲ διῃρημένα συντιθέντες· μὴ οὕτω δὲ ἐχόντων οὐκ ἂν ἔχοι ᾗ δεῖ. δίαιταν ἀνθρωπίνην μιμέεται· τὰ μὲν ξηρὰ ὑγραίνοντες, τὰ δὲ ὑγρὰ ξηραίνοντες, τὰ μὲν ὅλα διαιρέουσι, τὰ δὲ διῃρημένα συντιθέασι.
>
> Hippocratic Corpus, *On Regimen* 1[1]

This study approached the problem of the unity of Galenic physiology with the question of how Galen divides the body into parts and how those divisions help him to construct his account of the functioning of various vital systems. In other words, the ways in which he takes the body apart and then puts it back together again.

The first chapter was dedicated not only to outlining some of the more prevalent and informative divisions of parts in the Galenic corpus but also to showing that Galen's key preoccupation in discussing part-whole relationships within the body is activity, including such aspects as the type of governance a part is capable of (whether a part self-manages, governs or is governed by other parts). The subsequent chapters explore the ways in which the parts come together to fulfil the key vital activities, on the basis of their respective physiological domains: vegetative and nutrition, spirited and breathing, nervous and voluntary motion as well as perception. Moving from simpler and more fundamental towards more complex animal physiology, I argue that the preoccupation with unity is built into Galen's reflection on vitality. The vegetative life entails a complex type of self-sufficiency that unifies living organisms and differentiates them from non-living entities. The discussion of the spirited domain in Chapter 3 showed that the presence of this domain not only renders a living being an animal rather than a plant but also changes the vegetative capacities of that living being. However, it is the presence of the nervous system that has an especially dramatic effect: the

[1] *Vict.* 1.17 (Littré 6.492).

sensory and the motor capacities obviously enable the interaction with the external environment, but, equally importantly, the sensory capacity can be directed internally, registering pain or hunger. It enables an animal to 'perceive' itself, physiologically: it is a mechanism by means of which one tissue can register changes in another tissue, without being affected by the same process. In other words: the nervous system allows an animal to 'sense' itself as a single body constituted of different parts and move itself with intention and design, acting in its own interest and preservation. The final chapter deals with a problem of tripartition as it applies to physiology, arguing that three physiological domains are unified by focus on activity too, allowing to construct vitality as a cohesive cause, with tripartition acting as a single, central 'capacity' for vitality.

Living is constituted by vital activities. For the body to be unified and not fall apart, all of them need to be carried out. The unity of the body, therefore, ought to be understood in terms of process, not the presence of a specific part or even the structural connection between those parts, but the activities that such structures enable. The body parts themselves are understood primarily through the lenses of functional rather than normative parthood. And if Galen takes the body apart by using various notions of a body part, he puts it back together using the theorisations of an activity. In analysing and conceptualising the vital activity, he draws from the rich philosophical tradition, although his contemporary Middle Platonism is an especially important influence because some of its central preoccupations inform Galen's understanding of his philosophical heritage too. At the same time, he uses philosophical tools in odd contexts, with unique results. Most importantly, they help to theorise physiological processes. Galen treats process as goal-oriented, which ultimately leads to the idea that purpose, supported by the capacity and instruments, is the unifying force of the body.

His understanding of the originally Aristotelian idea that the final cause is of primary importance when it comes to explanations is filtered through the preoccupations of his contemporary Platonists, and comes with a strong commitment to providential design. It finds its way into Galen's analyses of bodily processes not only by means of emphasis on the teleological explanations of the functioning of various body parts but also by means of his own treatment of such notions as the cohesive cause. When discussing the processes of the body, he also uses the scheme of the cohesive cause, consisting of a purpose, a capacity and instruments, noting that the first is the most important one. Thus, Galen consistently picks out those theoretical tools that help him to account for the bodily functions as processes guided by a purpose of maintaining life in the most efficient and providential way.

The problem of the originality of Galen's thought is complex. In many respects, Galenic 'philosophy' is very much a product of his time: he shares similar commitments and assumptions with many of his contemporary Middle Platonists. At the same time, he certainly innovates, even though his contribution comes from his preoccupation with medicine. In other words, his acute awareness of the problems that pertain to the living body and its parts makes him push conceptual boundaries beyond what is typical in philosophical discourses. In this way, Galen's innovations are not entirely intended. He does not set out to be a philosopher, let alone an innovative philosopher; he sets out to be an extremely well-informed and learned doctor. He uses philosophical concepts and theories primarily to study the human body, to treat its illnesses and to maintain its health. But neither the philosophical concepts nor theories he uses were ever genuinely intended for such a study. Ancient philosophers are certainly preoccupied with the study of the body in general and they may have even drawn from the knowledge of medical practitioners, but this kind of study was not really aimed at application. Philosophers do not have patients, at least not the patients of the body. However elaborate Empedocles' account of respiration might have been, there is hardly any reason to suppose that anyone went to him with a cough.[2] Galen, meanwhile, did treat people with coughs and much else. The body in his works is not an abstract entity. It comprises many different parts, and most of which – ideally all – need to be kept in working order.

[2] Although doxographical sources show that Empedocles had substantial interest in medical topics, he is by no means an ordinary practitioner. Aëtius reports his views on a number of medical issues, including breathing (4.22.1 Mansfeld and Runia), sleep (5.24.2), nourishment (5.27.1), mixtures that constitute body parts (5.22.1) and especially embryology (5.7.1; 5.8.1; 5.11.1; 5.12.2; 5.14.2; 5.18.1; 5.21.1). He is certainly one of the most important proponents of *phusiologia* (see section 2 in the Introduction). However, another doxographer, Diogenes Laertius, preserves descriptions of Empedocles' medical endeavours as extraordinary, nearly divine, acts of healing, hardly ordinary medical practice. Diogenes provides two accounts, one by Heraclides and another one by Hermippus, of Empedocles' resurrecting a woman considered dead. In both accounts, this act is connected to a sacrifice the Presocratic philosopher performed. The resurrection of the dead has close associations with divinity, especially with the god Asclepius (see Plato *R.* 3.408B–C which references Pindar's *Pythian Ode* 3.55 (esp. line 55)). Heraclides' report, in particular, makes a connection with the deification of Empedocles (Diogenes Laertius 8.67–9). Similarly, Diogenes reports Diodorus of Ephesus' account of Empedocles ending a plague by figuring out that it was caused by the nearby river. He then diverts the stream to merge it with another one at his own expense, thus ending the plague. The event leads to the worship of Empedocles as if he were a deity (Diogenes Laertius 8.70). At least in these doxographical anecdotes, Empedocles is not portrayed as an ordinary doctor: his medical springs from a higher kind of knowledge that is comparable to the divine, and this knowledge is Empedocles' key preoccupation: if he finds himself in a situation when this knowledge can be applied for the sake of healing, that is a piece of good luck for people affected, but Empedocles is not portrayed as someone who undertakes to heal in general.

This study showed that preoccupation with activity is evident in many aspects of Galenic thought: in the way he reflects on and defines parthood, the interaction between the physiological domains and especially the relation between the three governing parts. When it comes to the latter, his interest in not just psychological conflict but also physiological consilience reveals an intricate picture of the levels of different types of vitality that build upon each other and come together to form a unified whole by means of their co-dependent activities: eating, breathing, moving and perceiving.

It was presumably the urgency of his experience as a doctor that led Galen to produce nuanced reflections on the nature of the living wholes and their parts. Indeed, his contribution in this area of philosophy is often overlooked. It does, however, deserve much more scholarly attention, partly because of its legacy. After all, Galenic medicine did not end with Galen's own life. It flourished centuries after his death and dominates medical discourses in both Europe and Western Asia.[3] Understanding the ways in which he theorised the unity of the body helps to understand this long, rich and multifaceted tradition that dominated the region almost until the modern period.

Having said that, Galen's works arguably ought to be read primarily for their own sake. There is an enduring sense of wonder preserved in his texts. He uses pronounced aesthetic vocabulary not only to describe the nerves but also the complexity of the human body in general.[4] What lies below the noses of the stargazers is no less complex or intricately made and no less worthy of awe and wonder. And perhaps this sense of wonder is a significant background to Galen's account of the functioning of the human body: even some questions that philosophers concern themselves with must remain unanswered, the body is marvellously moving and supporting life, and it is clear that there is not only immense coherence and unity in those movements but also beauty.

[3] See the papers collected in Bouras-Vallianatos and Zipser (2019); for the reception of Galen in the Renaissance, see Nutton (2008; 2020, chapter 6); Salas (2020: chapter 8); Temkin (1973); for Galen's reception in antiquity, see Nutton (2005) and Slaveva-Griffin (manuscript in preparation). For the development of the disciplines of physiology and anatomy after Galen, see Cunningham (2002, 2003, 2010).

[4] *UP* 2.15 (1.107 Helmreich=3.146K); 10.14 (2.107 Helmreich=3.833K); see also the comparison between the animal's body and the universe, stating that the best thing is the universe, but an animal's body is a reflection of it in miniature (*UP* 3.10 (1.177, 9–11 Helmreich=3.241K)). See also Hankinson (2022b: 155–7) for more examples of beauty of human anatomy. Galen's use of aesthetic vocabulary has some Stoic resonances, see Čelkytė (2020b: 182–6).

References

Adamson, P. 2014. 'Galen on Void'. In *Philosophical Themes in Galen,* ed P. Adamson, R. Hansberger and J. Wilberding. London: Institute of Classical Studies: 197–211.

Adamson, P., R. Hansberger and J. Wilberding (eds.). 2014. *Philosophical Themes in Galen*. London: Institute of Classical Studies.

Allen, J. 2001. *Inference from Signs: Ancient Debates about the Nature of Evidence.* Oxford: Oxford University Press.

von Arnim, J. (ed.). 1903–5. *Stoicorum veterum fragmenta.* 3 vols. Leipzig: Teubner.

Barnes, J. 1982. *The Presocratic Philosophers*. London: Routledge.

(ed.). 1984. *The Complete Works of Aristotle: The Revised Oxford Translation.* Princeton, NJ: Princeton University Press.

1988. 'Bits and Pieces'. In *Matter and Metaphysics*, ed. J. Barnes and M. Mignucci. Rome: Bibliopolis: 225–94.

Berman, B. 2015. 'Aristotle on Like-Partedness and the Like-Parted Bodies'. *Early Science and Medicine* 20: 27–47.

Berryman, S. 1997. 'Horror Vacui in the Third Century BC: When Is a Theory Not a Theory?' *Bulletin of the Institute of Classical Studies* Supplement no. 68: 147–57.

2002. 'Aristotle on Pneuma and Animal Self-Motion'. *Oxford Studies in Ancient Philosophy* 23: 85–97.

2009. *The Mechanical Hypothesis in Ancient Greek Natural Philosophy.* Cambridge: Cambridge University Press.

Betegh, G. 2019. 'Fire Heat and Motive Force in Early Greek Philosophy and Medicine'. In *Heat, Pneuma and Soul in Ancient Philosophy and Science*, ed. H. Bartos and C. G. King. Cambridge: Cambridge University Press: 35–60.

Bett, R. 2012. *Sextus Empiricus: 'Against the Physicists'.* Cambridge: Cambridge University Press.

Blank, D. 2000. 'Ammonius Hermeiou and His School'. In *The Cambridge History of Philosophy in Late Antiquity*, ed. L. Gerson. Cambridge: Cambridge University Press: 654–66.

Bobzien, S. 1998. '"Chrysippus" Theory of Causes'. In *Topics in Stoic Philosophy*, ed. K. Ierodiakonou. Oxford: Oxford University Press: 196–242.

de Boer, W. 1937. *De propriorum animi cuiuslibet affectuum dignotione et curatione, De animi cuiuslibet peccatorum dignotione et curatione and De atra bile, CMG V 4, 1, 1*. Berlin: AkademieVerlag.

Bonazzi, M. 2016. 'The Perfidious Strategy; or, the Platonists against Stoicism' In *Strategies of Polemics in Greek and Roman Philosophy*, ed. S. Weisser and N. Thaler. Leiden: Brill: 166–84.

Boudon-Millot, V. (ed.). 2000. *Galien. Tome ii: Exhortation à l'étude de la médecine; Art médical*. Paris: Belles Lettres.

2007. *Galien, Tome 1, Introduction générale. Sur l' Ordre des ses propres Livres. Sur ses propres Livres. Que l' excellent Médecin est aussi Philosophe*. Paris: Les Belles Lettres.

2012. 'Vision and Vision Disorders: Galen's Physiology of Sight'. In *Blood, Sweat and Tears: The Changing Concepts of Physiology from Antiquity into Early Modern Europe*, ed. H. Horstmanshoff, H. King and C. Zittel. Leiden: Brill: 551–68.

Boudon-Millot, V., and A. Pietrobelli (eds.). 2005. 'Galien ressuscité: édition princeps du texte Grec du De Propriis Placitis'. *Revue des Etudes Grecques* 118: 168–213.

Bouras-Vallianatos, P., and B. Zipser. (eds.). 2019. *Brill's Companion to the Reception of Galen*. Leiden: Brill.

Bowersock, G. W. (ed.). 1974. *Approaches to the Second Sophistic: Papers Presented at the 105th Annual Meeting of the American Philological Association*. University Park: American Philological Association, Pennsylvania State University.

Boylan, M. 1984. 'The Galenic and Hippocratic Challenges to Aristotle's Conception Theory'. *Journal of the History of Biology* 17(1): 83–112.

1986. 'Galen's Conception Theory'. *Journal of the History of Biology* 19(1): 47–77.

Boys-Stones, G. 2018. *Platonist Philosophy 80 BC to AD 250: An Introduction and Collection of Sources in Translation*. Cambridge: Cambridge University Press.

Brain, P. 1986. *Galen on Bloodletting: A Study of the Origins, Development and Validity of His Opinions, with a Translation of the Three Works*. Cambridge: Cambridge University Press.

Broadie, S. 1987. 'Nature, Craft and Phronesis in Aristotle'. *Philosophical Topics* 15(2): 35–50.

2007. 'Why No Platonistic Ideas of Artefacts?' In *Maieusis: Essays in Ancient Philosophy in Honour of Myles Burnyeat*, ed. D. Scott. Oxford: Oxford University Press: 232–53.

Brock, A. J. 1916. *Galen: On the Natural Faculties*. Cambridge, MA: Harvard University Press.

Brunschön, C. W. 2021. *Galeni De locis affectis V–VI, CMG V 6, 1, 3*. Berlin: De Gruyter.

Caston, V. 1997. 'Epiphenomenalism, Ancient and Modern'. *The Philosophical Review* 106(3): 309–63.

Čelkytė, A. 2020a. 'The Soul and Personal Identity in Early Stoicism: Two Theories?' *Apeiron* 53(4): 463–86.

2020b. *The Stoic Theory of Beauty*. Edinburgh: Edinburgh University Press.

2023. 'The Medico-Oikonomic Model of Human Nature in Bryson's *Oikonomikos*'. *Phronesis* 68(2): 206–35.

Chiaradonna, R. 2009. 'Galen and Middle Platonism'. In *Galen and the World of Knowledge*, ed. C. Gill, T. Whitmarsh and J. Wilkins. Cambridge: Cambridge University Press: 243–60.

2014. 'Galen on What Is Persuasive (*Pithanon*) and What Approximates to Truth'. In *Philosophical Themes in Galen*, ed. P. Adamson, R. Hansberger and J. Wilberding. London: Institute of Classical Studies: 61–88.

2015. 'Plotinus' Account of Demiurgic Causation and Its Philosophical Background'. In *Causation and Creation in Late Antiquity*, ed. A. Marmadoro and B. D. Prince. Oxford: Oxford University Press: 31–50.

Clark, S. 1975. *Aristotle's Man: Speculations upon Aristotelian Anthropology*. Oxford: Oxford University Press.

Connell, S. 2016. *Aristotle on Female Animals: A Study of the Generation of Animals*. Cambridge: Cambridge University Press.

Corcilius, K., and P. Gregoric. 2013. 'Aristotle's Model of Animal Motion.' *Phronesis* 58(1): 52–97.

Coughlin, S. 2020. 'Cohesive Causes in Ancient Greek Philosophy and Medicine'. In *Holism in Ancient Medicine and Its Reception*, ed. C. Thumiger. Brill: Leiden: 237–67.

Cunningham, A. 1997. *The Anatomical Renaissance: The Resurrection of the Anatomical Projects of the Ancients*. London: Routledge.

2010. *The Anatomists Anatomis'd: An Experimental Discipline in Enlightenment Europe*. Farnham: Ashgate.

2003. 'The Pen and the Sword: Recovering the Disciplinary Identity of Physiology and Anatomy before 1800 II: Old Anatomy – the Sword'. *Studies in History and Philosophy of Biological and Biomedical Sciences* 34: 51–76.

2002. 'The Pen and the Sword: Recovering the Disciplinary Identity of Physiology and Anatomy before 1800 I: Old Physiology – the Pen'. *Studies in History and Philosophy of Biological and Biomedical Sciences* 33: 631–65.

Curd, P. 1998. *The Legacy of Parmenides: Eleatic Monism and Later Presocratic Thought*. Princeton, NJ: Princeton University Press.

Curtis, T. 2010. *Rhetorical Strategies and Generic Conventions in the Galenic Corpus*. PhD dissertation, Newcastle University, Newcastle.

Daremberg, C., and C. É. Ruelle. 1963 (1879). *Oeuvres de Rufus d'Éphèse*. Amsterdam: Hakkert (original Paris: Imprimerie Nationale).

Das, A. 2020. *Galen and the Arabic Reception of Plato's "Timaeus"*. Cambridge: Cambridge University Press.

Debru, A. 1996. *Le Corps Respirant*. Leiden: Brill.

1997. 'Philosophie et Pharmacologie: La Dynamique des Substances *Leptomeres* Chez Galen'. *Galen on Pharmacology: Philosophy, History, and Medicine: Proceedings of the 5th International Galen Colloquium, Lille, 16–18 March 1995*, ed. A. Debru. Leiden: Brill: 85–102.

2008. 'Physiology'. In *The Cambridge Companion to Galen*, ed. R. J. Hankinson. Cambridge: Cambridge University Press: 263–82.

Destrée, P. 2007. 'Aristotle on the Causes of *Akrasia*'. In *Akrasia in Greek Philosophy*. Leiden: Brill: 139–65.

Devinant, J. 2020. *Les troubles psychiques selon Galien: Étude d'un système de pensée*. Paris: Les Belles Lettres.

Diels, H. 1893. 'Uber das physikalische System des Straton'. *Sitzungsberichte der Preussischen Akademie der Wissenschaften* 12: 101–27.

Diels, H., and W. Kranz (eds.). 1951–2. *Die Fragmente der Vorsokratiker*. 6th edn. 3 vols. Berlin: Weidmann.

Diller, H. 1999. *Hippocratis De aere aquis locis, CMG I 1, 2*. Berlin: Akademie Verlag.

Donini, P. 2008. 'Psychology'. *The Cambridge Companion to Galen*, ed. R. J. Hankinson. Cambridge: Cambridge University Press: 184–209.

Duckworth, W. L. H. (tr.). 1962. *Galen on Anatomical Procedures, the Later Books*, ed. M. C. Lyons and B. Towers. Cambridge: Cambridge University Press.

Duncombe, M. 2015. 'The Role of Relatives in Plato's Partition Argument, *Republic* 4, 436b9–439c9'. *Oxford Studies in Ancient Philosophy* 48: 37–60.

Durling, R. J. 1988. 'The Innate Heat in Galen'. *Medizinhistorisches Journal* 23(3/4): 210–12.

van der Eijk, P. 1997. 'Galen's Use of the Concept of "Qualified Experience" in His Dietetic and Pharmacological Works'. In *Galen on Pharmacology: Philosophy, History, and Medicine*, ed. A. Debru. Leiden: Brill: 35–57.

2000–1. *Diocles of Carystus: A Collection of the Fragments with Translation and Commentary*. 2 vols. Leiden: Brill.

2005. *Medicine and Philosophy in Classical Antiquity: Doctors and Philosophers on Nature, Soul, Health and Disease*. Cambridge: Cambridge University Press.

2009. 'Aristotle! What a Thing for You to Say!' Galen's Engagement with Aristotle and Aristotelians'. In *Galen and the World of Knowledge*, ed. C. Gill, T. Whitmarsh and J. Wilkins. Cambridge: Cambridge University Press: 261–81.

2014. 'Galen on the Nature of Human Beings'. In *Philosophical Themes in Galen*, ed. P. Adamson, R. Hansberger and J. Wilberding. London: Institute of Classical Studies: 89–134.

2017. 'The Place of Disease in a Teleological World-view: Plato, Aristotle, Galen'. In *Teleology in the Ancient World: Philosophical and Medical Approaches*, ed. J. Rocca. Cambridge: Cambridge University Press: 217–41.

2020. 'Galen on Soul, Mixture, Pneuma'. In *Body and Soul in Hellenistic Philosophy*, ed. B. Inwood and J. Warren. Cambridge: Cambridge University Press: 62–88.

Falcon, A. 2021. 'The Reception of Aristotle's Biology in Late Antiquity and Beyond'. In *The Cambridge Companion to Aristotle's Biology*, ed. S. Connell. Cambridge: Cambridge University Press: 246–60.

Flemming, R. 2000. *Medicine and the Making of Roman Women: Gender, Nature, and Authority from Celsus to Galen*. Oxford: Oxford University Press.

Fortuna, S. 1997. *Galeni de Constitutione Artis Medicae ad Patrophilum, CMG V 1, 3*. Berlin: Akademie Verlag.

Frede, M. 1987. *Essays in Ancient Philosophy*. Minneapolis: University of Minnesota Press.

Furley, D. J., and J. S. Wilkie. 1984. *Galen: On Respiration and the Arteries*. Princeton, NJ: Princeton University Press.

Garofalo, I. 1991. *Procedimenti anatomici*. Milan: Rizzoli.

Garofalo, I., and A. Lami. 2012 *Galeno, l'anima e il dolore. De Indolentia; De Propriis Placitis*. Milan: Rizzoli.

Gärtner, F. 2015. *Galenus. De locis affectis I–II*. Berlin: De Gruyter.

Gelber, J. 2010. 'Form and Inheritance in Aristotle's Embryology'. *Oxford Studies in Ancient Philosophy* 39: 183–212.

Gemelli Marciano, M. L. 2007. *Democrito e l'Accademia: studi sulla trasmissione dell'atomismo antico da Aristotele a Simplicio*. Berlin: De Gruyter.

Gill, C. J. 2006. *The Structured Self in Hellenistic and Roman Thought*. Oxford: Oxford University Press.

2010. *Naturalistic Psychology in Galen and Stoicism*. Oxford: Oxford University Press.

Gill, C. J., T. Whitmarsh and J. Wilkins (eds.). 2009. *Galen and the World of Knowledge*. Cambridge: Cambridge University Press.

Glare, P. (ed.). 1982. *Oxford Latin Dictionary*. Oxford: Oxford University Press.

Gotthelf, A. 2012. *Teleology, First Principles, and Scientific Method in Aristotle's Biology*. Oxford: Oxford University Press.

Gottschalk, H. B. 1987. 'Aristotelian philosophy in the Roman world from the time of Cicero to the end of the second century AD.' In *Aufstieg Und Niedergang Der Römischen Welt. Tel Ii: Teilband: Philosophie (Platonismus (Fortsetzung) Aristotelismus) Band 36: Philosophie, Wissenschaften, Technik*, ed. W. Haase. Berlin: De Gruyter: 1079–175.

Gourinat, J.-B. 2007. '*Akrasia* and *Enkrateia* in Ancient Stoicism: Minor Vice and Minor Virtue?' In *Akrasia in Greek Philosophy*, ed. C. Bobonich and P. Destrée. Leiden: Brill: 215–47.

Grensemann, H. 1968. *Die hippokratische Schrift 'Über die heilige Krankheit'*. Berlin: De Gruyter.

Gundert, B. 1992. 'Parts and Their Roles in Hippocratic Medicine'. *Isis* 83(3): 453–65.

2000. 'Soma and Psyche in Hippocratic Medicine'. In *Psyche and Soma: Physicians and Metaphysicians on the Mind-Body Problem from Antiquity to Enlightenment*, ed. J. Wright and P. Potter. Oxford: Oxford University Press: 13–35.

2009. *Galeni De Symptomatum Differentiis, CMG V 5, 1*. Berlin: Akademie Verlag.

Guthrie, W. K. C. 1965. *A History of Greek Philosophy: Vol. 2, The Presocratic Tradition from Parmenides to Democritus*. Cambridge: Cambridge University Press.

Hankinson, R. 1989. 'Galen and the Best of All Possible Worlds'. *The Classical Quarterly* 39(1): 206–27.

1991a. 'Galen's Anatomy of the Soul'. *Phronesis* 36(2): 197–233.

1991b. 'A Purely Verbal Dispute? Galen on Stoic and Academic Epistemology'. *Revue Internationale de Philosophie* 45(178(3)): 267–300.

1993. 'Actions and Passions: Affection, Emotion, and Moral Self-Management in Galen's Philosophical Psychology'. In *Passions and Perceptions: Studies in Hellenistic Philosophy of Mind*, ed. J. Brunschwig and M. Nussbaum. Cambridge: Cambridge University Press: 184–222.

1994. 'Galen's Theory of Causation'. *ANRW II*, 37(2): 1757–74.

1998. *Cause and Explanation in Ancient Greek Thought*. Oxford: Oxford University Press.

2003. 'Causation in Galen'. In *Galien et la Philosophie Entretiens sur l'antiquite classique, vol. 49*, ed. J. Barnes and J. Jouanna. Vandoeuvres-Geneva: Fondation Hardt: 31–72.

2006. 'Body and Soul in Galen'. In *Common to Body and Soul: Philosophical Approaches to Explaining Living Behaviour in Greco-Roman Antiquity*, ed. R. A. H. King. Berlin: De Gruyter: 232–58.

2008a. 'Philosophy of Nature'. In *The Cambridge Companion to Galen*, ed. R. J. Hankinson. Cambridge: Cambridge University Press: 210–41.

2008b. 'The Man and His Work'. In *The Cambridge Companion to Galen*, ed. R. J. Hankinson. Cambridge: Cambridge University Press: 1–33.

(ed.) 2008c. *The Cambridge Companion to Galen*. Cambridge: Cambridge University Press.

2009. 'Galen on the Limitations of Knowledge'. In *Galen and The World of Knowledge*, ed. C. Gill, T. Whitmarsh and J. Wilkins. Cambridge: Cambridge University Press: 206–42.

2014. 'Partitioning the Soul: Galen on the Anatomy of the Psychic Functions and Mental Illness'. In *Partitioning the Soul: Debates from Plato to Leibniz*, ed. K. Corcilius and D. Perler. Berlin: De Gruyter: 85–106.

2016. 'Galen's Reception of Aristotle'. In *Brill's Companion to the Reception of Aristotle in Antiquity*, ed. A. Falcon. Leiden: Brill: 238–57.

2017a. 'Substance, Element, Quality, Mixture: Galen's Physics and His Hippocratic Inheritance'. *Aitia* 7(2).

2017b. 'Teleology and Necessity in Greek Embryology'. In *Teleology in the Ancient World*, ed. J. Rocca. Cambridge: Cambridge University Press: 242–71.

2022a. 'Discovery, Method, and Justification: Galen and the Determination of Therapy'. In *Galen's Epistemology: Experience, Reason, and Method in Ancient Medicine*, ed. R. Hankinson and M. Havrda. Cambridge: Cambridge University Press: 79–115.

2022b. 'A Hymn to Nature: Structure, Function, Design and Beauty in Galen's Biology'. In *Poikile Physis: Biological Literature in Greek during the Roman Empire: Genres, Scopes, and Problems*, ed. D. de Brasi and F. Fronterotta. Berlin: De Gruyter: 145–66.

Harder, R. 1926. *Ocellus Lucanus: Neue philologische Untersuchungen, vol. 1*. Berlin: Weidmann.

Hardie, R. P., and R. K. Gaye (tr.) 1984. 'Aristotle's *Physics*'. In *The Complete Works of Aristotle*, ed. J. Barnes. Princeton, NJ: Princeton University Press: 315–446.

Harris, C. R. S. 1973. *The Heart and the Vascular System in Ancient Greek Medicine: From Alcmaeon to Galen*. Oxford: Clarendon Press.

Harte, V. 2002. *Plato on Parts and Wholes: The Metaphysics of Structure*. Oxford: Oxford University Press.

Havrda, M. 2015. 'The Purpose of Galen's Treatise *On Demonstration*'. *Early Science and Medicine* 20: 265–87.

2017. 'Body and Cosmos in Galen's Account of the Soul'. *Phronesis* 62(1): 69–89.

Helle, R. 2021. 'Self-causation and Unity in Stoicism'. *Phronesis* 66(2): 178–213.

Heiberg, J. L. 1927. *Hippocratis Indices librorum, Iusiurandum, Lex, De arte, De medico, De decente habitu, Praeceptiones, De prisca medicina, De aere locis aquis, De alimento, De liquidorum usu, De flatibus, CMG I 1*. Leipzig: Teubner.

Helmreich, G. 1893. *Claudii Galeni scripta minora*. 3 vols. Leipzig: Teubner.

1901. *Galenus de optima corporis constitutione. Idem de bono habitu*. Programm des Königlichen humanistischen Gymnasiums: Hof.

1968 (1907–1909). *De Usu Partium*. 2 vols. Amsterdam: Hakkert (original Leipzig: Bibliotheca Teubneriana.

Hensley, I. 2020. 'The Physics of Pneuma in Early Stoicism'. In *The Concept of Pneuma after Aristotle*, ed. S. Coughlin, D. Leith and O. Lewis. Berlin: Topoi: 171–202.

Holmes, B. 2012. 'Sympathy between Hippocrates and Galen: The Case of Galen's Commentary on Epidemics II'. In *Epidemics in Context: Hippocrates, Galen and Hunayn between East and West*, ed. P. E. Pormann. Berlin: De Gruyter: 49–70.

2015. 'Reflection: Galen's Sympathy'. In *Sympathy: A History*, ed. E. Schliesser. Oxford: Oxford University Press: 61–9.

2017. 'Pure Life: The Limits of the Vegetal Analogy in the Hippocratics and Galen'. In *The Comparable Body: Analogy and Metaphor in Ancient Mesopotamian, Egyptian, and Greco-Roman Medicine*, ed. J. Wee. Leiden: Brill: 358–86.

2020. 'Holism, Sympathy, and the Living Being in Ancient Greek Medicine and Philosophy'. In *Holism in Ancient Medicine and Its Reception*, ed. C. Thumiger. Leiden: Brill: 47–83.

Horstmanshoff, H. F. J., H. King and C. Zittel (eds.). 2012. *Blood, Sweat and Tears: The Changing Concepts of Physiology from Antiquity into Early Modern Europe*. Leiden: Brill.

Hort, A. (tr.). 2015. *Theophrastus: Enquiry into Plants*. Cambridge, MA: Harvard University Press.

Ierodiakonou, K. 1999. 'Galen's Criticism of the Aristotelian Theory of Colour Vision'. In *Antiaristotelismo*, ed. C. Natali and S. Maso. Amsterdam: Hakkert: 123–41.

2014. 'On Galen's Theory of Vision'. In *Philosophical Themes in Galen*, ed. P. Adamson, R. Hansberger and J. Wilberding. London: Institute of Classical Studies: 235–48.

2015. 'Wholes and Parts: M 9.331–358'. In *Sextus Empiricus and Ancient Physics*, ed. K. Algra and K. Ierodiakonou. Cambridge: Cambridge University Press: 105–29.

2022. 'On Sense-Perception: Galen in Dialogue with Plato and the Stoics'. In *Galen's Epistemology: Experience, Reason, and Method in Ancient Medicine*, ed. R. Hankinson and M. Havrda. Cambridge: Cambridge University Press: 218–31.

Ilberg, J. 1927. *Sorani Gynaeciorum libri iv, de signis fracturarum, de fasciis, vita Hippocratis secundum Soranum, CMG 4*. Leipzig: Teubner.

Jaeger, W. W. 1938. *Diokles von Karystos: Die griechische Medizin und die Schule des Aristoteles*. Berlin: Weidmann.

Johnston, I. 2006. *Galen on Diseases and Symptoms (tr. of 'On the Differentiae of Diseases', 'On the Causes of Diseases' 'On the Differentiae of Symptoms', 'On the Causes of Symptoms')*. Cambridge: Cambridge University Press.

2016. *Galen: On the Constitution of the Art of Medicine; The Art of Medicine; A Method of Medicine to Glaucon*. Cambridge, MA: Harvard University Press.

(ed. and tr.). 2018. *Galen: Hygiene*. Cambridge, MA: Harvard University Press.

Johnston, I., and G. H. R. Horsley. 2011. *Galen: Method of Medicine*. Cambridge, MA: Harvard University Press.

Joly, R., and S. Byl. 1984. *Hippocrate: Du regime, CMG I 2, 4*. Berlin: Akademie Verlag.

Jouanna, J. 1990. *Hippocrate II I: De l'ancienne médecine*. Paris: Les Belles Lettres.

2002. *Hippocratis De natura hominis, CMG I 1, 3*. Berlin: Akademie Verlag.

2009. 'Does Galen Have a Medical Programme for Intellectuals and the Faculties of the Intellect?' In *Galen and the World of Knowledge*, ed. C. Gill, T. Whitmarsh and J. Wilkins. Cambridge: Cambridge University Press: 190–205.

2013. *Greek Medicine from Hippocrates to Galen: Selected Papers*. Leiden: Brill.

Joyce, R. 1995. 'Early Stoicism and Akrasia'. *Phronesis* 40(3): 315–35.

Kalbfleisch, K. 1896. *Galeni Institutio logica*. Leipzig: Teubner.

Kamtekar, R. 2017. *Plato's Moral Psychology: Intellectualism, the Divided Soul, and the Desire for Good*. Oxford: Oxford University Press.

Katayama, E. G. 1999. *Aristotle on Artifacts: A Metaphysical Puzzle*. Albany: State University of New York Press.

Kaufman, D. 2017. 'Galen on Reason and Appetite: A Study of the *De 6*'. *Apeiron* 50(3): 367–92.

King, D. 2018. *Experiencing Pain in Imperial Greek Culture*. Oxford: Oxford University Press.

King, H. 1998. *Hippocrates' Women: Reading the Female Body in Ancient Greece*. London: Routledge.

Koch, K., G. Helmreich, K. Kalbfleisch and O. Hartlich. 1923. *Galeni de Sanitate Tuenda [Koch]; de Alimentorum Facultatibus [Helmreich]; de Bonis et Malis Alimentorum Sucis [Helmreich]; de Victu Attenuante [Kalbfleisch]; de Ptisana [Hartlich], CMG V 4, 2*. Berlin: Teubner.

Kollesch, J. 1964. *De Instrumento Odoratus, CMG V*. Berlin: Akademie Verlag.

1981. 'Galen und die Zweite Sophistik'. In *Galen: Problems and Prospects*, ed. V. Nutton. London: The Wellcome Institute for the History of Medicine: 1–11.

Koslicki, K. 2008. *The Structure of Things*. Oxford: Oxford University Press.

Kovačić, F. 2001. *Der Begriff der Physis bei Galen vor dem Hintergrund seiner Vorgänger*. Stuttgart: Steiner.

Kress, E. 2023. 'How the Soul Uses Its Tools: Flexible Agency in Aristotle's Account of Animal Generation'. *Phronesis* 68(3): 293–325.

Kühn, K. G. (ed.). 1821–33. *Claudii Galeni Opera Omnia*. 22 vols. Leipzig: Knobloch.

Kupreeva, I. 2014. 'Galen's Theory of Elements'. *Bulletin of the Institute of Classical Studies* Supplement no. 114: 153–96.

2022. 'Galen's Empiricist Background: A Study of the Argument in *On Medical Experience*'. In *Galen's Epistemology: Experience, Reason, and Method in Ancient Medicine*, ed. R. Hankinson and M. Havrda. Cambridge: Cambridge University Press: 32–78.

de Lacy, P. 1972. 'Galen's Platonism'. *The American Journal of Philology* 93(1): 27–39.

1978–84. *Galen: De Placitis Hippocratis et Platonis, CMG V 4, 1, 2*. 3 vols. Berlin: Akademie Verlag.

1979. 'Galen's Concept of Continuity'. *Greek, Roman and Byzantine Studies* 20(4): 355–69.

1992. *Galen: De Semine, CMG V 3, 1*. Berlin: Akademie Verlag.

1996. *Galen: On the Elements According to Hippocrates, CMG V 1, 2*. Berlin: Akademie Verlag.

Larrain, C. J. 1992. *Galens Kommentar zu Platons Timaios*. Stuttgart: Teubner.

Leith, D. 2012. 'Pores and Void in Asclepiades' Physical Theory'. *Phronesis* 57(2): 164–91.

2014. 'Galen's Refutation of Atomism'. *Bulletin of the Institute of Classical Studies* Supplement no. 114: 213–34.

2015. 'Elements and Uniform Parts in Early Alexandrian Medicine'. *Phronesis* 60(4): 462–91.

2020. 'Herophilus and Erasistratus on the Hēgemonikon'. In *Body and Soul in Hellenistic Philosophy*, ed. B. Inwood and J. Warren. Cambridge: Cambridge University Press: 30–61.

Lennox, J. 2001. *Aristotle's Philosophy of Biology*. Cambridge: Cambridge University Press.

Leunissen, M. 2010. *Explanation and Teleology in Aristotle's Science of Nature*. Cambridge: Cambridge University Press.

Lewis, E. 1995. 'The Stoics on Identity and Individuation'. *Phronesis* 40(1): 89–108.

Lewis, O. 2017. *Praxagoras of Cos on Arteries, Pulse and Pneuma.* Leiden: Brill.

Lewis, O., and P. Gregoric. 2015. 'The Context of "De Spiritu."' *Early Science and Medicine* 20(2): 125–49.

Liddell, H. G., Scott, R., and Jones, H. S. 1996 (1940). *A Greek–English Lexicon.* 9th edn. Oxford: Oxford University Press.

Littré, É. (ed.). 1839–61. *Oeuvres complètes d'Hippocrate.* 10 vols. Paris: J. B. Baillière.

Lloyd, G. E. R. 1991. *Methods and Problems in Greek Science.* Cambridge: Cambridge University Press.

1996. 'Theories and Practises of Demonstration in Galen'. In *Rationality in Greek Thought,* ed. M. Frede and G. Striker. Oxford: Clarendon Press: 255–77.

2007. 'Pneuma between Body and Soul'. *The Journal of the Royal Anthropological Institute* 13: S135–46.

2008. 'Galen and His Contemporaries'. In *The Cambridge Companion to Galen,* ed. R. J. Hankinson. Cambridge: Cambridge University Press: 34–48.

Long, A. A., and D. Sedley (eds.). 1987. *The Hellenistic Philosophers.* 2 vols. Cambridge: Cambridge University Press.

Longrigg, J. 1993. *Greek Rational Medicine: Philosophy and Medicine from Alcmaeon to the Alexandrians.* London: Routledge.

Lyons, M. C. 1969. *Galeni de Partibus Artibus Medicativae, de Causis Contentivis, de Diaeta in Morbis Acutis Secundum Hippocratem, CMG Suppl. Or. II.* Berlin: Akademie Verlag.

Makin, S. 2014. 'Parmenides, Zeno, and Melissus.' In *The Routledge Companion to Ancient Philosophy,* ed. J. Warren and F. Sheffield. London: Routledge: 34–48.

Manetti, D. 2011. *Anonymi Londiniensis. De medicina.* Berlin: De Gruyter.

Mansfeld, J. 1991. 'The Idea of the Will in Chrysippus, Posidonius, and Galen'. *Proceedings of the Boston Area Colloquium in Ancient Philosophy* 7: 107–45.

Mansfeld, J., and D. Runia. 2020. *Aëtiana V: An Edition of the Reconstructed Text of the Placita with a Commentary and a Collection of Related Texts.* 4 vols. Boston: Brill.

Marechal, P. 2019. 'Galen's Constitutive Materialism'. *Ancient Philosophy* 39(1): 191–209.

Mattern, S. P. 2008. *Galen and the Rhetoric of Healing.* Baltimore: The Johns Hopkins University Press.

May, M. T. 1968. *Galen, On the Usefulness of the Parts of the Body.* Ithaca, NY: Cornell University Press.

Mayhew, R. 2010. *The Female in Aristotle's Biology: Reason or Rationalization.* Chicago: University of Chicago Press.

Meeusen, M. 2020. 'Ps.-Alexander of Aphrodisias on Unsayable Properties in Medical Puzzles and Natural Problems'. In *Ancient Greek Medicine in Questions and Answers,* ed. M. Meeusen. Leiden: Brill: 80–107.

Mendelsohn, E. 1964. *Heat and Life: The Development of the Theory of Animal Heat.* Cambridge, MA: Harvard University Press.

Moraux, P. 1984. *Der Aristotelismus bei den Griechen von Andronikos bis Alexander von Aphrodisias, Band II: Der Aristotelismus im I. und II. Jr. n. Chr.* Berlin: De Gruyter.

Morison, B. 2008. 'Logic'. In *The Cambridge Companion to Galen*, ed. R. J. Hankinson. Cambridge: Cambridge University Press: 66–115.

Müller, J. 1891. *Galeni Pergameni Scripta Minora*, vol. 2. Leipzig: Teubner.

Nickel, D. 2001. *Galeni De foetuum formatione, CMG V 3, 3*. Berlin: Akademie Verlag.

van Nuffelen, P. 2014. 'Galen, Divination and the Status of Medicine'. *Classical Quarterly* 64(1): 337–52.

Nussbaum, M. C. 1978. *Aristotle's De motu animalium: Text with Translation, Commentary, and Interpretive Essays*. Princeton, NJ: Princeton University Press.

Nutton, V. 1999. *Galen: On my Own Opinions, CMG 3, 2*. Berlin: Akademie Verlag.

2005. 'The Fatal Embrace: Galen and the History of Ancient Medicine'. *Science in Context* 18(1): 111–21.

2008. 'The Fortunes of Galen'. In *The Cambridge Companion to Galen*, ed. J. Hankinson. Cambridge: Cambridge University Press: 355–90.

2012a. *Ancient Medicine*. 2nd edn. Hoboken, NJ: Taylor and Francis.

2012b. '*Physiologia* from Galen to Jacob Bording'. In *Blood, Sweat and Tears: The Changing Concepts of Physiology from Antiquity into Early Modern Europe*, ed. M. Horstmanshoff, H. King and C. Zittel. Leiden: Brill: 25–40.

2020. *Galen: A Thinking Doctor in Imperial Rome*. London: Routledge.

Nutton, V., and G. Bos. 2011. *Galen: On Problematical Movements*. Cambridge: Cambridge University Press..

O'Brien, C. S. 2015. *The Demiurge in Ancient Thought. Secondary Gods and Divine Mediators*. Cambridge: Cambridge University Press.

Ochs, S. 2004. *A History of Nerve Functions: From Animal Spirits to Molecular Mechanisms*. Cambridge: Cambridge University Press.

Opsomer, J. 2005. 'Demiurges in Early Imperial Platonism'. In *Gott und die Gotter bei Plutarch*, ed. R. Hirsch-Luipold. Berlin: De Gruyter: 51–99.

Overwien, O. 2014. *Hippocratis De humoribus, CMG I 3, 1*. Berlin: De Gruyter.

Petit, C. 2009. *Galien. Œuvres. Tome III: Le médecin. Introduction*. Paris: Les Belles Lettres.

2018. *Galien de Pergame ou la rhétorique de la Providence: Médecine, Littérature et Pouvoir à Rome*. Leiden: Brill.

(ed.). 2019. *Galen's Treatise Περὶ Ἀλυπίας (De indolentia) in Context*. Leiden: Brill.

Polito, R. 2006. 'Matter. Medicine and the Mind: Asclepiades versus Epicurus'. *OSAP* 30: 285–336.

Powers, N. 2013. 'Plato's Demiurge as Precursor to the Stoic Providential God'. *The Classical Quarterly* 63(2): 713–22.

Prager, F. D. 1974. *Pneumatica: The Treatise on Experimental Physics, Western Version and Eastern Version: Facs. and Transcript of the Latin manuscript,*

CLM 534, Bayer. Staatsbibliothek, Munich: transl. and ill. of the Arabic manuscript, A.S. 3713, Aya-Sofya, Istanbul. Wiesbaden: Reichert.

Reydams-Schils, G. 1997. 'Posidonius and the *Timaeus*: Off to Rhodes and Back to Plato?' *The Classical Quarterly* 47(2): 455–76.

Rhetorical Strategies and Generic Conventions in the Galenic Corpus' (PhD dissertation. Newcastle University).

Rocca, J. 2003. *Galen on the Brain: Anatomical Knowledge and Physiological Speculation in the Second Century AD.* Leiden: Brill.

2006. '"Plato Will Tell You": Galen's Use of the *Phaedrus* in *De Placitis Hippcoratis et Platonis* IX'. In *Reading Plato in Antiquity*, ed. H. Tarrant and D. Baltzly. London: Bloomsbury Publishing: 49–60.

2012. 'From Doubt to Certainty: Aspects of the Conceptualisation and Interpretation of Galen's Natural Pneuma'. In *Blood, Sweat and Tears: The Changing Concepts of Physiology from Antiquity into Early Modern Europe*, ed. M. Horstmanshoff, H. King and C. Zittel. Brill: Leiden: 627–59.

2017. 'Galen and Middle Platonism: The Case of the Demiurge'. In *Brill's Companion to the Reception of Plato in Antiquity*. Leiden: Brill: 206–22.

2020. 'Pneuma as a Holistic Concept in Galen'. In *Holism in Ancient Medicine and Its Reception*, ed. C. Thumiger. Brill: Leiden: 268–91.

Rosen, R. 2013. 'Galen, Plato, and the Physiology of Eros'. In *Eros in Ancient Greece*, ed. E. Sanders, C. Thumiger, C. Carey and N. Lowe. Oxford: Oxford University Press: 111–27.

Salas, L. A. 2020a. 'Galen on the Definition of Disease'. *American Journal of Philology* 141(4): 603–34.

2020b. *Cutting words: Polemical Dimensions of Galen's Anatomical Experiments*. Leiden: Brill.

Sauvé Meyer, S. 2009. 'Chain of Causes: What Is Stoic Fate?' In *God and Cosmos in Stoicism*, ed. R. Salles. Oxford: Oxford University Press: 71–92.

Scade, P. 2010. 'Stoic Cosmological Limits and Their Platonic Background'. *Bulletin of the Institute of Classical Studies* Supplement 107: 143–83.

Schiefsky, M. J. 2007. 'Galen's Teleology and Functional Explanation'. *Oxford Studies in Ancient Philosophy* 33: 369–400.

2012. 'Galen and the Tripartite Soul'. In *Plato and the Divided Self*, ed. R. Barney, T. Brennan and C. Brittain. Cambridge: Cambridge University Press: 331–49.

Schmidt, W. 1899. *Heronis Alexandrini opera quae supersunt omnia, vol. 1.* Leipzig: Teubner.

Schmitz, T. 1997. *Bildung und Macht: zur sozialen und politische Funktion der zweiten Sophistik in der griechischen Welt der Kaiserzeit.* Munich: Beck.

Schröder, H. O., and P. Kahle. 1934. *Galeni in Platonis Timaeum Commentarii Fragmenta, CMG 1.* Berlin: Akademie-Verlag.

Sedley, D. 1982. 'The Stoic Criterion of Identity'. *Phronesis* 27(3): 255–75.

2005. 'Stoic Metaphysics at Rome'. In *Metaphysics, Soul and Ethics: Themes from the Work of Richard Sorabji*, ed. R. Salles. Oxford: Oxford University Press: 117–42.

2007. *Creationism and Its Critics in Antiquity.* Berkeley: University of California Press.

2008. 'Atomism's Eleatic Roots'. In *The Oxford Handbook of Presocratic Philosophy*, ed. P. Curd and D. W. Graham. Oxford: Oxford University Press: 305–32.
Shields, C. 2007. 'Unified Agency and Akrasia in Plato's Republic'. In *Akrasia in Greek Philosophy: From Socrates to Plotinus*, ed. C. Bobonich and P. Destrée. Leiden: Brill: 61–8.
2008. 'Substance and Life in Aristotle'. *Apeiron* 41(3): 129–51.
Sider, D., and M. McVaugh. 1979. 'Galen, on Tremor, Palpitation, Spasm and Rigor'. *Transactions and Studies of the College of Physicians of Philadelphia* 1: 183–210.
Siegel, R. E. 1968–73. *Galen's System of Physiology and Medicine*. Basel: Karger.
1976. *Galen: On the Affected Parts*. Basel: Karger.
Singer, C. 1956. *Galen On Anatomical Procedures: De Anatomicis Administrationibus*. Oxford: Oxford University Press.
Singer, P. 1991. 'Aspects of Galen's Platonism'. In *Galeno: obra, pensamiento e influencia: Coloquio internacional, Madrid, 1988*, ed. López Férez. Madrid: Universidad Nacional de Educación a Distancia: 41–56.
1996. 'Notes on Galen's Hippocrates'. In *Studi Storia Della Medicina Antica E Medievale*, ed. M. Vegetti and S. Gastaldi. Florence: La Nuova Italia: 66–76.
1997. *Galen: Selected Works*. Oxford: Oxford University Press.
2013a. 'General Introduction'. In *Galen: Psychological Writings*, ed. P. N. Singer. Cambridge: Cambridge University Press: 1–40.
2013b. 'Introduction to The Capacities of the Soul Depend on the Mixture of the Body'. In *Galen: Psychological Writings*, ed. P. N. Singer. Cambridge: Cambridge University Press: 335–70.
2014. 'Galen and the Philosophers: Philosophical Engagement, Shadowy Contemporaries, Aristotelian Transformations'. In *Philosophical Themes in Galen*, ed. P. Adamson, R. Hansberger and J. Wilberding. London: Institute of Classical Studies: 7–38.
2017. 'The Essence of Rage: Galen on Emotional Disturbances and Their PhysicalS Correlates'. In *Selfhood and the Soul*, ed. R. Seaford, J. Wilkins and M. Wright. Oxford: Oxford University Press: 161–96.
2018. 'Galen's Pathological Soul: Diagnosis and Therapy in Ethical Medical Texts and Contexts'. In *Mental Illness in Ancient Medicine*, ed. C. Thumiger and P. Singer. Leiden: Brill: 381–420.
2020. 'Galen on Pneuma: Between Metaphysical Speculation and Anatomical Theory'. In *The Concept of Pneuma after Aristotle*, ed. S. Coughlin, D. Leith and O. Lewis. Berlin: De Gruyter: 237–82.
Slaveva-Griffin, S. Manuscript in preparation. *Medical Interest of the Neoplatonists: From Plotinus to Proclus*.
Sorabji, R. 2000. *Emotion and Peace of Mind: From Stoic Agitation to Christian Temptation*. Oxford: Oxford University Press.
von Staden, H. 1989. *Herophilus: The Art of Medicine in Early Alexandria*. Cambridge: Cambridge University Press.

1992. 'Jaeger's "Skandalon der historischen Vernunft": Diocles, Aristotle, and Theophrastus'. In *Werner Jaeger Reconsidered*, ed. W. M. Calder III. Atlanta: Scholars Press: 227–65.

1995. 'Anatomy as Rhetoric: Galen on Dissection and Persuasion'. *Journal of the History of Medicine and Allied Sciences* 50(1): 47–66.

1997a. 'Galen and the "Second Sophistic."' *Bulletin of the Institute of Classical Studies* Supplement 68: 33–54.

1997b. 'Teleology and Mechanism: Aristotelian Biology and Early Hellenistic Medicine'. In *Aristotelische Biologie: Intentionen, Methoden, Ergebnisse*, ed. W. Pullman and S. Follinger. Stuttgart: Steiner: 183–208.

2000. 'Body, Soul, and Nerves: Epicurus, Herophilus, Erasistratus, the Stoics, and Galen'. In *Psyche and Soma: Physicians and Metaphysicians on the Mind-Body Problem from Antiquity to Enlightenment*, ed. J. Wright and P. Potter. Oxford: Oxford University Press: 79–116.

Stewart, K. A. 2018. *Galen's Theory of Black Bile: Hippocratic Tradition, Manipulation, Innovation*. Leiden: Brill.

Swain, S. 1996. *Hellenism and Empire: Language, Classicism and Power in the Greek World AD 50–250*. Oxford: Oxford University Press.

Tarrant, H. 2017. 'Teleology and Names in the Platonic and Anaxogorean Tradition'. In *Teleology in the Ancient World*, ed. J. Rocca. Cambridge: Cambridge University Press: 58–75.

Tecusan, M. 2004. *The Fragments of the Methodists: Methodism outside Soranus: Volume 1: Text and Translation*. Leiden: Brill.

Temkin, O. 1973. *Galenism: Rise and Decline of a Medical Philosophy*. Ithaca, NY: Cornell University Press.

Thumiger, C., and P. N. Singer (eds.). 2018. *Mental Illness in Ancient Medicine: From Celsus to Paul of Aegina*. Leiden: Brill.

Tieleman, T. 1995. 'Dialectic and Science: Galen, Herophilus and Aristotle on Phenomena. Vol. 2'. In *Ancient Medicine in Its Socio-cultural Context*, ed. P. van der Eijk, H. Horstmanshoff and P. Schrijvers. Amsterdam: Rodopi: 487–95.

1996. *Galen and Chrysippus on the Soul: Argument and Refutation on the De Placitis Books II–III*. Leiden: Brill.

2003a. *Chrysippus' On Affections: Reconstruction and Interpretation*. Leiden: Brill.

2003b. 'Galen's Psychology'. In *Galien et la Philosophie Entretiens sur l'antiquite classique, vol. 49*, ed. J. Barnes and J. Jouanna. Vandoeuvres-Geneva: Fondation Hardt: 131–61.

2005. 'Galen and Genesis'. In *The Creation of Heaven and Earth: Re-interpretations of Genesis I in the Context of Judaism, Ancient Philosophy, Christianity, and Modern Physics*, ed. George H. van Kooten. Leiden: Brill: 125–45.

2008. 'Methodology'. In *The Cambridge Companion to Galen*, ed. J. Hankinson. Cambridge: Cambridge University Press: 49–65.

2009. 'Galen and the Stoics: On the Art of Not Naming'. In *Galen and the World of Knowledge*, ed. C. Gill, T. Whitmarsh and J. Wilkins. Cambridge: Cambrdige University Press: 282–99.

2016. 'Religion and Therapy in Galen'. In *Religion and Illness*, ed. G. Etzelmüller and A. Weissenrieder. Eugene, OR: Wipf and Stock Publishers: 15–31.

2020. 'Galen's Self-understanding and the Platonic *Phaedrus*'. In *The Reception of Plato's 'Phaedrus' from Antiquity to the Renaissance*, ed. S. Delcomminette, P. D'Hoine and M.-A. Gavray. Berlin: De Gruyter: 25–39.

2022. 'Galen's Notion of Dialectic'. In *Galen's Epistemology: Experience, Reason, and Method in Ancient Medicine*, ed. R. Hankinson and M. Havrda. Cambridge: Cambridge University Press: 136–55.

Forthcoming. 'Galen and Academic Scepticism'. In *Galen aus Pergamon: Philosophie in der römischen Kaiserzeit, Philosophie der Antike, hrsg. W. Kullmann*, ed. K.-H. Leven. Stuttgart: Steiner.

Trompeter, J. 2018. 'The Actions of Spirit and Appetite: Voluntary Motion in Galen'. *Phronesis* 63(2): 176–207.

2025. *Galen on Ethics and Human Nature*. Leiden: Brill.

Vallance, J. T. 1990. *The Lost Theory of Asclepiades of Bithynia*. Oxford: Oxford University Press.

Vasallo, C. (ed.). 2017. *Physiologia: Topics in Presocratic Philosophy and Its Reception in Antiquity (= AKAN-Einzelschriften, 12)*. Trier: Wissenschaftlicher Verlag.

Vegetti, M. 2000. 'De caelo in terram. Il Timeo in Galeno (De placitis, Quod animi)'. In *La filosofia in età imperiale: Le scuole e le tradizione filosofiche*, ed. A. Brancacci. Rome: Bibliopolis: 69–84.

Vinkesteijn, R. 2022. *Philosophical Perspectives on Galen of Pergamum: Four Case-Studies on Human Nature and the Relation between Body and Soul.* Leiden: Brill.

Walzer, R. 1949. *Galen on Jews and Christians*. Oxford: Oxford University Press.

Waterlow, S. 1982. *Nature, Change, and Agency in Aristotle's Physics*. Oxford: Oxford University Press.

Wenkebach, E. 1951. *Galeni Adversus Lycum et Adversus Iulianum, CMG V 10, 3*. Berlin: Akademie Verlag.

White, M. 2003. 'Stoic Natural Philosophy (Physics and Cosmology)'. In *The Cambridge Companion to the Stoics*, ed. B. Inwood. Cambridge: Cambridge University Press: 124–52.

Wilberding, J. 2014. 'The Secret of Sentient Vegetative Life in Galen'. *Bulletin of the Institute of Classical Studies* Supplement, no. 114: 249–68.

Wills, A. 1999. 'Herophilus, Erasistratus and the birth of Neuroscience'. *Lancet* 354: 1719–20.

Witt, C. 2012. 'Aristotle on Deformed Animal Kinds'. *Oxford Studies in Ancient Philosophy* 43: 83–106.

Yeo, I.-S. 2002. 'Hippocrates in the Context of Galen: Galen's Commentary on the Classification of Fevers'. In *Epidemics VI: In Hippocrates in Contexts*, ed. P. van der Eijk. Leiden: Brill: 433–44.

General Index

Index Locorum

Printed by Integrated Books International,
United States of America